Autism and Child Psychopathology Series

Series Editor

Johnny L. Matson
Department of Psychology, Louisiana State University,
Baton Rouge, LA, USA

For further volumes:
http://www.springer.com/series/8665

Johnny L. Matson

Editor

Functional Assessment for Challenging Behaviors

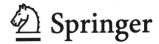 Springer

Editor
Johnny L. Matson
Department of Psychology
Louisiana State University
Baton Rouge, LA, USA

ISSN 2192-922X   e-ISSN 2192-9238
ISBN 978-1-4939-4127-8   ISBN 978-1-4614-3037-7 (eBook)
DOI 10.1007/978-1-4614-3037-7
Springer New York Dordrecht Heidelberg London

Springer is part of Springer Science+Business Media (www.springer.com)

Contents

Contributors

Jennifer L. Austin School of Psychology, University of Glamorgan, Pontypridd, UK

R. Justin Boyd Department of Behavioral Psychology, Kennedy Krieger Institute and The Johns Hopkins University School of Medicine, Baltimore, MD, USA

Holly Brown Hillside Children's Center, Rochester, NY, USA
University of Rochester School of Nursing, Rochester, NY, USA

Robert Didden Behavioural Science Institute, Radboud University Nijmegen, Nijmegen, The Netherlands

Dennis R. Dixon Center for Autism and Related Disorders Inc., Tarzana, CA, USA

Wayne W. Fisher Center for Autism Spectrum Disorders, Munroe-Meyer Institute, University of Nebraska Medical Center, 985450 Nebraska Medical Center, Omaha, NE, USA

Max Horovitz Louisiana State University, Baton Rouge, LA, USA

John M. Huete Department of Behavioral Psychology, Kennedy Krieger Institute and The Johns Hopkins University School of Medicine, Baltimore, MD, USA

Sarah Hurwitz Department of Psychiatry, Indiana University School of Medicine, Indianapolis, IN, USA
Christian Sarkine Autism Treatment Center, James Whitcomb Riley Hospital for Children, Indiana University School of Medicine, Indianapolis, IN, USA

Michael E. Kelley Center for Autism Spectrum Disorders, Munroe-Meyer Institute, University of Nebraska Medical Center, 985450 Nebraska Medical Center, Omaha, NE, USA

Vicki Madaus Knapp Summit Educational Resources, Getzville, NY, USA

Alison M. Kozlowski Louisiana State University, Baton Rouge, LA, USA

Patricia F. Kurtz Department of Behavioral Psychology, Kennedy Krieger Institute and The Johns Hopkins University School of Medicine, Baltimore, MD, USA

Giulio E. Lancioni Department of Psychology, University of Bari, Bary, Italy

Russell Lang College of Education, Texas State University, San Marcos, TX, USA

Amanda Mahoney Department of Psychology, Western Michigan University, Kalamazoo, MI, USA

Johnny L. Matson Department of Psychology, Louisiana State University, Baton Rouge, LA, USA

David B. McAdam University of Rochester School of Medicine, Rochester, NY, USA

Noha F. Minshawi Department of Psychiatry, Indiana University School of Medicine, Indianapolis, IN, USA

Christian Sarkine Autism Treatment Center, James Whitcomb Riley Hospital for Children, Indiana University School of Medicine, Indianapolis, IN, USA

Deborah A. Napolitano University of Rochester School of Medicine, Rochester, NY, USA

Mark F. O'Reilly Department of Special Education, College of Education, The University of Texas at Austin, Austin, TX, USA

Stephanie M. Peterson Department of Psychology, Western Michigan University, Kalamazoo, MI, USA

Alan Poling Department of Psychology, Western Michigan University, Kalamazoo, MI, USA

Henry S. Roane State University of New York Upstate Medical University, Syracuse, NY, USA

Nicole M. Rodriguez Center for Autism Spectrum Disorders, Munroe-Meyer Institute, University of Nebraska Medical Center, 985450 Nebraska Medical Center, Omaha, NE, USA

Amanda B. Rone Psychology Department, University of Florida, Gainesville, FL, USA

Jeff Sigafoos School of Educational Psychology and Pedagogy, Victoria University of Wellington, Wellington, New Zealand

Nirbhay N. Singh American Health and Wellness Institute, Raleigh, NC, USA

Megan Sipes Louisiana State University, Baton Rouge, LA, USA

Elizabeth Speares Hillside Children's Center, Rochester, NY, USA

Peter Sturmey Department of Psychology, Queens College, City University of New York, Flushing, NY, USA

Jonathan Tarbox Center for Autism and Related Disorders Inc., Tarzana, CA, USA

Talya Vogel Center for Autism and Related Disorders Inc., Tarzana, CA, USA

Timothy R. Vollmer Psychology Department, University of Florida, Gainesville, FL, USA

Marc Weeden Department of Psychology, Western Michigan University, Kalamazoo, MI, USA

Department of Special Education and Literacy Studies, Western Michigan University, Kalamazoo, MI, USA

Introduction

Johnny L. Matson

Functional assessment has become a heavily studied and frequently used method in the field of applied behavior analysis. The literature as a result has grown rapidly, and thus, a volume on the topic is timely. This book consists of chapters that cover the major issues in the field. The book begins with a historical overview that highlights the roots of functional assessment in the beginning of applied behavior analysis and the focus on antecedent events. Since functional assessment is used primarily for challenging behaviors such as self-injury and aggression, three chapters are devoted to the nature, prevalence, characteristics, and functions of these behaviors. Also, the populations studied and most likely to benefit from these interventions are discussed at length.

The second section of the book is a review of specific methods and procedures that are routinely used in a functional assessment. Methods of defining and observing behaviors are the first building blocks in functional assessment and thus constitute the first chapter in this section. This section is followed by four chapters on specific methods of assessment. These methods include interviews, observations, experimental functional analysis, in vivo assessment, and different scaling methods. The third and final section is comprised of four chapters. These include practical considerations such as treatment methods and planning, methods and procedures to clarify ambiguous functional assessment results, and ethical considerations.

The overall purpose of our book is to provide an up-to-date resource for clinicians and researchers, covering all the major issues on functional assessment. The book should serve as a reference and hopefully a guide for persons working in the field of applied behavior analysis.

J.L. Matson (✉)
Department of Psychology, Louisiana State University,
Baton Rouge, LA 70803, USA
e-mail: johnmatson@aol.com

J.L. Matson (ed.), *Functional Assessment for Challenging Behaviors*,
Autism and Child Psychopathology Series, DOI 10.1007/978-1-4614-3037-7_1,
© Springer Science+Business Media, LLC 2012

A Brief History of Functional Analysis and Applied Behavior Analysis

Dennis R. Dixon, Talya Vogel, and Jonathan Tarbox

The history of functional analysis, as both a concept and a procedure, can be traced back to the earliest days of the discipline of applied behavior analysis (ABA) and even to the earliest days of basic research in behavior analysis that formed the foundation for ABA. Indeed, it is not unreasonable to state that the history of functional analysis is inextricably linked to the history of the discipline of ABA. The general discipline of ABA and the concepts and methods of functional analysis have been built upon the conceptual foundation of operant conditioning, and as advancements have been made in the basic and conceptual arenas of behavior analysis, new refinements have been made in the area of application.

It is sometimes said that the development of experimental functional analysis methodology by Iwata, among others, led to a major shift in focus in the field of ABA toward an acknowledgment of the need for understanding the root causes of behavior before simply applying potent consequences. Some call this a transition from "behavior modification" to "applied behavior analysis" (Mace, 1994). Appreciating the function of behavior when planning treatment is now widely regarded as best practice (as evidenced by the

publication of this volume), but it was not always so. Early applications of behavioral principles to problematic behaviors in humans often failed to acknowledge the underlying function of behavior (Mace, 1994). In this model, the application of potent reinforcers and punishers were effective when they simply overcame the ongoing contingencies with which they were juxtaposed, not because they addressed the core underlying cause or function of the behavior. The shift in focus to understanding the operant function of behavior before treating it marked a major evolution in ABA, but to say such a perspective was not present until standardized experimental assessment methodology had been published is an overstatement. As discussed in this chapter, the importance of understanding the environmental contingencies responsible for maintaining *all* behavior, aberrant or adaptive, was present since the beginnings of the field, in Skinner's writings and elsewhere. But little in the way of practical procedures was available for directly addressing the functions of behavior in clinical settings. As we outline in this chapter, the pioneering work of Bijou, Lovaas, Iwata, and Carr, among others, spurred a revolution in applied behavioral research by developing a basic experimental format for functional analysis that continues to thrive decades later.

In this chapter, we start by briefly outlining the history of behavior analysis, the development of ABA, and the origins of procedures designed to ascertain the function of challenging behavior. We then describe the landmark paper by Iwata,

D.R. Dixon (✉) • T. Vogel • J. Tarbox
Center for Autism and Related Disorders Inc.,
19019 Ventura Blvd., Tarzana, CA 91356, USA
e-mail: d.dixon@centerforautism.com;
t.vogel@centerforautism.com;
j.tarbox@centerforautism.com

J.L. Matson (ed.), *Functional Assessment for Challenging Behaviors*,
Autism and Child Psychopathology Series, DOI 10.1007/978-1-4614-3037-7_2,
© Springer Science+Business Media, LLC 2012

Dorsey, Slifer, Bauman, and Richman (1982), the influence of which is evidenced in that, to date, it has been cited by 235 publications indexed in PsycINFO (plus an additional 533 publications that cite its 1994 reprint). The remainder of the chapter is dedicated to a brief overview of procedural refinements which have been developed up to the current day, the majority of which are described in greater detail in other chapters within this volume.

Historical Roots of Behavior Analysis

A bit of historical background will set the stage for a description of the beginnings of behavior analysis, a thoroughly natural science of psychology. Psychology in the early 1900s was dominated by the study of mental processes and introspection. Carefully observing one's own conscious mental, emotional, or feeling states was the primary method of investigation (Wolf, 1978). Until the introduction of behaviorism, introspective psychology dominated American psychological thinking (Watson, 1913). Even within this context, though, psychologists were grappling with the causes of behavior. Early functionalists, such as William James (1890), posited that mental processes had evolved to serve useful functions for individuals struggling to cope in complex environments.

Watson (1913) argued for an objective study of behavior as a natural science, consisting of direct observation of the relationships between environmental stimuli and behavioral responses. In doing so, he laid the groundwork for an analysis of how the environment determined behavior. He was confident in stimulus–response (S–R) psychology's ability to predict and control human behavior, so much so that many would argue he overstated the potential significantly (Skinner, 1974). Even so, Watson's insistence upon studying relations between behavior and environment, in their own right, was critical in establishing the belief that behavior could be studied as a natural science, on par with biology, physics, and the other natural sciences (Cooper, Heron, & Heward, 2007).

B. F. Skinner's first major treatise, *The Behavior of Organisms* (1938), spurred the development of what would come to be known as the "experimental analysis of behavior," now known simply as "behavior analysis." Like Watson, Skinner was interested in giving a scientific account for all behavior, but unlike other psychologists of his time, he found the S–R paradigm insufficient to explain the majority of behavior, especially for those behaviors for which there appeared to be no obvious antecedent environmental causes (Cooper et al., 2007). Somewhat serendipitously, while studying the ingestive behavior of rats, Skinner observed that environmental events that immediately followed behaviors had as much or more influence on the future occurrence of those behaviors as did the antecedents. Skinner then promoted the idea that the traditional model of S–R cause-and-effect should be abandoned and replaced by a more descriptive, functional analysis of the relationship between independent and dependent variable (Sturmey & Bernstein, 2004), consisting of the three-term contingency (antecedent–behavior–consequence or stimulus–response–stimulus). It was soon found that Skinner's S–R–S model was able to account for behaviors that the S–R model did not sufficiently explain—behaviors that did not have apparent antecedent causes or for which the consequences figured more prominently. He called these behaviors "operant," that is, those behaviors are influenced by the consequences of similar behaviors in an organism's past (Cooper et al., 2007).

The three-term contingency provided a model for studying behavior in a new way. Rather than searching for inner psychic causes of behavior, as traditional psychologists had done, and rather than searching for simplistic antecedent causes, as S–R psychologists had done, the task of the behaviorist was now to identify reliable three-term contingencies that describe behavior/environment relations. Scientific understanding of behavior, then, was achieved by identifying and manipulating the environmental variables that change the probability of its occurrence. Through repeated manipulation of environmental variables, a functional relationship between environment (independent variable) and behavior (dependent variable) can be discovered. For Skinner, the term "functional relationship," which describes the relationship between behavior and environment, essentially became synonymous with "cause-and-effect" relationship (Skinner, 1953). In Skinner's words, "the external variables of which behavior is a function provide for what may be called a causal or functional analysis. We undertake to predict and control the behavior of the individual organism" (Skinner, 1953, p. 35).

The term "functional analysis," in its original use, simply meant an activity that shed light upon the potential ways in which the environment may control behavior (Skinner, 1953). It did not originally connote an experimental analysis, as it often does today, although Skinner always preferred experimental over descriptive analyses. In *Verbal Behavior* (1957), Skinner described the book, an almost entirely conceptual treatment of language, as a "functional analysis of language," clearly not referring to an experimental procedure. In the most general sense, the term retains the same meaning today, although, practically speaking, many people are referring to an experimental functional analysis when they use the term "functional analysis."

Skinner's early work described essential methods, concepts, and functional relations that would serve as the foundation for the development of a functional analysis of behavior. These included the focus on a single organism, the rate of response as the main dependent variable, the operant–respondent distinction with related difference between conditioned stimulus and discriminative stimulus, and the effects of various kinds of intermittent reinforcement (Michael, 1980). In its most simplistic form, Skinner recorded the rate at which a single animal emitted a given behavior in a controlled operant chamber. His investigative procedures evolved into an experimental approach that "enabled clear and powerful demonstrations of orderly and reliable functional relations between behavior and various types of environmental events" (Cooper et al., 2007, p. 11). However, behavior analysis was never intended as a science of animal behavior. In *Science and Human Behavior* (1953), Skinner proposed that the techniques of behavior analysis

should be extended to explain and change the behavior of people in everyday arenas such as education, work, clinical problems, and social behavior. While most experimental psychologists were inherently conservative in describing the generalizability of their work to practical situations, Skinner managed to address a wide array of human situations from an entirely behavioral point of view. In the 1950s and 1960s, research on application of behavior analysis began in earnest.

Applying Behavioral Principles to Humans

Research during the 1950s and 1960s utilized the methods of the experimental analysis of behavior to examine whether the principles of behavior derived from experimentation with nonhumans could be replicated with human subjects (Cooper et al., 2007). Early researchers established that the principles of behavior observed in animal studies were applicable to human behavior (Baer, 1960; Bijou, 1955; Ferster & DeMyer, 1961, 1962; Lindsley, 1956, 1960) and provided the foundation for the development of ABA in general and the functional analysis of clinically relevant behavior in particular (Cooper et al., 2007).

One of the first studies to apply operant principles to human behavior was conducted by Fuller (1949), who used positive reinforcement (sugar solution) to teach an 18-year-old man with profound intellectual disabilities to raise his hand. Prior to this, it was widely assumed that individuals with severe intellectual disabilities were not capable of learning. Indeed, Fuller wrote that in regard to the specific participant, doctors "thought it was impossible for him to learn anything," but the results of this study demonstrated that "if time permitted, other responses could be conditioned and discriminations learned" (Fuller, 1949, p. 590). A few years later, Lindsley, Skinner, and Solomon (1953) applied the principles of operant conditioning to inpatients at a psychiatric state hospital, further establishing the basic concept that the behavior of all individuals is subject to behavioral principles of learning and motivation.

While a variety of methods and procedures were available for use within the animal studies, little had been done to extend these procedures to human subjects. Sidney Bijou's early work (e.g., Bijou, 1955, 1957, 1958) was fundamental in extending the methods and findings of animal research so that the behavior of humans could be experimentally analyzed. He proposed descriptions of methodologies for "a systematic approach to an experimental analysis of child behavior" (Bijou, 1957, p. 250). He described specific instrumentation, how data was to be recorded, and how to maximize control over independent variables. He said that once the methodology was properly refined, it would enable researchers to study behavior "by relating the direct effect of one variable upon another" (Bijou, 1957, p. 243). These publications were seminal in establishing a methodology through which the functional relationships of human behavior could be analyzed in a well-controlled environment.

Ogden Lindsley was another pioneer in adapting the methods of animal studies to the study of human behavior and was among the first to apply free-operant procedures to studying the behavior of chronic and acute psychotic children and adults. Addressing the methodological limitations of the emerging field, Lindsley (1956) described how American psychologists had used a "confusing variety of apparatuses" (p. 120) to measure behavior, and psychology as an experimental field had not yet agreed upon a universal instrument to measure behavior; thus, researchers were constantly designing new instruments or modifying old ones. Lindsley cited Pavlov's studies as exhibiting a higher degree of experimental control than any other researcher in the early 1900s, and while more contemporary researchers described their various apparatuses, they failed to design well-controlled experimental situations. He argued that "American psychologists in the early part of this century imitated Pavlov's verbal behavior, but they did not imitate his experimental behavior" (Lindsley, 1956, p. 124).

A significant step toward applying the methods developed in animal studies to address abnormal behavior among humans was made by Ferster (1958), who was one of the first to recognize that aberrant behaviors were often maintained by other individuals. In other words, Ferster conceptualized that a deficient behavioral repertoire is a social problem. He argued that problem behaviors may arise because of (a) an inadequate reinforcement history, (b) the schedule of reinforcement, or (c) punishment that may distort a performance which otherwise would be reinforced (Ferster, 1958). In order to treat an individual's inadequate behavioral repertoire, Ferster promoted the use of a "functional program of therapy" (Ferster, 1958, p. 105) in which the therapist manipulates variables in the patient's environment to identify potential reinforcers that maintain the problem behavior. Thus, Ferster was one of the first to acknowledge the importance of functional relations between problematic behaviors and environmental events.

The studies in the 1940s and 1950s did not attempt to make clinically meaningful behavior changes in the individuals they studied, but they served to establish further the notion that behavior change in severely challenged populations was possible and that human behavior, too, was a function of the environment (Wilkins & Matson, 2009). By demonstrating that operant principles could be applied to the behavior of humans, the groundwork was laid for the development of a discipline centered on using behavioral principals to bring about socially meaningful behavior change.

The Birth of Applied Behavior Analysis

The late 1950s through the 1960s saw the birth of what came to be known as the field or discipline of ABA. Ayllon & Michael's, 1959 paper is often cited as the first ABA publication. In "The Psychiatric Nurse as a Behavioral Engineer," personnel in a state hospital were trained to use techniques that were derived from behavioral principles to improve the functioning of residents with schizophrenia and other psychiatric diagnoses. While no systematic approach to studying such problems was in existence, the authors stated that the aim of their research was "an attempt to discover and manipulate some of the environmental variables for the purpose of modifying problem behavior" (Ayllon & Michael, 1959, p. 323). Over the next decade, the researchers began to apply these same principles of behavior to a variety of socially problematic behavior and developmental disabilities (Jacobson & Holburn, 2004). This new line of research represented a major advance in how severe behavior problems were conceptualized. Studies were able to demonstrate experimentally that maladaptive behaviors, such as self-injury or aggression, could be explained as functional responses to environmental stimuli (Durand, 1987).

The application of operant principles and experimental method to the analysis of human behavior emerged as its own discipline in the 1960s with a mission to solve important social problems in a systematic and individualized manner (Jacobson & Holburn, 2004). In the inaugural issue of the *Journal of Applied Behavior Analysis,* Baer, Wolf, and Risley (1968) described some of the defining features of ABA, distinct from the experimental analysis of behavior. They outlined seven dimensions of ABA: applied, behavioral, analytic, technological, conceptually systematic, effective, and generalizable. Baer et al. (1968) described ABA as a discipline which "will make obvious the importance of the behavior changed, the experimental manipulations which analyze with clarity what was responsible for the change, the technologically exact description of all procedures contributing to that change, the effectiveness of those procedures in making sufficient change for value, and the generality of that change" (Baer et al., 1968, p. 97). Of particular relevance to the current chapter is the dimension of ABA referred to as "analytic." The analytic component stressed the importance of using valid single-subject experimental designs to manipulate environmental variables and observe the effects such variables have on behavior, a practice at the very heart of experimental functional analysis methodology.

A Focus on the Function of Challenging Behaviors

Early research in ABA attempted to reduce the frequency and severity of challenging behaviors and facilitate the acquisition of adaptive skills (Wilkins & Matson, 2009). While much early research demonstrated that mere management of behavioral consequences could effectively decrease challenging behaviors, behavior analysts have long had concerns about unnecessary use of punishment-based procedures. Skinner and many early behaviorists warned that punishment may bring about undesirable side effects and that striving to promote control of behavior through positive reinforcement as much as possible was a valuable goal in and of itself. In addition, the operant perspective assumes that different behaviors have different functions for different people, and even multiple functions within the same person, and so a prior understanding of the cause or function of the behavior will inevitably aid in designing an effective treatment. This belief was implicit from the beginning, but it was not until the 1960s that research began which attempted to directly identify the function of challenging behavior.

An early study on the function of self-injurious behavior (SIB) in a child with schizophrenia was conducted by Lovaas, Freitag, Gold, and Kassorla (1965). This study is noteworthy because it was the first to systematically investigate a problem behavior wherein "the investigator has attempted control over self-destruction by systematically manipulating the variables of which it might be a function" (Lovaas et al., 1965, p. 68). In the first phase of the study, the participant initially received social approval for appropriate behaviors, and following a period of acquisition, the behavior was then extinguished by withholding the social reinforcers. The second study occurred in a different experimental setting than the first but procedurally was very similar. Social approval was delivered contingent upon the subject pressing a lever, and once the lever-pressing rate had stabilized, the behavior was then again extinguished by withholding the social attention. In the third phase, the authors demonstrated that delivering verbal attention contingent upon SIB resulted in an increase in the frequency of the behavior (Lovaas, et al., 1965).

Carr (1977) was among the first researchers in ABA to promote a system in which interventionists would develop hypotheses for conditions that maintain problem behavior and then develop treatment strategies on the basis of those hypotheses. Carr's, 1977 review of the functions of self-injury greatly influenced the development of a method of conducting functional analysis (Sturmey & Bernstein, 2004). His review concluded that self-injury could be maintained by three general classes of environmental contingencies: positive reinforcement, negative reinforcement, and sensory or automatic consequences of the behavior (Carr, 1977). As noted by Sturmey and Bernstein (2004), Carr and his colleagues conducted a series of important studies demonstrating functional relationships between the occurrence of certain events and SIB, all of which developed experimental conditions that could be used to experimentally identify the functions of maladaptive behaviors (Carr, Newsom, & Binkoff, 1980; Rincover, Newsom, & Carr, 1979).

Early Research on Specific Functions of Challenging Behavior

Before the landmark paper by Iwata et al. (1982) was published, several early studies focused on individual functions of behavior. These papers helped establish the foundations upon which more comprehensive experimental assessments were later developed.

Positive Reinforcement

One of the most prominent theories presented in the early literature on functions of aberrant behavior was that maladaptive behaviors were shaped and maintained by socially mediated positive reinforcement (Carr, 1977). One of the first empirical demonstrations of how attention can positively reinforce aberrant behavior was conducted by Ayllon and Michael (1959). An informal analysis led the authors to suggest that attention from nursing staff was inadvertently positively reinforcing the psychotic speech of a psychiatric inpatient. When the nurses ceased replying to the patient's statements, the rate of aberrant speech dropped dramatically. The authors observed that within the overcrowded,

understaffed wards of mental hospitals, outbursts of problem behavior were often the only way for individuals to attract a nurse's attention. Unfortunately, the more adaptive, socially acceptable behaviors often went unnoticed or were even punished by overworked hospital orderlies, a circumstance that many clinicians sadly still observe to this day in residential settings for individuals with developmental and other disabilities.

Many studies in the 1960s applied this same principle of adjusting the contingencies of adult attention in seeking to modify challenging behaviors of children. Hart, Allen, Buell, Harris, and Wolf (1964) treated the frequent crying of two preschool children, starting with the hypothesis that the behavior was reinforced by teacher attention. The authors successfully extinguished crying by training teachers to give no attention to excessive crying and to provide immediate positive attention for more appropriate responses. Subsequent studies found the same mediating effects of attention on the presence of problem behavior in both the classroom (Harris, Wolf, & Baer, 1964; Thomas, Becker, & Armstrong, 1968) and the home (Baskett & Johnson, 1982; Budd, Green, & Baer, 1976; Hawkins, Peterson, Schweid, & Bijou, 1966). A substantial body of literature published in the 1960s and 1970s supported the positive reinforcement hypothesis, indicating that the complete removal of social consequences greatly reduced or eliminated SIB (Jones, Simmons, & Frankel, 1974; Lovaas & Simmons, 1969; Tate & Baroff, 1966; Wolf, Risley, Johnston, Harris, & Allen, 1967; Wolf, Risley, & Mees, 1964).

Lovaas et al. (1965) experimentally investigated variables that controlled self-destructive behavior in a child with schizophrenia. In a series of three studies, it was found that, following several sessions of social extinction, reinstatement of social attention contingent on self-destructive behavior produced the highest magnitude and frequency of the problem behavior. A later study by Lovaas and Simmons (1969) built upon this work in an attempt to isolate some of the environmental conditions that controlled the self-destructive behavior of three children with severe developmental disabilities. Similar to Lovass and colleagues' earlier study, when the children were placed in a room where they were allowed to engage in SIB, isolated from interpersonal contact and social consequences, they eventually ceased to hurt themselves (Lovaas & Simmons, 1969).

While a significant amount of evidence supported the concept of an attention function for challenging behavior, some early work also suggested that aberrant behavior may be maintained by other types of socially mediated positive reinforcement. For example, Patterson, Littman, and Bricker (1967) conducted an early descriptive analysis of aggressive behavior and discussed the possibility that access to food, candy, or preferred toys may maintain it. They described cases in which children emitted aggressive behavior, resulting in their victims relinquishing toys or other preferred materials.

Negative Reinforcement

In addition to investigating socially mediated positive reinforcement as a potential function of challenging behavior, early work on behavioral function hypothesized that aberrant behavior may be maintained by negative reinforcement. The negative reinforcement hypothesis stated that aberrant behavior was learned behavior, reinforced by escape or avoidance of an aversive stimulus or situation (Carr, Newsom, & Binkoff, 1976). Much early work on the negative reinforcement hypothesis focused on SIB. Early anecdotal reports noted that children who engaged in SIB often did so in order to terminate an aversive situation. For example, Freud and Burlingham (1944) described a girl living in an institution who would bang her head against her crib when she was put to bed, noting that this behavior resulted in being removed from the crib.

Ferster (1958) recognized that the problem behaviors of many psychiatric patients were inadvertently maintained by negative reinforcement. He noted that, rather than providing an individual with an adaptive behavioral repertoire, attempts at punishment often reinforced aberrant behaviors by allowing the individual to avoid or escape aversive consequences (Ferster, 1958).

Other descriptive reports noted that demands were very likely to increase SIB in children (e.g., Jones et al., 1974; Myers & Deibert, 1971; Wolf et al., 1967). In these early papers, it was observed that following such self-destructive behavior, the adults who were working with the children would often terminate the demands they were placing upon the children. Taken together, these reports suggested that demands may constitute aversive stimuli, and SIB functioned as an escape response maintained by the termination of demands; however, no studies had yet attempted to experimentally manipulate environmental variables to confirm this hypothesis.

The first attempt at experimentally manipulating the environment to evaluate the negative reinforcement hypothesis appeared in Carr, Newsom, and Binkoff's seminal paper (1976). Carr and colleagues focused their experimental analysis on the *antecedent* stimuli that would likely control escape-maintained SIB. The study demonstrated that levels of SIB were high in demand situations (such as a classroom) and low in situations that did not contain demands (such as conversation or freeplay). In addition, they manipulated the occurrence of stimuli which had historically been paired with removal of demands, hypothesizing that SIB should decrease upon the onset of the stimulus correlated with the termination of demands. When the child, who was engaging in SIB, was presented with the vocal prompt "O.K., let's go," a cue that normally terminated the demand period, the child abruptly stopped the self-destructive behavior. In contrast, when a neutral vocal stimulus was presented to the child, such as "The sky is blue" (a cue that had never been paired with the termination of demands), the child's rate of SIB remained high. By manipulating antecedent events that should be correlated with escape-maintained behavior, and by demonstrating that the occurrence of the behavior varied in a predictable way with the manipulation, Carr provided a convincing early experimental demonstration of maladaptive behavior with a negative reinforcement function, albeit without yet manipulating the actual consequences of which the behavior was thought to be a function.

SIB was not the only behavior thought to serve an escape function. Carr et al. (1980) sought to identify the variables controlling severe aggressive behavior in two children. In a series of four experiments, aggression was frequent in demand conditions and rare in nondemand situations. Like SIB, aggression was shown to function sometimes as an escape response. While previous investigations had implied that aggression could serve the function of an escape response to terminate demands or other aversive stimuli (Ludwig, Marx, Hill, & Browning, 1969; Patterson et al., 1967), Carr et al. (1980) was the first experimental study to systematically investigate the possible role of escape factors in the maintenance of aggression.

Weeks and Gaylord-Ross (1981) examined the relationship between task characteristics and problem behavior and provided additional experimental support for the negative reinforcement hypothesis of aberrant behaviors. It was conceptualized that severely handicapped children, when presented with a difficult task, would emit aberrant responses to terminate the aversive stimulus. Three experimental conditions were created to test this possibility in which the students would be presented with difficult tasks, easy tasks, and no tasks. As predicted, the highest frequency of aberrant behavior was associated with difficult demands, and near-zero levels of problem behavior occurred in settings that were free of demands, thereby providing further support for the negative reinforcement hypothesis.

Automatic Reinforcement

The concept of automatic reinforcement has early roots in behavior analysis, dating back at least as far as Skinner's analysis of verbal behavior (1957). Automatic reinforcement is reinforcement that is produced automatically when a behavior occurs. That is, it is reinforcement that is *not* dependent on the behavior of someone else to deliver it. Automatic reinforcement is sometimes described as reinforcement that is inherent in the behavior itself. Everyday examples include the relief of the itching sensation that the behavior of scratching an insect bite produces or the

pleasant odor that the behavior of smelling a flower produces. It is also important to note that stereotyped behaviors, behaviors which occur repeatedly in the same manner, are often assumed to be automatically reinforced. For this reason, it is likely that stereotypy is often referred to as "self-stimulatory" behavior, a term that assumes that the behavior is maintained by automatic reinforcement. However, it is important to note that the topography of a behavior (e.g., stereotypy) does not necessarily indicate function (e.g., automatic reinforcement). It is for this reason that the term stereotypy is generally preferred over "self-stimulatory" or "self-stim" behavior.

Early animal research on automatically reinforced behaviors addressed stereotypy across several species (Berkson, Mason, & Saxon, 1963). Experiments in the 1960s examined the effects of environments that were "deprived" of stimulation. In particular, social isolation was studied in primates because "it is difficult or impossible to study scientifically the impacts of culturally produced social isolation at the human level" (Harlow, Dodsworth, & Harlow, 1965). Researchers noted that the same behavioral principles seemed to operate for both humans and primates and that "social conditions which produce abnormality in one species will have comparable effects on the other" (Harlow et al., 1965, p. 90). Behaviors such as thumb sucking, unusual limb postures, and self-clasping were observed as common primate stereotypies.

A study by Berkson et al. (1963) examined stimulus and situational factors affecting the stereotyped behaviors characteristic of primates raised without their mothers. They observed that the level of stereotypy was highest in an environment in which vision, locomotion, and opportunities to manipulate objects were restricted. The authors argued that it was very likely that the absence of environmental stimulation was an important factor in the presence of such behavior, as the stereotyped responses were reduced when alternative activities were evoked (Berkson et al., 1963). These early animal studies reflected a basic hypothesis that automatically reinforced behavior is more likely to occur when an organism is deprived of stimulation because the behavior may be one of the only sources of environmental stimulation available to the organism.

Residential facilities were conceptualized as one type of setting in which individuals with disabilities may be deprived of stimulation, and researchers began to conceptualize environmental deprivation as a factor that may contribute to the maintenance of automatically reinforced maladaptive behaviors in humans (Green, 1967; McKinney, 1962; Murphy, 1982). For example, early researchers noted several cases of problem behavior among children who were restricted to their cribs without toys (Dennis & Najarian, 1957). Collins (1965) treated head banging in an isolated, severely intellectually disabled adult by exposing the individual to a high level of sensory stimulation. The consequent decrease in SIB was attributed to the increased tactile and kinesthetic stimulation that was provided in treatment. Green (1967) was another researcher to propose that the stereotypy often seen in children living in institutional settings occurred as an adaptive response to a decreased level of environmental stimulation. He postulated that, in the overall absence of stimulation, operant responses, such as self-destructive behaviors, develop into persistent behavior as a function of the increased sensory input they provide.

Experimental investigations of the effects of noncontingent stimuli on stereotypies provided additional foundation for the hypothesis that some aberrant behaviors have an automatic reinforcement function. Early studies demonstrated that vibration significantly decreased the stereotyped behavior of intellectually disabled children (Bailey & Meyerson, 1969, 1970; Meyerson, Kerr, & Michael, 1967). Maisto, Baumeister, and Maisto (1978) noted that individuals who lacked adaptive modes of behavior or appropriate opportunities to increase stimulation often resorted to activities that involved direct contact or manipulation of the body.

Wolery (1978) assessed the effects of experimenter-applied sensory stimulation that was comparable to the child's stereotypic behavior. Results from this study demonstrated that contingent trainer-applied sensory stimulation (which duplicated the child's stereotypy) functioned as a powerful positive reinforcer. An additional study conducted by Rincover (1978) investigated the self-stimulatory behavior of psychotic children in order to identify possible maintaining/supporting variables. The results showed that the self-stimulatory behavior was "reliably decreased when a certain sensory consequence was removed, then increased when that consequence was permitted" (p. 307), thereby supporting the notion that the behavior was maintained by operant reinforcement in the form of sensory stimulation. Furthermore, Rincover stated that then-current theories holding that stereotypy is a result of understimulation did "not easily account for these data, primarily because the suppressive effect of removing sensory consequences was specific to a particular sensory modality" (p. 307).

The First Comprehensive Experimental Functional Analysis

The studies described thus far provided ample evidence for three possible functions of challenging behavior: (1) socially mediated positive reinforcement (e.g., attention), (2) negative reinforcement (e.g., escape from nonpreferred tasks), and (3) automatic reinforcement. Substantial evidence existed to support each hypothesis, but little or no research had been published on attempts at evaluating more than one potential function for the same behavior of one individual. In addition, although a substantial amount of literature had been published which had implications for how to identify the functions of challenging behavior, no standard set of comprehensive functional analysis procedures had yet been proposed, and several researchers acknowledged the need for it (Carr, 1977; Weeks & Gaylord-Ross, 1981). In particular, Weeks and Gaylord-Ross (1981) wrote that "a useful contribution to the burgeoning field of behavioral assessment would be the development of clear criteria for determining whether aberrant behavior is maintained by positive reinforcement, negative reinforcement, or intrinsic reinforcement (self-stimulation)" (p. 461).

One year later, Iwata et al. published their seminal paper, "Toward a Functional Analysis of

Self-Injurious Behavior" (1982), which was reprinted in 1994 in the *Journal of Applied Behavior Analysis*. The study included nine children and adolescents with developmental disabilities and SIB. A randomized multielement design (rapid alternation between 15-min sessions of each condition) was used to compare the occurrence of SIB under four experimental conditions: (1) academic, (2) alone, (3) social disapproval, and (4) play. The first three conditions were selected to represent the three general functions of behavior that had been hypothesized up to that point (positive, negative, and automatic reinforcement) and the fourth served as a control condition.

In the academic condition (now usually referred to as the "demand" or "escape" condition), the experimenter and participant sat at a desk. The experimenter presented tasks to the participant, using a graduated "three-step" prompting sequence. The sequence began with the experimenter presenting the task vocally. If the participant did not respond within 5 s, the experimenter repeated the vocal instruction and provided a model prompt. If the participant did not respond appropriately after 5 s, the experimenter physically guided the participant to respond, after which the next task was presented vocally. If the participant responded appropriately, the experimenter responded with brief praise. If, at any time, the participant engaged in SIB, the experimenter turned away from the participant and ceased task demands for 30 s. This condition was designed to test for a negative reinforcement function because escape from demands was systematically presented, contingent on the occurrence of the target behavior.

In the alone condition, the participant was placed in a therapy room alone, with no toys or items of any kind. This condition was designed to test for automatic reinforcement and mimicked the types of "deprived" environments hypothesized to contribute to automatically reinforced behavior that were discussed in earlier research on automatic reinforcement.

In the social disapproval condition (now usually referred to as the "attention" condition), the experimenter and the participant entered a therapy room that was equipped with a variety of toys. The experimenter then told the participant to play with the toys while the experimenter "did some work." Contingent on each occurrence of SIB, or burst of occurrences, the experimenter delivered brief statements of concern (e.g., "Don't do that, you will hurt yourself") while also delivering brief physical attention (e.g., patting the person on the shoulder). All other participant behaviors were ignored. The purpose of this condition was to test for a possible function of positive reinforcement in the form of access to attention from others.

In the play condition (sometimes referred to as the "toy play" or "control" condition), the therapy room was equipped with a variety of toys, and no demands were placed on the child. The experimenter delivered brief social and physical attention to the participant, contingent on the absence of SIB, at least every 30 s. SIB was ignored. This condition was included to serve as a control condition. It served as a suitable control condition for the attention condition because the antecedent for attention-maintained behavior was absent (i.e., the participant was not deprived of attention), and attention was not delivered as a consequence of SIB. Similarly, the play condition served as a suitable control condition for escape-maintained behavior because the relevant antecedent was not present (i.e., presentation of demands), nor was the putative maintaining consequence (escape was not delivered contingent on SIB). It is difficult to construct a control condition that withholds the consequence for automatically reinforced behavior because the consequence is automatically produced, but the relevant antecedent (general deprivation of stimulation) is not present.

The analysis continued to be conducted until (1) stability in the level of SIB was observed, (2) unstable levels of SIB continued for 5 days, or (3) sessions had been conducted for 12 days. No assessment lasted longer than 11 days, and the number of 15-min sessions that were required ranged from 24 to 53. The results demonstrated significant variability in responding, both across various conditions within each participant and across patterns of responding between participants. These results provided strong support for the position that particular topographies of challenging behavior do not have singular causes but, rather, are learned behaviors that differ in their relationship to environmental events, depending on the unique learning history of each individual person. In particular, the results of some participants strongly suggested that their SIB was maintained by attention, while others appeared to be maintained by escape from demands, and still others appeared to be maintained by automatic reinforcement. Another important finding was that the function of the SIB did not appear to be correlated in any significant way with the rate or severity of the behavior. All of these results strongly supported the notion developed in the functional assessment literature that the function and topography of any given behavior are distinct and, more importantly, that clinicians cannot, therefore, assume a cause of behavior by simply looking at the topography or severity.

Another important contribution of the paper by Iwata et al. (2000) was that it set forth a simple format for experimentally investigating the function of any behavior. By pitting one or more test conditions, each of which tests one potential consequence as a reinforcer, against a single control condition that reverses or eliminates each of the contingencies being manipulated in the test conditions, multiple potential functions could be assessed during the course of a single assessment. Furthermore, the variety of potential functions that could be assessed within this format was limited only by the imagination and ability of the assessor to control environmental conditions. As we will see in the coming section of this chapter, this basic format has changed little in the last 30 years, but a considerable variety of different behaviors and functions have been assessed.

After 1982

The seminal 1982 paper by Iwata et al. offered an elegant yet powerful format for conducting experimental assessments of the function of maladaptive behaviors, and the three decades that have passed since its publication have seen the basic format used across a variety of other populations, settings, and behaviors. In addition, alterations to the basic format have been researched in order to accommodate a variety of different behaviors, idiosyncratic environmental variables, and other behavioral functions, among others. A complete description of the history of experimental functional analysis research post-1982 would likely require several volumes in itself, and other chapters in the current volume provide additional details in multiple areas. In what follows, we provide descriptions of some of the major highlights in terms of how the basic experimental functional analysis format has been used to study many additional phenomena, as well as how it has been modified to expand its scope further, and we will conclude the chapter with a discussion of future directions for research.

The "standard" functional analysis methodology proposed by Iwata et al. (2000) has proven to be robust and widely applicable, as described above. Indeed, reviews of functional analysis methodology have suggested that functional analyses result in a determination of behavioral function in about 94% of the cases in which they are applied (Hanley, Iwata, & McCord, 2003; Iwata, Pace, et al., 1994). While some functional analyses may result in undifferentiated or ambiguous outcomes, this does not necessarily mean that the assessment process has failed or that the contingencies maintaining the problem behavior cannot be understood (Tiger, Fisher, Toussaint, & Kodak, 2009). Many authors have noted that the traditional functional analysis methods developed by Iwata et al. (1982) occasionally require modifications to assess behavioral function more accurately across distinct populations, response topographies, and settings, especially when an initial conventional functional analysis proves to be inconclusive (Bowman, Fisher, Thompson, & Piazza, 1997; Cooper, Wacker, Sasso, Reimers, & Donn, 1990; Tiger et al., 2009). In what follows, we review some of the highlights of studies that have sought to modify some aspect of the basic approach in order to experimentally assess the function of behavior that may be difficult to assess using the standard approach.

Expansion Across Populations

The majority of functional analysis research has been conducted with individuals with developmental disabilities, which is not surprising, given the increased prevalence of challenging behaviors in this population (Hanley et al., 2003). Additionally, functional analysis methodology has been expanded to young children with challenging behavior. For example, Wacker et al. (1998) trained parents to conduct functional analyses and Functional Communication Training (FCT) for 28 children, ages 1–6, with developmental disabilities who displayed aberrant behavior. Results indicated that problem behavior served socially mediated functions for the majority of children. Twenty-one percent of participants exhibited problem behavior maintained by positive reinforcement, 46% exhibited aberrant behavior maintained by negative reinforcement, and 18% engaged in problem behavior that was multiply controlled. Kurtz et al. (2003) further extended functional analysis research by conducting functional analyses across 30 very young children (ages 10 months to 4 years and 11 months) with SIB and other forms of challenging behaviors. The mean age of emergence of SIB was 17 months, and head banging was the most common topography. Functional analyses succeeded in identifying a function in 87.5% of cases, and successful function-based treatments were implemented in most cases, as well.

In addition to expansion of functional analysis methodology to very young children with developmental disabilities, research has demonstrated its efficacy with a variety of other populations, including children with attention deficit hyperactivity disorder (DuPaul & Ervin, 1996) and typically developing children with conduct disorders (Cooper et al., 1990).

Expansion Across Behaviors

Multiple Topographies

Iwata et al.'s, 1982 article was able to build upon previous theoretical papers (e.g., Carr, 1977) and research methods (e.g., Bijou, Peterson, & Ault,

1968; Thomas et al., 1968) to formulate the first standardized functional analysis methodology. Although initially applied to the analysis of self-injurious behavior, the methodology was quickly adapted to analyze environment–behavior relationships that maintained a wide array of problem behaviors, such as aggression (Day, Horner, & O'Neill, 1994; Lalli & Casey, 1996; Mace, Page, Ivancic, & O'Brien, 1986; Wacker et al., 1990), destructive behavior (Bowman et al., 1997; Slifer, Ivancic, Parrish, Page, & Burgio, 1986), stereotypy (Durand & Carr, 1987; Mace, Browder, & Lin, 1987; Wacker et al., 1990), pica (Mace & Knight, 1986; Piazza et al., 1998), and tantrums (Carr & Newsom, 1985).

The majority of functional analyses conducted in the 1980s and early 1990s focused on single functions that maintained one or more aberrant responses (e.g., Carr & Durand, 1985; Iwata et al., 1982; Northup et al., 1991; Wacker et al., 1990). However, some researchers noted that, on occasion, multiple functions of distinct topographies of aberrant behavior interfered with the analysis of those behaviors (Derby et al., 1994). While many investigators noted the existence of different topographies of behavior serving different functions for a single client (e.g., Durand, 1982; Mace et al., 1986; Slifer et al., 1986; Smith, Iwata, Vollmer, & Pace, 1992; Sturmey, Carlsen, Crisp, & Newton, 1988), the majority of research conducted prior to 1994 combined separate topographies of problem behavior and conducted one functional analysis on an aggregate class of target behavior (e.g., Durand & Carr, 1991; Wacker et al., 1990). Conducting separate functional analyses for several distinct topographies presented huge time and cost constraints, leading researchers to develop alternative strategies to accurately and efficiently measure these separate topographies. Derby et al. (1994) suggested conducting a single functional analysis, initially graphing all presenting target behaviors in an aggregate fashion and subsequently analyzing each topography of behavior on separate graphs. This approach offered investigators the practical advantage of conducting a single functional analysis while still allowing them to separate each topography in order to generate specific hypotheses about the function of each behavior (Derby et al., 1994). The results of this study demonstrated how separate functions could be hidden by an aggregate analysis but could be accurately identified when the results for each target behavior were plotted separately.

Precursor Behaviors

Experimental Functional Analysis (EFA) of behavior disorders often produces temporary increases in problem behavior and has led to concerns over the potentially reinforcing consequences of evoking such behavior during the assessment procedures (Najdowski, Wallace, Ellsworth, MacAleese, & Cleveland, 2008). To reduce risk associated with an experimental functional analysis, some investigators have conducted a functional analysis of precursor behavior in order to *indirectly* infer the variables that maintain problem behavior (Najdowski et al., 2008; Smith & Churchill, 2002). Lalli, Mace, Wohn, and Livezey (1995) provided a foundation for this approach by showing that three problem behaviors displayed by a 15-year-old girl typically occurred in a predictable sequence (referred to as a response hierarchy), and when reinforcement contingencies were applied to the first of these responses, later ones in the sequence were suppressed. Based on this information, subsequent studies demonstrated that it was possible to infer the maintaining variables for more severe behaviors based on the outcomes of analyzing the more benign, precursor behavior (Smith & Churchill, 2002). Furthermore, interventions based on the outcomes of such analyses reduced precursor behavior and were associated with zero levels of severe problem behavior (Najdowski et al., 2008). These results represent a promising alternative to assessing the operant function of severe problem behavior directly.

Low-Rate Behaviors

Clinicians have often noted that high-frequency behavior appears to be easier to functionally assess than low-frequency behavior (Sprague & Horner, 1999). Since low-rate behavior occurs infrequently, it may be difficult to observe during descriptive analyses, and it may not occur at all during traditional experimental functional analyses (Kahng, Abt, & Schonbachler, 2001). In an early study on functional analysis of low-rate behavior, Kahng et al. (2001) conducted a modified functional analysis of low-rate aggression, extending the session duration to 7 h per day and conducting sessions 5 days per week, with each day representing a different analogue condition. The modified functional analysis produced clear results, whereas a previous functional analysis with standard session durations did not. The Kahng et al. procedural modification succeeded in producing clear assessment results for low-rate behavior, but two possible limitations are of note. First, many may be uncomfortable with exposing participants to the experimental conditions for such extended periods of time (especially in the attention condition, which essentially amounted to ignoring appropriate behavior all day), and second, some organizations may have difficulty allocating the large number of highly trained staff that is needed for such an extended functional analysis.

Tarbox, Wallace, Tarbox, Landaburu, and Williams (2004) evaluated an additional modification to functional analysis methodology for assessing low-rate behavior. In particular, functional analysis sessions were initiated contingent upon the occurrence of challenging behavior. This modification resulted in clear results in three adults with intellectual disabilities and low-rate challenging behaviors who had not engaged in a sufficient amount of challenging behavior during prior standard functional analyses. Furthermore, treatment analyses were conducted on the basis of the functional analysis outcomes for the two participants who were available for treatment, and both resulted in successful reductions in challenging behavior.

Expansion Across Settings

The immediate success of functional analysis within hospital settings led researchers to work on transferring the use of the technology across other settings, and the results have been encouraging. A common misconception seems to remain that successful experimental functional analyses require a highly controlled hospital or university setting, consisting of two or three staff members, laptop computers for data collection, and padded session rooms with one-way mirrors, but published research shows this is clearly not the case. A significant amount of research has demonstrated that functional analysis techniques are useful in less-controlled much shorter-term outpatient clinical settings (Derby et al., 1992; Wacker et al., 1990). A still-common misconception among educators is that functional analysis methodology is not appropriate or not practical for schools, and this notion is cited as justification for often implementing only indirect and descriptive assessments in school settings (Weber, Killu, Derby, & Barretto, 2005). However, a very substantial amount of research has been published on the successful application of functional analysis methodology within schools. Hanley et al. (2003) found that just over 31% of published research on experimental functional analyses was conducted in school settings. In addition, a small but significant amount of research has demonstrated the use of functional analysis methodology in homes. For example, Arndorfer, Miltenberger, Woster, Rortvedt, and Gaffaney (1994) conducted brief experimental functional analyses with six children in their homes and found conclusive results in each case. Finally, the large amount of research on functional analyses in schools and homes described above clearly shows that contrived settings are not necessary to produce clear results, but little research has directly compared contrived and naturalistic settings. One recent study by Lang et al. (2008) directly compared the results of functional analyses conducted in therapy rooms versus classrooms for two children with autism. The results were somewhat inconsistent, but generally speaking, clearer results were obtained in the therapy room. More research is needed which directly compares contrived versus natural settings.

Expansion to Other Functions of Behavior

It should not be surprising that the original article by Iwata et al. (2000), and the earlier developments leading up to it, could not possibly have identified all possible operant functions for challenging behavior. From a purely operant standpoint, all functions can be classified under either positive or negative reinforcement and either automatic or socially mediated. However, a small but significant number of additional subdivisions of these categories have been identified in the past 30 years, the highlights of which are reviewed next.

Tangible

Perhaps the most substantial and enduring addition to the standard functional analysis methodology is the addition of a condition to assess for the "tangible" function, that is, maintenance of behavior by forms of positive reinforcement, such as food, toys, or other items or activities. The tangible condition amounts to a minor modification to the attention condition. That is, positive reinforcement is still addressed as a potential function of behavior, but the form of positive reinforcement delivered is some form of preferred item or activity, and no physical or verbal attention is delivered. Mace and West (1986) were the first to include an experimental condition that assessed the effects of tangible reinforcement on problem behavior. However, the condition which provided access to preferred items/activities contingent upon challenging behavior also provided simultaneous escape from demands as a consequence. The first study to isolate access to preferred items/activities as a consequence for behavior during an experimental functional analysis was conducted by Day, Rea, Schussler, Larsen, & Johnson, (1988). This study included a condition that provided only access to preferred items/activities for 20–30 s contingent on problem behavior and is, therefore, often cited as the earliest demonstration of behavioral maintenance by access to tangible items (Hanley et al., 2003). However, the Day et al. study also included participant peers present in the condition, which represents another possible antecedent variable which may set the occasion for challenging behavior. One of the earliest studies to implement what is now considered the "standard" tangible condition was conducted by Vollmer, Marcus, Ringdahl, and Roane (1995).

In this study, tangible sessions were preceded by a brief period of access to preferred items that caregivers reported were correlated with challenging behavior. At the start of the session, the preferred items were removed and returned to the participant for approximately 20 s, contingent on each occurrence of the target behavior.

It is also interesting to note that, although the term "tangible" implies that the reinforcer for problem behavior is a physical item that can be grasped, this is not always the case. Significant creativity and flexibility may be needed to accommodate the full range of items or activities that may serve as positive reinforcers for challenging behavior. For example, one recent study demonstrated that the opportunity to go for walks was the maintained reinforcer of behavior, a consequence that was initially overlooked when more conventional consequences were first evaluated (Ringdahl, Christensen, & Boelter, 2009).

The tangible condition has become common over the last two decades of functional analysis research, and it is generally considered a "standard" condition. Indeed, in their review, Hanley et al. (2003) found that 38% of articles included a tangible condition and that the problem behavior of 10% of participants was reported to have a tangible function (as opposed to 34% for escape and 25% for attention). However, many researchers caution against including a tangible condition in a functional analysis unless caregivers report that the target behavior is associated with a preferred item or activity, because of the potential for "shaping up" a false tangible function (Thompson & Iwata, 2001). Little research has suggested that functional analyses create false positive results, but Shirley, Iwata, and Kahng (1999) found that it is possible to unintentionally "create" or "shape up" a false function for challenging behavior in the tangible condition. The findings of Shirley and colleagues support the general practice of excluding the tangible condition unless caregivers provide information that may suggest a possible tangible function.

Control

The role of "control" in the maintenance of challenging behavior is a potential function that is commonly discussed but has thus far been the subject of relatively little research. The general idea is that maintaining consequence of some challenging behavior is access to the opportunity to be in control. For example, a study by Bowman et al. (1997) demonstrated that the maintaining consequence of challenging behavior for children with developmental disabilities was the caregiver complying with the requests (i.e., "mands") of the participant, regardless of what those requests were. This is to be distinguished from a standard tangible condition in that the particular item or activity being requested was not relevant as long as the request was fulfilled. Similar findings were replicated in a controlled case study by O'Connor, Sorensen-Burnworth, Rush, and Eidman (2003) in which the destructive behavior of a 14-year-old boy with developmental disabilities was found to be maintained by adult compliance with mands. More research is needed to identify exactly what "control" is from a behavioral perspective and how it participates in the maintenance of challenging behavior.

Access to Stereotypy

Preliminary research has documented challenging behaviors whose functions appear to be positive reinforcement in the form of the opportunity to engage in ritualistic behavior, routines of some sort, or to engage in stereotyped behavior of some kind. For example, Fisher, Lindauer, Alterson, and Thompson (1998) assessed the property destruction of two boys with intellectual disabilities and found that the behavior was maintained by the opportunity which it afforded to engage in stereotypy with the destroyed property. Specifically, the participants destroyed plastic items and then engaged in stereotypy with the broken pieces of the items. Treatments based on these results successfully reduced the property destruction.

Idiosyncratic Variables

Numerous studies have identified potential idiosyncratic antecedent variables that can affect the outcomes of functional analyses. O'Reilly (1996) evaluated the influence of the location where a participant resided the night previous to the day in which functional analysis sessions were conducted. The participant was a 25-year-old man with moderate intellectual disabilities who exhibited intermittent SIB. The results of the analyses demonstrated clearly that SIB occurred on days following nights spent with respite care and did not occur on days following nights spent at home. A successful treatment for the behavior was designed in which an alternative respite placement was implemented.

Carr, Yarbrough, and Langdon (1997) evaluated the effects of idiosyncratic variables on functional analysis outcomes in three individuals with developmental disabilities. In each case, the presence or absence of highly idiosyncratic stimuli (large vs. small balls, magazines, and puzzles) determined whether the target behavior occurred during assessment conditions, regardless of the particular programmed consequence for the condition.

Ringdahl and Sellers (2000) examined the differential effects on problem behavior of caregivers and inpatient staff members as therapists, finding that aberrant behavior varied not only as a function of environmental contingencies but also as a function of therapist. Specifically, the aberrant behavior was more prevalent when the caregiver served as therapist during a functional analysis than when a staff member implemented the same procedures.

The effects of a multitude of other idiosyncratic variables have been studied as well, including the number of therapists present during the attention condition (Taylor, Sisson, McKelvey, & Trefelner, 1993), quality of attention delivered contingent on behavior (Fisher, Ninness, Piazza, & Owen-DeSchryver, 1996), and establishment of operations for escape-maintained behavior (McComas, Hoch, Paone, & El-Roy, 2000), among many others. Taken together, these studies further reinforce the basic philosophical assumptions behind functional analysis, specifically, that it is a general format which is useful for identifying behavior/environment relations at the level of the individual client and that these relations are assumed to vary, as each individual is unique.

Functional analysis, no matter how well developed, still requires the "analysis" component; it is not a universal cookbook approach to assessment, nor was it ever intended to be.

Experimental Designs

The functional analyses in the 1982 paper by Iwata et al. were carried out in the context of multielement experimental designs, and this design remains the most prevalent (Hanley et al., 2003). However, several alternatives have been shown to be effective. One such alternative is to match one test condition with the control condition in a "pair-wise" fashion in order to minimize potential carryover effects that may result from alternating multiple test conditions at once (Iwata, Duncan, Zarcone, Lerman, & Shore, 1994). The reversal design has also been used in favor of the multielement design in several studies, also with the intention of minimizing carryover effects (Vollmer et al., 1995). Finally, multiple studies have conducted what has come to be known as an "extended alone" condition in which multiple successive sessions of the alone condition are conducted for behaviors that are suspected to be maintained by automatic reinforcement (Vollmer et al., 1995).

Functional Analysis Duration

A commonly stated potential limitation to experimental functional analyses is that they are said to require lengthy durations of time to complete. There is little research to suggest that other equally reliable functional assessment options exist that require less time; however, maximizing efficiency of any clinical procedure is always valuable. A significant amount of research has been done on ways to shorten the overall duration of time required for functional analyses. One option for shortening the time required for a functional analysis is to shorten the duration of each session, from the usual 10–15 to 1–5 min. Wallace and Iwata (1999) retrospectively evaluated the effects of analyzing only the first 10 min, versus the first 5 min, versus the entire 15-min duration of functional analysis sessions, and found that 5-min session durations produced clear results in a majority of cases. A 90-min assessment, based on Iwata et al.'s (1982) model, has been developed for use in brief outpatient clinic visits. In this model, usually referred to as the "brief functional analysis," only one or two sessions of each condition are conducted, followed by a brief treatment assessment in which a replacement communication response is usually trained. The brief nature of the assessment does not always allow the target behavior to be observed successfully, but the model can be useful nonetheless (Cooper et al., 1990; Derby et al., 1992; Northup et al., 1991).

Interpreting Functional Analysis Data

Iwata et al.'s original functional analysis paper (1982) utilized visual inspection, without any formal criterion, to interpret data produced by the assessment. Visual inspection is the standard in single-case experimental design (Kazdin, 2010) and continues to be adequate in the vast majority of functional analyses. However, some researchers have expressed concern about the potential for subjectivity in the interpretation of functional analysis results, particularly in less-controlled settings. In order to increase both the validity and reliability of visual inspection for interpreting functional analysis results, Hagopian et al. (1997) developed a set of structured criteria and trained individuals to apply these rules when analyzing functional analysis data. The results suggested that, when applied correctly, the criteria improved the reliability of interpretations of functional analysis results.

Antecedent-Only Functional Analysis

An early study on experimental functional analysis by Carr and Durand (1985) used a methodology in which only the antecedents of challenging behavior were experimentally manipulated between conditions, whereas no programmed

consequences were delivered for challenging behavior in any conditions. That is, there was no contingency between target behavior and consequence, and therefore the target behavior was putatively on extinction throughout the assessment. Carr and Durand (1985) and many subsequent studies have obtained clear results using this methodology. Indeed, the review by Hanley et al. (2003) cited 56 studies which had been published using this antecedent-only methodology. A major potential limitation to this model is that, since challenging behavior is on extinction during the assessment, it may decrease before clear results are obtained. However, a major potential strength of the approach is that many caregivers (e.g., teachers, parents, etc.) who are not familiar with standard functional analysis methodology may not approve of the idea of intentionally reinforcing challenging behavior during assessment. In any case, the antecedent-only model is a significant contribution to the traditional model and should be considered as one possible alternative.

Training Others to Conduct Functional Analyses

One criticism of traditional functional analysis methodology is that the precision required to conduct such an analysis necessitates extensive training and clinical expertise (Wallace, Doney, Mintz-Resudek, & Tarbox, 2004). However, recent studies have demonstrated that individuals with no prior experience with functional analysis procedures could be trained to implement functional analyses with a high degree of fidelity (Iwata et al., 2000; Moore et al., 2002; Wallace et al., 2004). With the use of a training package that included reading materials, watching a videotaped simulation, passing a written test, and receiving feedback, Iwata et al. (2000) effectively trained undergraduate students to implement three functional analysis conditions (attention, demand, and play). Moore and colleagues (Moore et al., 2002; Moore & Fisher, 2007) trained individuals through video modeling. Recent studies have demonstrated that, using video modeling, undergraduate students and teachers could be

trained to implement functional analysis procedures with high fidelity (Iwata et al., 2000; Moore
et al., 2002; Wallace et al., 2004).

Nonexperimental Methods for Functional Assessment

Experimental functional analysis has become one
of the most widely used technologies in ABA
research on assessment and treatment of challenging behavior. However, the vast majority of clinical and educational settings do not conduct
experimental analyses prior to treatment. Based
upon the most commonly described methods for
conducting an EFA (e.g., Iwata, Dorsey et al.,
1994), determining the clear function of a target
behavior may take several weeks to complete,
depending on how many sessions can be conducted per day. As noted previously, researchers
have made efforts to create abbreviated analyses
(e.g., Northup et al., 1991). However, as discussed,
these procedures have a number of limitations
such as lower probability of observing the target
behavior during the shortened observation time.
Another limitation of EFA procedures is that several trained staff members are required to conduct
the analysis, again adding to the resources required
to conduct the analysis. Most clinical and educational settings simply do not have the staff available to conduct EFAs. In addition, many have
concerns regarding the practice of intentionally
reinforcing challenging behavior during EFAs.

Despite the large amount of research demonstrating the reliability of EFAs, one must wonder
why the procedure has not been adopted on a
wide scale in real-life clinical and educational
settings. Although there is no simple answer to
this question, it seems likely that all the potential
limitations described above play a part. Based
upon these limitations, a large amount of research
has been done on nonexperimental methods for
functional assessment. These methods are commonly classified as either indirect or descriptive
assessment (Tarbox et al., 2009). Indirect assessments consist of interviewing caregivers who
have previously observed the target behavior.
Interviews may be open-ended or structured.
Major advantages of indirect assessments are that

they are rapid, easy to administer, and do not
require direct observation of the target behavior.
Further, most require less than an hour to conduct. Descriptive assessments involve direct
observation and measurement of the target behavior as well as environmental variables that are
presumed to be functionally related (Cooper
et al., 2007). In light of the resource-intensive
nature of EFA, it is not surprising that Desrochers
et al. (1997) found that clinicians reported indirect and descriptive assessments as more useful
than experimental assessments. In cases where
resources (e.g., availability of trained staff) do
not permit experimental analyses, or the low-rate
of severe behavior requires an inordinate amount
of time to observe the behavior within an analogue setting, a significant amount of research
has demonstrated that various indirect and
descriptive methods of functional assessment can
yield useful information.

A more thorough review of indirect and
descriptive methods is outside of the scope of
this chapter. Readers are advised to see the
chapter titled, "Scaling Methods of Functional
Assessment," in this volume for a thorough treatment of the topic.

Concerns and Future Directions

Ecological Validity

Over the years, some studies have focused on a
descriptive analysis under natural settings (e.g.,
Bijou et al., 1968), while others have emphasized
the experimental analysis of aberrant behavior
within controlled laboratory conditions (e.g.,
Iwata et al., 1982). Throughout this time,
researchers have questioned the ecological validity of the procedures employed in functional
analyses, arguing that the results of such assessments are not reflective of the types of functional
relationships operating in an individual's natural
setting (Emerson, 1992).

While experimental functional analyses help
ensure careful control over the environment,
critics have raised questions regarding the
ecological validity of the procedures employed
(Emerson, 1992). The requirement of demonstrating

experimental control over a problem behavior may lead to artificial situations in which results are not reflective of the types of functional relationships operating in an individual's natural settings (Emerson, 1992).

References

Arndorfer, R. E., Miltenberger, R. G., Woster, S. H., Rortvedt, A. K., & Gaffaney, T. (1994). Home-based descriptive and experimental analysis of problem behaviors in children. *Topics in Early Childhood Special Education, 14,* 64–87.

Ayllon, T., & Michael, J. (1959). The psychiatric nurse as a behavioral engineer. *Journal of the Experimental Analysis of Behavior, 2,* 323–334.

Baer, D. M. (1960). Escape and avoidance response of pre-school children to two schedules of reinforcement withdrawal. *Journal of the Experimental Analysis of Behavior, 3,* 155–159.

Baer, D. M., Wolf, M. M., & Risley, T. R. (1968). Some still-current dimensions of applied behavior analysis. *Journal of Applied Behavior Analysis, 1,* 91–97.

Bailey, J., & Meyerson, L. (1969). Vibration as a reinforcer with a profoundly retarded child. *Journal of Applied Behavior Analysis, 2,* 135–137.

Bailey, J., & Meyerson, L. (1970). Effect of vibratory stimulation on a retardate's self-injurious behavior. *Psychological Aspects of Disability, 17,* 133–137.

Baskett, L. M., & Johnson, S. M. (1982). The young child's interactions with parents versus siblings: A behavioral analysis. *Child Development, 53,* 643–650.

Berkson, G., Mason, W. A., & Saxon, S. V. (1963). Situation and stimulus effects on stereotyped behaviors of chimpanzees. *Journal of Comparative and Physiological Psychology, 56,* 786–792.

Bijou, S. W. (1955). A systematic approach to an experimental analysis of young children. *Child Development, 26,* 161–168.

Bijou, S. W. (1957). Methodology for an experimental analysis of child behavior. *Psychological Reports, 3,* 243–250.

Bijou, S. W. (1958). A child study laboratory on wheels. *Child Development, 29,* 425–427.

Bijou, S. W., Peterson, R. F., & Ault, M. H. (1968). A method to integrate descriptive and experimental field studies at the level of data and empirical concepts. *Journal of Applied Behavior Analysis, 1,* 175–191.

Bowman, L. G., Fisher, W. W., Thompson, R. H., & Piazza, C. C. (1997). On the relation of mands and the function of destructive behavior. *Journal of Applied Behavior Analysis, 30,* 251–265.

Budd, K. S., Green, D. R., & Baer, D. M. (1976). An analysis of multiple misplaced parental social contingencies. *Journal of Applied Behavior Analysis, 9,* 459–470.

Carr, E. G. (1977). The motivation of self-injurious behavior: A review of some hypotheses. *Psychological Bulletin, 84,* 800–816.

Carr, E. G., & Durand, V. M. (1985). Reducing behavior problems through functional communication training. *Journal of Applied Behavior Analysis, 18,* 111–126.

Carr, E. G., & Newsom, C. (1985). Demand-related tantrums: Conceptualization and treatment. *Behavior Modification, 9,* 403–426.

Carr, E. G., Newsom, C. D., & Binkoff, J. A. (1976). Stimulus control of self-destructive behavior in a psychotic child. *Journal of Abnormal Child Psychology, 4,* 139–153.

Carr, E. G., Newsom, C. D., & Binkoff, J. A. (1980). Escape as a factor in the aggressive behavior of two retarded children. *Journal of Applied Behavior Analysis, 13,* 101–117.

Carr, E. G., Yarbrough, S. C., & Langdon, N. A. (1997). Effects of idiosyncratic stimuli variables on functional analysis outcomes. *Journal of Applied Behavior Analysis, 30,* 673–686.

Collins, D. T. (1965). Head-banging: Its meaning and management in the severely retarded adult. *Bulletin of the Menninger Clinic, 4,* 205–211.

Cooper, J. O., Heron, T. E., & Heward, W. L. (2007). *Applied behavior analysis* (2nd ed.). Upper Saddle River: Pearson Education.

Cooper, L. J., Wacker, D. P., Sasso, G. M., Reimers, T. M., & Donn, L. K. (1990). Using parents as therapists to evaluate appropriate behavior of their children: Application to a tertiary diagnostic clinic. *Journal of Applied Behavior Analysis, 23,* 285–296.

Day, H. M., Horner, R. H., & O'Neill, R. E. (1994). Multiple functions of problem behaviors: Assessment and intervention. *Journal of Applied Behavior Analysis, 27,* 279–289.

Day, R. M., Rea, J. A., Schussler, N. G., Larsen, S. E., & Johnson, W. L. (1988). A functionally based approach to the treatment of self-injurious behavior. *Behavior Modification, 12,* 565–588.

Dennis, W., & Najarian, P. (1957). Infant development under environmental handicap. *Psychological Monograph, 71*(436), 1–13.

Derby, K. M., Wacker, D. P., Peck, S., Sasso, G., DeRaad, A., Berg, W., et al. (1994). Functional analysis of separate topographies of aberrant behavior. *Journal of Applied Behavior Analysis, 27,* 267–278.

Derby, K. M., Wacker, D. P., Sasso, G., Steege, M., Northup, J., Cigrand, K., et al. (1992). Brief functional assessment techniques to evaluate aberrant behavior in an outpatient setting: A summary of 79 cases. *Journal of Applied Behavior Analysis, 25,* 713–721.

Desrochers, M. N., Hile, M. G., & Williams-Mosely, T. (1997). A survey of functional assessment procedures used with individuals with severe problem behaviors and mental retardation. *American Journal on Mental Retardation, 101,* 535–546.

DuPaul, G. J., & Ervin, R. A. (1996). Functional assessment of behaviors related to attention-deficit/hyperactivity disorder: Linking assessment to intervention design. *Behavior Therapy, 27,* 601–622.

Durand, V. M. (1982). Analysis and intervention of self-injurious behavior. *The Journal of the Association for the Severely Handicapped, 7,* 44–54.

Durand, V. M. (1987). "Look homeward angel": A call to return to our (functional) roots. *Behavior Analyst, 10*, 299–302.

Durand, V. M., & Carr, E. G. (1987). Social influences on "self-stimulatory" behavior: Analysis and treatment application. *Journal of Applied Behavior Analysis, 20*, 119–132.

Durand, V. M., & Carr, E. G. (1991). Functional communication training to reduce challenging behavior: Maintenance and application in new settings. *Journal of Applied Behavior Analysis, 24*, 251–264.

Emerson, E. (1992). Self-injurious behaviour: An overview of recent trends in epidemiological and behavioural research. *Mental Handicap Research, 5*, 49–81.

Ferster, C. B. (1958). Reinforcement and punishment in the control of human behavior of social agencies. *Psychiatric Research Reports, 10*, 101–118.

Ferster, C. B., & DeMyer, M. K. (1961). The development of performances in autistic children in an automatically controlled environment. *Journal of Chronic Diseases, 13*, 312–345.

Ferster, C. B., & DeMyer, M. K. (1962). A method for the experimental analysis of the behavior of autistic children. *The American Journal of Orthopsychiatry, 32*, 89–98.

Fisher, W. W., Lindauer, S. E., Alterson, C. J., & Thompson, R. H. (1998). Assessment and treatment of destructive behavior maintained by stereotypic object manipulation. *Journal of Applied Behavior Analysis, 31*, 513–527.

Fisher, W. W., Ninness, H. A., Piazza, C. C., & Owen-DeSchryver, J. S. (1996). On the reinforcing effects on the content of verbal attention. *Journal of Applied Behavior Analysis, 29*, 235–238.

Freud, A., & Burlingham, D. T. (1944). *Infants without families*. New York: International Universities Press.

Fuller, P. R. (1949). Operant conditioning of a vegetative human organism. *The American Journal of Psychology, 62*, 587–590.

Green, A. H. (1967). Self-mutilation in schizophrenic children. *Archives of General Psychiatry, 17*, 234–244.

Hagopian, L. P., Fisher, W. W., Thompson, R. H., Owen-DeSchryver, J., Iwata, B. A., & Wacker, D. P. (1997). Toward the development of structured criteria for interpretation of functional analysis data. *Journal of Applied Behavior Analysis, 30*, 313–326.

Hanley, G. P., Iwata, B. A., & McCord, B. E. (2003). Functional analysis of problem behavior: A review. *Journal of Applied Behavior Analysis, 36*, 147–185.

Harlow, H. F., Dodsworth, R. O., & Harlow, M. K. (1965). Total social isolation in monkeys. *Proceedings of the National Academy of Sciences of the United States of America, 54*, 90–97.

Harris, F. R., Wolf, M. M., & Baer, D. M. (1964). Effects of adult social reinforcement on child behavior. *Journal of Nursery Education, 20*, 8–17.

Hart, B. M., Allen, E. K., Buell, J. S., Harris, F. R., & Wolf, M. M. (1964). Effects of social reinforcement on operant crying. *Journal of Experimental Child Psychology, 1*, 145–153.

Hawkins, R. P., Peterson, R. F., Schweid, E., & Bijou, S. W. (1966). Behavior therapy in the home: Amelioration of problem parent-child relations with a parent in a therapeutic role. *Journal of Experimental Child Psychology, 3*, 99–107.

Iwata, B. A., Dorsey, M. F., Slifer, K. J., Bauman, K. E., & Richman, G. S. (1982). Toward a functional analysis of self-injury. *Analysis and Intervention in Developmental Disabilities, 2*, 3–20.

Iwata, B. A., Dorsey, M. F., Slifer, K. J., Bauman, K. E., & Richman, G. S. (1994). Toward a functional analysis of self-injury. *Journal of Applied Behavior Analysis, 27*, 197–209.

Iwata, B. A., Duncan, B. A., Zarcone, J. R., Lerman, D. C., & Shore, B. A. (1994). A sequential, test-control methodology for conducting functional analyses of self-injurious behavior. *Behavior Modification, 18*, 289–306.

Iwata, B. A., Pace, G. M., Dorsey, M. F., Zarcone, J. R., Vollmer, T. R., Smith, R. G., et al. (1994). The functions of self-injurious behavior: An experimental-epidemiological analysis. *Journal of Applied Behavior Analysis, 27*, 215–240.

Iwata, B. A., Wallace, M. D., Kahng, S., Lindberg, J. S., Roscoe, E. M., Conners, J., et al. (2000). Skill acquisition in the implementation of functional analysis methodology. *Journal of Applied Behavior Analysis, 33*, 181–194.

Jacobson, J. W., & Holburn, S. (2004). History and current status of applied behavior analysis in developmental disabilities. In J. L. Matson, R. B. Laud, & M. L. Matson (Eds.), *Behavior modification for persons with developmental disabilities: Treatments and supports* (Vol. 1, pp. 1–32). Kingston: NADD Press.

James, W. (1890). *Principles of psychology* (Vol. 1 & 2). New York: Dover.

Jones, F. H., Simmons, J. Q., & Frankel, F. (1974). An extinction procedure for eliminating self-destructive behavior in a 9-year-old autistic girl. *Journal of Autism and Childhood Schizophrenia, 4*, 241–250.

Kahng, S. W., Abt, K. A., & Schonbachler, H. E. (2001). Assessment and treatment of low-rate high-intensity problem behavior. *Journal of Applied Behavior Analysis, 34*, 225–228.

Kazdin, A. E. (2010). *Single-case research designs: Methods for clinical and applied settings* (2nd ed.). New York: Oxford University Press.

Kurtz, P. F., Chin, M. D., Huete, J. M., Tarbox, R. S. F., O'Connor, J. T., Paclawskyj, T. R., et al. (2003). Functional analysis and treatment of self-injurious behavior in young children: A summary of 30 cases. *Journal of Applied Behavior Analysis, 36*, 205–219.

Lalli, J. S., & Casey, S. D. (1996). Treatment of multiply controlled problem behavior. *Journal of Applied Behavior Analysis, 29*, 391–395.

Lalli, J. S., Mace, F. C., Wohn, T., & Livezey, K. (1995). Identification and modification of a response-class hierarchy. *Journal of Applied Behavior Analysis, 28*, 551–559.

Lang, R., O'Reilly, M., Machalicek, W., Lancioni, G., Rispoli, M., & Chan, J. M. (2008). A preliminary comparison of functional analysis results when conducted in contrived versus natural settings. *Journal of Applied Behavior Analysis, 41*, 441–445.

Lindsley, O. R. (1956). Operant conditioning methods applied to research in chronic schizophrenia. *Psychiatric Research Reports, 5*, 118–139.

Lindsley, O. R. (1960). Characteristics of the behavior of chronic psychotics as revealed by free-operant conditioning methods. *Diseases of the Nervous System, 21*, 66–78.

Lindsley, O. R., Skinner, B. F., & Solomon, H. C. (1953). *Studies in behavior therapy (Status Report I)*. Walthama: Metropolitan State Hospital.

Lovaas, O. I., Freitag, G., Gold, V. J., & Kassorla, I. C. (1965). Experimental studies in childhood schizophrenia: Analysis of self-destructive behavior. *Journal of Experimental Child Psychology, 2*, 67–84.

Lovaas, O. I., & Simmons, J. Q. (1969). Manipulation of self-destruction in three retarded children. *Journal of Applied Behavior Analysis, 2*, 143–157.

Ludwig, A. M., Marx, A. J., Hill, P. A., & Browning, R. M. (1969). Control of violent behavior through faradic shock: A case study. *The Journal of Nervous and Mental Disease, 148*, 624–637.

Mace, F. C. (1994). The significance and future of functional analysis methodologies. *Journal of Applied Behavior Analysis, 27*, 385–392.

Mace, F. C., Browder, D. M., & Lin, Y. (1987). Analysis of demand conditions associated with stereotypy. *Journal of Behavior Therapy and Experimental Psychiatry, 18*, 25–31.

Mace, F. C., & Knight, D. (1986). Functional analysis and the treatment of severe pica. *Journal of Applied Behavior Analysis, 19*, 411–416.

Mace, F. C., Page, T. J., Ivancic, M. T., & O'Brien, S. (1986). Analysis of environmental determinants of aggression and disruption in mentally retarded children. *Applied Research in Mental Retardation, 7*, 203–221.

Mace, F. C., & West, B. J. (1986). Analysis of demand conditions associated with reluctant speech. *Journal of Behavior Therapy and Experimental Psychiatry, 17*, 285–294.

Maisto, C. R., Baumeister, A. A., & Maisto, A. A. (1978). An analysis of variables related to self-injurious behaviour among institutionalised retarded persons. *Journal of Intellectual Disability Research, 22*, 27–36.

McComas, J., Hoch, H., Paone, D., & El-Roy, D. (2000). Escape behavior during academic tasks: A preliminary analysis of idiosyncratic establishing operations. *Journal of Applied Behavior Analysis, 33*, 479–493.

McKinney, J. P. (1962). A multidimensional study of the behavior of severely retarded boys. *Child Development, 33*, 923–938.

Meyerson, L., Kerr, N., & Michael, J. L. (1967). Behavior modification in rehabilitation. In S. W. Bijou & D. M. Baer (Eds.), *Child development: Readings in experimental analysis* (pp. 214–239). New York: Appleton.

Moore, J. W., Edwards, R. P., Sterling-Turner, H. E., Riley, J., DuBard, M., & McGeorge, A. (2002). Teaching acquisition of functional analysis methodology. *Journal of Applied Behavior Analysis, 35*, 73–77.

Moore, J. W., & Fisher, W. W. (2007). The effects of videotape modeling on staff acquisition of functional analysis methodology. *Journal of Applied Behavior Analysis, 40*, 197–202.

Michael, J. (1980). Flight from behavior analysis. *Behavior Analyst, 3*, 1–22.

Murphy, G. (1982). Sensory reinforcement in the mentally handicapped and autistic child: A review. *Journal of Autism and Developmental Disorders, 12*, 265–278.

Myers, J. J., & Deibert, A. N. (1971). Reduction of self-abusive behavior in a blind child by using a feeding response. *Journal of Behavior Therapy and Experimental Psychiatry, 2*, 141–144.

Najdowski, A. C., Wallace, M. D., Ellsworth, C. L., MacAleese, A. N., & Cleveland, J. M. (2008). Functional analyses and treatment of precursor behaviors. *Journal of Applied Behavior Analysis, 1*, 97–105.

Northup, J., Wacker, D., Sasso, G., Steege, M., Cigrand, K., Cook, J., et al. (1991). A brief functional analysis of aggressive and alternative behavior in an outclinic setting. *Journal of Applied Behavior Analysis, 24*, 509–522.

O'Connor, J. T., Sorensen-Burnworth, R. J., Rush, K. S., & Eidman, S. L. (2003). A mand analysis and levels of treatment in an outpatient clinic. *Behavioral Interventions, 18*, 139–150.

O'Reilly, M. F. (1996). Assessment and treatment of episodic self-injury: A case study. *Research in Developmental Disabilities, 17*, 349–361.

Patterson, G. R., Littman, R. A., & Bricker, W. (1967). Assertive behavior in children: A step toward a theory of aggression. *Monographs of the Society for Research in Child Development, 32*, iii–43.

Piazza, C. C., Fisher, W. W., Hanley, G. P., LeBlanc, L. A., Worsdell, A. S., Lindauer, S. E., et al. (1998). Treatment of pica through multiple analyses of its reinforcing functions. *Journal of Applied Behavior Analysis, 31*, 165–189.

Rincover, A. (1978). Sensory extinction: A procedure for eliminating self-stimulatory behavior in developmentally disabled children. *Journal of Abnormal Child Psychology, 6*, 299–310.

Rincover, A., Newsom, C. D., & Carr, E. G. (1979). Using sensory extinction procedures in the treatment of compulsive like behavior of developmentally disabled children. *Journal of Consulting and Clinical Psychology, 47*, 695–701.

Ringdahl, J. E., Christensen, T. J., & Boelter, E. W. (2009). Further evaluation of idiosyncratic functions for severe problem behavior: Aggression maintained by access to walks. *Behavioral Interventions, 24*, 275–283.

Ringdahl, J. E., & Sellers, J. A. (2000). The effects of different adults as therapists during functional analyses. *Journal of Applied Behavioral Analysis, 33*, 247–250.

Shirley, M. J., Iwata, B. A., & Kahng, S. W. (1999). False-positive maintenance of self-injurious behavior by access to tangible reinforcers. *Journal of Applied Behavior Analysis, 32*, 201–204.

Skinner, B. F. (1938). *The behavior of organisms: An experimental analysis*. Acton: Copley.

Skinner, B. F. (1953). *Science and human behavior*. New York: The Macmillan Company.

Skinner, B. F. (1957). *Verbal behavior*. Acton: Copley.

Skinner, B. F. (1974). *Beyond behaviorism*. New York: Vintage Books.

Slifer, K. J., Ivancic, M. T., Parrish, J. M., Page, T. J., & Burgio, L. D. (1986). Assessment and treatment of multiple behavior problems exhibited by a profoundly retarded adult. *Journal of Behavior Therapy and Experimental Psychiatry, 17*, 203–213.

Smith, R. G., & Churchill, R. M. (2002). Identification of environmental determinants of behavior disorders through functional analysis of precursor behaviors. *Journal of Applied Behavior Analysis, 35*, 125–136.

Smith, R. G., Iwata, B. A., Vollmer, T. R., & Pace, G. M. (1992). On the relationship between self-injurious behavior and self-restraint. *Journal of Applied Behavior Analysis, 25*, 433–445.

Sprague, J. R., & Horner, R. H. (1999). Low-frequency high-intensity problem behavior: Toward an applied technology of functional assessment and intervention. In A. C. Repp & R. H. Horner (Eds.), *Functional analysis of problem behavior: From effective assessment to effective support* (pp. 98–116). Belmont: Wadsworth.

Sturmey, P., & Bernstein, H. (2004). Functional analysis of maladaptive behaviors: Current status and future directions. In J. L. Matson, R. B. Laud, & M. L. Matson (Eds.), *Behavior modification for persons with developmental disabilities: Treatments and supports* (Vol. 1, pp. 1–32). Kingston: NADD Press.

Sturmey, P., Carlsen, A., Crisp, A. G., & Newton, J. T. (1988). A functional analysis of multiple aberrant responses: A refinement and extension of Iwata et al.'s (1982) methodology. *Journal of Intellectual Disability Research, 32*, 31–46.

Tarbox, J., Wallace, M. D., Tarbox, R. S., Landaburu, H. J., & Williams, W. L. (2004). Functional analysis and treatment of low rate problem behavior in individuals with developmental disabilities. *Behavioral Interventions, 19*, 187–204.

Tarbox, J., Wilke, A. E., Najdowski, A. C., Findel-Pyles, R. S., Balasanyan, S., Caveney, A. C., et al. (2009). Comparing indirect, descriptive, and experimental functional assessments of challenging behavior in children with autism. *Journal of Developmental and Physical Disabilities, 21*, 493–514.

Tate, B. G., & Baroff, G. S. (1966). Aversive control of self-injurious behavior in a psychotic boy. *Behaviour Research and Therapy, 4*, 281–287.

Taylor, J. C., Sisson, L. A., McKelvey, J. L., & Trefelner, M. F. (1993). Situation specificity in attention-seeking problem behavior: A case-study. *Behavior Modification, 17*, 474–497.

Thomas, D. R., Becker, W. C., & Armstrong, M. (1968). Production and elimination of disruptive classroom behavior by systematically varying teacher's behavior. *Journal of Applied Behavior Analysis, 1*, 35–45.

Thompson, R. H., & Iwata, B. A. (2001). A descriptive analysis of social consequences following problem behavior. *Journal of Applied Behavior Analysis, 34*, 169–178.

Tiger, J. H., Fisher, W. W., Toussaint, K. A., & Kodak, T. (2009). Progressing from initially ambiguous functional analyses: Three case examples. *Research in Developmental Disabilities, 30*, 910–926.

Vollmer, T. R., Marcus, B. A., Ringdahl, J. E., & Roane, H. S. (1995). Progressing from brief assessments to extended experimental analyses in the evaluation of aberrant behavior. *Journal of Applied Behavior Analysis, 28*, 561–576.

Wacker, D. P., Berg, W. K., Harding, J. W., Derby, K. M., Asmus, J. M., & Healy, A. (1998). Evaluation and long-term treatment of aberrant behavior displayed by young children with disabilities. *Developmental and Behavioral Pediatrics, 19*, 260–266.

Wacker, D. P., Steege, M. W., Northup, J., Sasso, G., Berg, W., Reimers, T., et al. (1990). A component analysis of functional communication training across three topographies of severe behavior problems. *Journal of Applied Behavior Analysis, 23*, 417–429.

Wallace, M. D., Doney, J. K., Mintz-Resudek, C. M., & Tarbox, R. S. F. (2004). Training educators to implement functional analyses. *Journal of Applied Behavior Analysis, 37*, 89–92.

Wallace, M. D., & Iwata, B. A. (1999). Effects of session duration on functional analysis outcomes. *Journal of Applied Behavior Analysis, 32*, 175–183.

Watson, J. B. (1913). Psychology as the behaviorist views it. *Psychological Review, 20*, 158–177.

Weber, K. P., Killu, K., Derby, K. M., & Barretto, A. (2005). The status of functional behavioral assessment (FBA): Adherence to standard practice in FBA methodology. *Psychology in the Schools, 42*, 737–744.

Weeks, M., & Gaylord-Ross, R. (1981). Task difficulty and aberrant behavior in severely handicapped students. *Journal of Applied Behavior Analysis, 14*, 449–463.

Wilkins, J., & Matson, J. L. (2009). History of treatment in children with developmental disabilities and psychopathology. In J. L. Matson, F. Andrasik, & M. L. Matson (Eds.), *Treating Childhood Psychopathology and Developmental Disabilities* (pp. 3–28). New York: Springer.

Wolery, M. (1978). Self-stimulatory behavior as a basis for devising reinforcers. *AAESPH Review, 3*, 23–29.

Wolf, M. M. (1978). Social validity: The case for subjective measurement or how applied behavior analysis is finding its heart. *Journal of Applied Behavior Analysis, 11*, 203–214.

Wolf, M., Risley, T., Johnston, M., Harris, F., & Allen, E. (1967). Application of operant conditioning procedures to the behavior problems of an autistic child: A follow-up and extension. *Behaviour Research and Therapy, 5*, 103–111.

Wolf, M. M., Risley, T., & Mees, H. (1964). Application of operant conditioning procedures to the behavior problems of an autistic child. *Behaviour Research and Therapy, 1*, 305–312.

Nature, Prevalence, and Characteristics of Challenging Behavior

Robert Didden, Peter Sturmey, Jeff Sigafoos,
Russell Lang, Mark F. O'Reilly, and Giulio E. Lancioni

Challenging behaviors are among the most serious and studied problems in the field of developmental disabilities (Matson, Kozlowski et al. 2011). An increasing number of studies are being published that have provided more insight

R. Didden (✉)
Behavioural Science Institute, Radboud University Nijmegen, 6500 HE, P.O. Box 9104, Nijmegen, The Netherlands
e-mail: r.didden@pwo.ru.nl

P. Sturmey
Department of Psychology, Queens College, City University of New York, A-315 Science Building, 6530 Kissina Blvd, Flushing, NY 11367, USA
e-mail: psturmey@gmail.com

J. Sigafoos
School of Educational Psychology and Pedagogy, Victoria University of Wellington, Karori Campus, PO Box 17-310, Wellington, New Zealand
e-mail: jeff.sigafoos@vuw.ac.nz

R. Lang
College of Education, Texas State University, San Marcos, TX 78666, USA
e-mail: russlang@txstate.edu

M.F. O'Reilly
Department of Special Education, College of Education, The University of Texas at Austin, Austin, TX 78712, USA
e-mail: markoreilly@mail.utexas.edu

G.E. Lancioni
Department of Psychology, University of Bari, Via QuintinoSella 268, Bary 70100, Italy
e-mail: g.lancioni@psico.uniba.it

into the nature, prevalence, and characteristics of challenging behaviors in this target group. Results of these studies have shown that challenging behaviors are common in children and adults with autism spectrum disorders (ASD) and/or intellectual disabilities (ID). Population studies have shown that between 5 and 15% of individuals with ID show some type of challenging behavior, like self-injury, aggression, stereotypic behavior, and other problem behaviors. Studies also show that rates of challenging behaviors are increased if individuals also have ASD. For example, Holden and Gitlesen (2006) found that among over 900 individuals with ID, 11% showed one or more types of challenging behavior. Of the study sample, 6% had been diagnosed with autism, and 36% of this subgroup showed challenging behavior. Rojahn, Matson, Lott, Esbensen, and Smalls (2001) employed the *Behavior Problem Inventory-01* (BPI-01) in a sample of individuals with ID ($n = 432$) who lived in a residential facility and who were between 14 and 19 years old. Results showed that individuals with ASD had higher rates of aggression, self-injury and stereotypy than those with ID without ASD. These findings were corroborated by results from a meta-analysis by McClintock, Hall, and Oliver (2003) who have explored risk factors for challenging behaviors in individuals with developmental disabilities. They have published a meta-analysis of 22 studies conducted over 30 years, and the results showed that children and adults with ASD were more likely than other

J.L. Matson (ed.), *Functional Assessment for Challenging Behaviors*,
Autism and Child Psychopathology Series, DOI 10.1007/978-1-4614-3037-7_3,
© Springer Science+Business Media, LLC 2012

individuals with ID to exhibit challenging behaviors such as self-injury and aggression. These results indicate that ASD itself may be a risk factor for challenging behavior in individuals with ID. However, other researchers failed to find an association between challenging behavior and ASD. For example, Tyrer et al. (2006) investigated prevalence rate of physical aggression in over 3,000 adults with profound to mild ID, and they failed to find a relationship between challenging behavior and the presence of autism.

During the last decades, several definitions of challenging behavior have been proposed. For example, Emerson (2005) defined challenging behavior as

> …culturally abnormal behaviour of such intensity, frequency or duration that the physical safety of the person or others is placed in serious jeopardy, or behaviour which is likely to seriously limit or deny access to the use of ordinary community facilities…

In this definition, there is no reference to specific topographies or causes of the challenging behavior, but it is defined in terms of its effects on the person's life. Other researchers have employed a definition of challenging behavior that distinguishes between more and less demanding behavior (e.g., Holden & Gitlesen, 2006). The former means that the person shows challenging behavior on a daily basis, that this behavior usually prevents the person from taking part in programs or activities, that more than one caregiver is needed to physically control the behavior, and that the behavior causes major bodily injury to the person or others. Less demanding behavior includes attacking others, self-injurious behaviors, destruction, or otherwise problematic behavior that does not meet these requirements.

Challenging behavior in individuals with ASD and/or ID has many adverse consequences for the person involved and his or her family members, professional carers, and society at large. It may result in rejection by peers and caregivers, exclusion from settings, restrictive and potential harmful treatment practices (such as polypharmacy), serious health risks, and distress to all involved. Challenging behavior interferes with learning adaptive skills, and it leads to additional costs of specialized services.

In the last two decades, major advances have been made in the treatment of challenging behaviors in individuals with ASD and/or ID. Results of numerous studies have shown that challenging behavior may be the result of a learning process in which this behavior acquires an operant function through its interaction with environmental events. In this view, challenging behavior is not conceptualized as a symptom of "underlying" psychopathology but as a response that has acquired one or more behavioral functions for the person. Effective behavioral intervention requires the identification of functional properties of the challenging behavior, a technology that is called functional assessment.

The most often addressed types of behavior in functional assessment in individuals with ASD and/or ID are SIB and aggression, followed by stereotypic behavior, tantrums, destruction, and, to a lesser extent, feeding problems, pica, and rumination, among others (Matson, Sipes et al., 2011). This chapter considers the nature, prevalence, and characteristics of most of these challenging behaviors among individuals with ASD and/or ID. We focus on self-injury, stereotypy, aggression, feeding disorders, pica, and rumination/vomiting. Each section begins with a definition of one of these behaviors. Afterwards, forms of the behavior that have been observed among individuals with ASD/ID are described and classified. We then provide a selective review of studies that have explored the prevalence of challenging behavior. The final sections consider risk factors and adverse consequences of that type of challenging behavior.

Self-Injurious Behavior

Definition

Researchers have adopted two general approaches to defining SIB. The first requires not only that the self-inflicted acts cause injury but also that they occur with deliberate intent. Winchel and Stanley (1991) defined SIB as

...the commission of deliberate harm to one's own body. The injury is done to oneself, without the aid of another person, and the injury is severe enough for tissue damage (such as scarring) to result. (p. 306)

In their elaboration of this definition, Winchel and Stanley excluded acts that occurred with "conscious suicidal intent or associated with sexual arousal" (p. 306). Klonsky and Meuhlenkamp (2007) also emphasized underlying intent and added reference to social norms when they defined SIB as the "intentional destruction of body tissue without suicidal intention and for purposes not socially sanctioned" (p. 1045). In line with these definitions, behaviors associated with suicide, sexual arousal, or sociocultural practices are excluded from our definition of SIB.

In contrast to the above approach, Rojahn, Whittaker, Hoch, and Gonzáles (2007) argued for defining SIB without reference to underlying intentions so as to prevent the formation of potentially misleading inferences regarding the causes of SIB. They endorsed the approach of Tate and Baroff (1966), who defined SIB as repetitive acts directed to one's own body that cause tissue damage or physical harm. Similarly, Smith, Vollmer, and St. Peter Pipkin (2007) defined SIB as "Behavior that produces or has the capacity to produce tissue damage to the individual's own body." (p. 188).

For the purpose of this chapter, these two definitional approaches have been integrated. SIB is defined as behavior directed towards oneself that causes—or has the potential to cause—tissue damage, exclusive of acts associated with suicide, sexual arousal, or socially sanctioned practices. This integrated definition reflects the common forms of SIB that have been observed among people with ASD and acknowledges that acts associated with suicide, sexual arousal, or socially sanctioned practices are often quite distinct from the forms of SIB most commonly seen in individuals with ASD and other developmental disabilities (Weiss, 2003).

Forms and Classification

Numerous specific forms or topographies of behavior can meet the above definition of SIB.

SIB forms documented in the repertoires of individuals with ASD and other developmental disabilities include head banging, head hitting, hair pulling, eye poking, face slapping, and biting, pinching, and scratching oneself (Fee & Matson, 1992; Matson, Fodstad, Mahan, & Rojahn, 2010; Sigafoos, Arthur, & O'Reilly, 2003; Smith et al., 2007). Many other forms of behavior can produce self-inflicted injury and/or serious health complications if they occur with sufficient frequency and/or severity (e.g., pica, rumination—also see section on "Pica, Vomiting, and Rumination").

Weiss (2003) reviewed several conceptually and empirically based schemes that have been used to classify these SIB forms. Fee and Matson (1992), for example, placed SIB behaviors on a continuum of severity ranging from mild forms (e.g., head rubbing, finger sucking, nail licking, thigh slapping) to more severe forms (e.g., eye poking, self-scratching, chronic rumination, head banging). Consideration of severity would seem a useful type of classification when prioritizing behaviors for treatment, and this approach might also provide cues to the development of severe SIB. Along these lines, data from Murphy, Hall, Oliver, and Kissi-Debra (1999) suggest that SIB may emerge from early and less severe (or proto-injurious) behaviors that are often present in the child's repertoire before 2 years of age.

In addition to severity, SIB could also be viewed along a continuum of frequency as proposed by Jones (1987). At one end of this continuum are high frequency/stereotyped acts that may cause injury over time, such as the almost constant hand rubbing seen in individuals with Rett syndrome (Deb, 1998). At the other end are high intensity acts that occur less frequently, such as bursts of head banging that might occur once or twice per day.

SIB has also been classified in terms of having a social versus nonsocial basis (Schroeder, Mulick, & Rojahn, 1980; Sigafoos, Reichle, & Light Shriner, 1994). Social SIB occurs because of past success in recruiting some type of social response from other people. SIB forms reported to be associated with a social basis include head banging, self-biting, self-scratching, gouging oneself, pinching oneself, and pulling out one's own hair. Nonsocial SIB, in contrast, appears to produce direct sensory stimulation that is automatically reinforcing. Such acts may include stuffing orifices, mouthing objects, and finger sucking. Experimental data have accumulated to support this social/nonsocial distinction. Specifically, it is now well established that for some individuals with ASD, SIB is often maintained by positive or negative reinforcement that is socially mediated, such as attention from a caregiver, access to preferred objects or activities, and/or being allowed to escape from a non-preferred task. For other individuals, however, SIB appears to be maintained by direct sensory consequences or automatic reinforcement (Iwata, Pace et al., 1994). However, the social versus nonsocial distinction does not necessarily follow precise topographical lines. Thus, some individuals could potentially develop seemingly nonsocial forms of SIB that are in fact socially motivated or that might acquire a social basis overtime and vice versa.

Prevalence

The prevalence of SIB has been more widely studied among individuals with ID than individuals with ASD. Overall, studies of individuals with ID indicate that SIB occurs in approximately 10–12% of this population (Bienstein & Nussbeck, 2009; Emerson et al., 2001; Holden & Gitlesen, 2006; Lowe et al., 2007; Murphy et al., 1993; Oliver, Murphy, & Corbett, 1987; van Ingen, Moore, Zaja, & Rojahn, 2010).

The 10–12% prevalence rate from studies of individuals with ID can be analyzed in relation to the results of three recent studies that have provided data on the extent and circumstances of SIB among individuals with ASD. One of these three studies included 222 young children from French service agencies for children with ASD (Baghdadli, Pascal, Grisi, & Aussilloux, 2003). These 222 children ranged from 2 to 7 years of age with a mean age of 5 years. The children met the ICD-10 criteria for infantile autism (World Health Organization, 1992). The children were

also assessed with the *Childhood Autism Rating Scale* (CARS: Schloper, Reichler, DeVellis, & Daly, 1988). The resulting mean total score for the group was 36, which corresponds to a classification of moderately autistic. Most of these 222 children also had an ID. In fact, 70% of the sample had severe ID, 5.9% had profound ID, 20.3% had mild ID, and only 4% had no ID. Other diagnoses included epilepsy (7.2%), genetic syndromes (3.2%), and perinatal conditions (5%). The boy to girl ratio was 4.7:1, which is consistent with reports that ASD is four to five times more common in boys than girls (American Psychiatric Association [APA], 2000).

To identify children with SIB, the researchers had care staff to complete a questionnaire regarding the presence or absence of SIB in each child's repertoire. When SIB was present, care staff also rated its severity in a three-point scale (mild, moderate, severe). Assessment was also undertaken of each child's expressive speech and adaptive behavior functioning using the *Autism Diagnostic Interview-Revised* (Lord, Rutter, & Lecoutteur, 1994) and the *Vineland Adaptive Behavior Scales* (Sparrow, Balla, & Cicchetti, 1984), respectively. These additional measures allowed the researchers to undertake analyses to identify risk factors for SIB among these 222 children. Based on the results of the care-staff questionnaire, the children were classified into two groups based on presence or absence of SIB. These two groups were then compared in terms of gender, age, parental social class, level of speech/adaptive behavior, and perinatal and medical conditions.

The results of these analyses were remarkable in terms of the relatively high percentage of children who were identified as having SIB. Specifically, 53% ($n = 109$) of the sample was reported by care staff to engage in SIB, with 14.6% reported to engage in severe SIB. Interestingly, there were no significant differences between the SIB and non-SIB groups in terms of age, gender, epilepsy, genetic syndromes, or parental social class. The SIB group did, however, differ significantly from the non-SIB group in terms of the severity of their autistic symptoms, their extent of speech and adaptive behavior deficits, and their birth complications (i.e., perinatal conditions). Younger age, severe autism, and greater daily living skill deficits were identified as increasing the likelihood that a child would be rated as having SIB.

Compared to the consistently reported 10–12% prevalence rate of SIB among individuals with ID, the 53% prevalence rate reported by Baghdadli et al. (2003) suggests that SIB could be up to five times more prevalent among individuals with ASD than for individuals with ID. However, the results of this study should be interpreted with caution because critical psychometric properties of the care-staff questionnaire (e.g., inter-rater reliability, content validity) were lacking. In addition, details on the definition and forms of SIB assessed were lacking, and descriptive anchors for the rating of SIB severity were not provided. The high prevalence rate might also reflect the fact that 70% of these children had ASD and severe ID. Among individuals with ID, SIB is more prevalent among those with severe, as compared to mild/moderate, ID (Schroeder, Tessel, Loupe, & Stodgell, 1997).

In a second relevant study, Matson and Rivet (2008a) studied 320 adults from two residential centers in Louisiana, USA. Participants ranged from 20 to 88 years of age with a mean age of 52 years. The sample included more males (56%) than females (44%). Most of these adults (75.5%) were reported to have a profound level of ID. The sample was divided into an ASD group, a PDD-NOS group, and an ID-only group. Sixty-two individuals (19%) had a diagnosis of autistic disorder, and 99 individuals (31%) were diagnosed with PDD-NOS. The remaining participants had ID only. The three groups did not differ in terms of gender, ethnicity, or length of time living in the centers, but they did differ in terms of their age and level of ID. Specifically the autistic and PDD-NOS groups had fewer individuals over 60 years of age, and the autistic group had more individuals with profound ID than the ID-only group.

In this study, Matson and Rivet (2008a) used a reliable and valid measure of problem behavior: the *Autism Spectrum Disorders-Behavior Problems for Adults* (ASD-BPA; Matson, Terlonge, & Gonzáles, 2006). The ASD-BPA has 19 items

and four subscales: (a) Aggression/Destruction, (b) Stereotypy, (c) SIB, and (d) Disruptive behavior. Items were rated as either 0 (not a problem, no impairment) or 1 (problem, impairment). The SIB subscale consisted of three items: (a) poking self in the eye; (b) harming self by hitting, pinching, or scratching, etc.; and (c) mouthing or swallowing objects causing bodily harm. As in Baghdadli et al. (2003), direct care staff served as informants. Additional ratings using standardized scales were made of autistic symptoms and comorbid conditions to identify risk factors.

The results of the Matson and Rivet (2008a) study showed that adults with autistic disorder had significantly higher mean total problem behavior scores (4.39) followed by the PDD-NOS (2.92), and ID-only (1.41) groups. Mean SIB ratings were also significantly different for the autism (0.61), PDD-NOS (0.40), and ID-only (0.13) groups. As is often found in studies of problem behavior among individuals with developmental disabilities, most individuals in this sample engaged in more than one type of problem behavior. For example, SIB and stereotypy were significantly correlated ($r=0.48$). Consistent with Baghdadli et al. (2003), Matson and Rivet also found that the frequency of problem behavior, including SIB, increased with the severity of autistic symptoms, suggesting that severe autism is a risk factor for SIB and other problem behaviors. However, this conclusion should be interpreted with caution because the sample consisted only of adults living in residential facilities. There are data suggesting that individuals with severe behavior problems, including SIB, are more likely to end up in more restrictive settings, such as residential centers (see Sigafoos et al., 2003, pp. 42–43 for a review). The Matson and Rivet (2008a) study is limited by the inclusion of only adults most of whom had profound ID. Still, the results point to a significantly higher prevalence of SIB among the autism group compared to the PDD-NOS and ID-only groups.

Murphy, Healy, and Leader (2009) studied 157 children with ASD. The children were recruited from Irish educational units. Their ages ranged from 3 to 14.2 years with a mean of 8.5 years. As is typical of the ASD population, the sample included more boys (82.8%) than girls (17.2%). The level of ID was reported for only 69% ($n = 109$) of the children. Of these 109, 20% had normal intelligence, 37.6% had mild ID, 23.8% had moderate ID, 17.4% had severe ID, and only one child had profound ID.

Data were provided by informants with a minimum of 1 year experience in working with the child. The researcher interviewed informants using the *Behavior Problems Inventory* (BPI-01; Rojahn, Matson, Lott, Esbensen, & Smalls, 2001). The BPI has 52 items covering various types of problem behaviors (e.g., aggression, stereotypy), including 14 SIB-specific items. Items are rated for frequency on a 5-point scale ranging from 0 (never) to 4 (hourly) and for severity on a 4-point scale ranging from 0 (no problem) to 3 (severe problem).

The resulting prevalence figure for SIB was lower than reported by Baghdadli et al. (2003), but roughly three times higher than the 10–12% reported in studies of individuals with ID. Specifically, 32.5% of the children were rated as having SIB, aggression, and stereotyped behavior, whereas 11% showed SIB and stereotyped behavior, and 4% showed SIB and aggression. Thus, most children showed more than one type of problem behavior. The most common form of SIB was self-biting, which was present in 22% of the children with SIB. There were no significant relations between age or gender and problem behavior. Children with severe ID had a higher median rating for severity of SIB. This is an important study due to the fact that there was a greater distribution of levels of ID among these 157 children when compared to the Baghdadli et al. (2003) and Matson and Rivet (2008a) studies. However, the study is limited by a relatively modest sample size and restricted age range. Still, the results are consistent with a general conclusion that SIB is more prevalent among individuals with ASD and severe ID than for individuals with less severe ID and less severe autistic symptoms.

Risk Factors

In a review chapter, Sigafoos et al. (2003) delineated a number of risk factors for SIB and other problem behaviors among individuals with developmental disabilities. Based on this review, and the results of Baghdadli et al. (2003), Matson and Rivet (2008a), and Murphy et al. (2009), a number of factors might be pointed out as responsible for increasing the risk of SIB among individuals with ASD. These are:

Severity of Intellectual Disability
SIB is more prevalent among those with ASD and severe ID, as compared to those with ASD and either mild/moderate levels of ID or no ID.

Severity of Autistic Symptoms
The prevalence of SIB is higher among individuals with more severe symptoms of autism when compared to individuals with less severe autism symptoms.

ASD Diagnosis
An ASD diagnosis increases the risk of SIB among individuals with ID.

Comorbid Conditions
SIB among individuals with ASD, severe ID, and comorbid psychopathology (e.g., depression, bipolar disorder) appears to be higher than for any other clinical group (Matson & LoVullo, 2008).

Placement
SIB is more prevalent among people with ID in institutional versus community settings (Holden & Gitlesen, 2006; Lowe et al., 2007). This could reflect a tendency for people with SIB to be placed in institutions, although Oliver et al. (1987) noted that the prevalence of SIB is more difficult to estimate among community samples. There is insufficient evidence regarding the relation between placement and SIB among individuals with ASD.

Genetic Syndromes
Certain genetic syndromes appear to predispose the individual to SIB (Percy et al., 2007). Lesch-Nyhan and Cornelia de Lange syndromes, for example, are associated with an increased risk of SIB, which often takes a precise, syndrome-specific form (Winchel &

Stanley, 1991). There also appears to be a relatively high prevalence of SIB among individuals with Fragile X syndrome, and many such individuals also meet diagnostic criteria for autism. However, Hall, Lighthouse, and Reiss (2008) reported that individuals with Fragile X and autism were no more likely to show SIB than individuals with Fragile X alone.

Age

There is conflicting evidence regarding the relation between age and SIB. Baghdadli et al. (2003) reported that younger children were more at risk for SIB, but Murphy et al. (2009) found no such relation. Currently, there is insufficient evidence on the influence of chronological age on SIB in persons with ASD.

Gender

Gender does not appear to be a risk factor for SIB among children with ASD.

Adaptive Behavior Functioning

Baghdadli et al. (2003) found that greater deficits in daily living skills were risk factors for SIB, but the evidence base is too meager at present to draw any firm conclusions.

Adverse Consequences

SIB is a major problem because of the associated injury and related health problems that can arise from this behavior. SIB can lead to long-term negative health consequences. Mandell (2008) noted that SIB is a significant antecedent to the hospitalization of children with ASD. In addition to serious injury, long-term health problems, and hospitalization risk, SIB is associated with a number of other side effects, such as increased risk of being placed on powerful medications that can cause serious side effects. SIB may also lead to social and physical isolation of the individuals. This in turn might restrict opportunities for learning, social development, and community participation. The use of mechanical restraints and other intrusive treatments for SIB raises ethical concerns (National Institutes of Health, 1989).

The National Institutes of Health (1989) noted the cost of SIB at up to $US100,000.00 per year for a person with severe SIB. In addition to the financial costs, there are likely to be significant social costs, such as institutionalization and reduced opportunities for social inclusion (Winchel & Stanley, 1991).

Stereotypic Behavior

Definition

The APA (2000) defined Stereotyped Movement Disorder (SMD) as "… motor behavior that is repetitive, often seemingly driven, and nonfunctional (Criterion A) … markedly interferes with normal activities … (Criterion B) … sufficiently severe to be a focus of treatment (Criterion C) no better accounted for by compulsion … a tic … a stereotypy that is part of a Pervasive Developmental Disorder, or hair pulling (Criterion D) … is not due to the direct effects of a substance or general medical condition (Criterion E) … [and] must persist for at least 4 weeks (Criterion F)."

In addition to SMD, DSM-IV's diagnostic criteria for Autistic Disorder include "restricted, repetitive, and stereotyped patterns of behavior, interests, and activities as manifested by at least one of the following: (a) encompassing preoccupation with one or more stereotyped and restricted patterns of interest that is abnormal either in intensity or focus (b) apparently inflexible adherence to specific, nonfunctional routines or rituals (c) stereotyped and repetitive motor mannerisms (e.g., hand or finger flapping or twisting or complex whole-body movements) (d) persistent preoccupation with parts of objects." Thus, there is overlap between the diagnostic criteria for SMD and Autistic Disorder related to repetitive motor behavior; however, the diagnostic criteria for Autistic Disorder placed stereotyped and repetitive motor mannerisms as only one of four kinds of restrictive, repetitive, and stereotyped behavior. (The

DSM-IV diagnostic criteria for Pervasive Developmental Disorders other than Autistic Disorder also reference repetitive motor behavior). Thus, when someone presents with repetitive motor behavior that is a focus of clinical attention and the person does not also meet criteria for Autistic Disorder, then a diagnosis of SDM may be made; however, if the person also displays other behavior that meets criteria for Autistic Disorder, then that diagnosis is appropriate.

The APA (2000) distinguishes SIB (see previous section) as one subtype of SMD. Although many forms of SIB are indeed repetitive, such as some examples of repeated head banging, face slapping, and hand mouthing, not all examples of SIB are indeed repetitive or appear to be stereotypical in topography. For example, in response to apparently minor social provocations, a person may slam their fingers into the wheels of their wheelchair resulting in tissue damage. Although such SIB is indeed clinically significant strictly speaking, it does not meet the criteria for *SMD, self-injurious type,* since the behavior is not repetitive.

Forms and Classification

Some of the most common topographies of SMD include body rocking, repetitive hand movements, finger flicking, spinning, twirling and mouthing objects, and repetitive posturing (Bodfish et al., 1995). Some common forms of SIB include head banging, face and head slapping, and self-biting.

Typically developing infants show many repetitive motor behaviors such as arm waving, kicking legs, and repetitive manipulation of objects (Thelen, 1981). Indeed, some typically developing infants also display SIB such as head banging (Sallustro & Atwell, 1978; Thelen, 1981). Typical adults also often engage in repetitive behavior such as hair twirling, body rocking, and repetitive object manipulation. These repetitive movements can be distinguished from SMD and those associated with ASDs because they do not come to dominate the child's behavioral repertoire, do not persist over time, and do not interfere with learning and daily functioning.

Prevalence

SMD is relatively common among people with developmental disabilities with perhaps as many of half of those diagnosed with ID displaying some form of stereotypy (Bodfish et al., 1995; Rojahn, 1986). People with ASD show even higher prevalence rates of SMD. A study by Goldman et al. (2009) illustrates this observation. Goldman et al. compared the prevalence of stereotypies in four groups of children: high or low functioning children with autism and high and low functioning children with other developmental disorders. Two hundred and seventy-seven children participated. They used an IQ cutoff of 80 to operationalize high and low functioning and assessed stereotypies with a checklist that the authors developed themselves for this study. The prevalence of stereotypies in the entire sample was 44%. However, the prevalence of stereotypies was 71 and 64% in the low and high functioning group of children with autism, respectively, and 31 and 18% for the low and high functioning non-autistic groups. Thus, the prevalence of stereotypies was a function of both the presence of autism and degree of ID.

Adverse Consequences

SMD has a number of adverse consequences, some of which are minor and some of which may be quite significant. Repetitive behaviors are often socially stigmatizing; thus, RMDs are often targeted in intervention studies, and reduction in stereotypic behavior had been used to validate staff-training procedures (Dib & Sturmey, 2007). SMD may also have adverse consequences as it may be related to other more directly harmful behavior, for example, it might function as a member of a response chain that terminates in a dangerous behavior such as elopement (Falcomata, Roane, Feeney, & Stephenson, 2010). The presence of SMD is also a risk marker for several other more serious challenging behaviors such as SIB and multiple challenging behaviors (Oliver, Petty, Ruddick, & Bacarese-Hamilton, 2011). Perhaps the most significant and insidious risk associated with SMD is that it may inhibit the expression of adaptive behavior and the acquisition of new skills.

Risk Factors

SMD is often more prevalent in people with autism, more severe ID, with sensory impairments, such as visual impairments, and limited mobility skills. Certain medical problems, such as otitis media, are also risk factors for head banging. Certain forms of stereotypy are also associated with genetic syndromes, for example, repetitive hand movements are associated with Rett disorder. Finally, a number of environmental variables also place an individual at greater risk, such as barren environments. Such environments may fail to provide the opportunities and contingencies to support acquisition and expression of adaptive behavior that may compete with the development and/or persistence of SMD and SIB. Additionally, some barren environments may inadvertently reinforce and shape repetitive and self-injurious behaviors or shape repetitive behavior into SIB (Guess & Carr, 1991).

Aggressive Behavior

Definition

There is no single accepted definition of aggression. Farmer and Aman (2011) review problems with defining aggression. In the psychology literature, aggression is defined as something along the lines of "intentional harm doing" and "behavior that is harming or injuring another person." In these "definitions," one implies that a certain behavior is directed to another person. Vitiello and Stoff (1997) broadened the definition to include also behavior directed at objects. They defined aggression as behavior deliberately aimed at inflicting damage to persons or property. An important element in these definitions is that there is an "attribution of intent" (Farmer & Aman, 2011; p. 318). This is problematic for use in people with ASD and/or ID. First, there is no

consensus about how to measure attribution of intent, and secondly, this term raises questions when applied to individuals with very limited cognitive skills or deficits in the ability to take the perspective of another person which is often the case in individuals with ASD and/or ID. Individuals with ASD and/or ID may engage in aggressive behavior despite having severe deficits in these areas. For our purposes, we "define" aggressive behavior as behavior that (potentially) results in injury or harm in another person or in property destruction without consideration of whether the aggressive behavior is "deliberately" exhibited or not.

Forms and Classification

The term "aggression" refers to a wide range of behavioral topographies. For example, Matson and Rivet (2008a) used the ASD-BPA, an informant-based 19-item rating scale consisting of four subscales derived from factor analysis. The Aggression/Destruction subscale contains seven behavioral topographies of aggression: kicking objects, throwing objects at others, banging on objects, aggression towards others, ripping clothes, yelling or shouting at others, and property destruction.

Usually, a distinction is made between aggressive behavior directed at objects (property destruction) and aggressive behavior directed at other people. Examples of topographies of aggression directed at objects are throwing, deliberately breaking, and hitting objects. Subcategories of aggression towards other people are physical aggression (e.g., hitting, kicking) and verbal aggression (e.g., yelling at someone, threatening someone). Some researchers distinguish a third category of aggression, namely, aggression directed towards the self or auto-aggression; this is also called SIB (see above section on SIB).

Aggressive behavior is often classified as a type of externalizing behavior as opposed to rumination, fearful behavior, and SIB that are examples of internalizing behaviors. Externalizing behaviors are directed towards the environment of the person, including other people, and these behaviors usually interfere with the behavior of others. By contrast, internalizing behaviors are directed towards the person himself and usually do not interfere with the behaviors of others. The *Child Behavior Checklist* (CBCL; Achenbach & Rescorla, 2000) is a well-researched measure of challenging behavior that addresses externalizing and internalizing behaviors. Scores are summed to form seven syndrome scales including the scale on aggression.

Another classification of aggressive behavior was proposed by Farmer and Aman (2011) who distinguish between "proactive" and "reactive" aggression. Proactive or instrumental aggression is characterized by instrumental goals, or the perception of a link between aggressive behavior and a desired outcome. Reactive aggression is characterized by behavior that results from external provocation or anger without thought of personal gain. The authors state that this distinction is clinically important because each subtype may have a different etiology. Farmer and Aman have developed the *Children's Scale of Hostility and Aggression: Reactive/Proactive* (C-SHARP) and recently used this scale with a sample of 121 children with ASD.

Another way to classify aggressive behavior is to look at the type of reinforcement that maintains this type of challenging behavior. For example, Matson, Sipes et al. (2011) reviewed 173 studies that used functional assessment with respect to type of challenging behavior and function(s) identified that maintained those behaviors. The most frequently studied type of challenging behavior after SIB was aggression. The most often reported function of aggression was avoidance of or escape from task demands, followed by access to tangibles and, to a lesser degree, nonsocial or sensory reinforcement. Results of this review suggest that aggressive behavior may be classified according to the type of environmental event that maintains it. While there are five functions for challenging behavior, aggression may primarily be maintained by escape from demand. So aggression may primarily be motivated by social events, while other types of challenging behavior may primarily be maintained by nonsocial ones. It should be noticed, however,

that aggression may also have one or more other functions for any given individual. For example, O'Reilly et al. (2010) have conducted functional analysis of challenging behavior in 10 children with ASD or PDD-NOS who were between 4 and 8 years old. Results showed that challenging behaviors, including aggression and SIB, were maintained by automatic reinforcement for 8 out of the 10 children and by multiple sources of reinforcement for the other 2 children. No data were presented for only aggressive behavior as each child engaged in a variety of challenging behaviors during functional analysis.

Prevalence

Several studies have reported high prevalence rates of aggressive behaviors in samples of children and adults with ASD. For example, Ming, Brimacombe, Chaaban, Zimmerman-Bier, and Wagner (2008) have used retrospective chart reviews to assess prevalence of aggressive behaviors in 160 children and youngsters who were consecutively admitted to a university-based center. All had received a diagnosis of ASD. Specifically, 48% had autism, 45% had PDD-NOS and the remaining 7% had Asperger disorder. Participants were between 2 and 18 years old. Results showed that 32% of the sample engaged in some type of aggressive behavior, and this behavior was significantly associated with mood disorder.

Hartley et al. (2008) investigated prevalence of challenging behaviors in a subgroup of children with ASD, namely, children with autism. Parents of 169 children who were between 1.5 and 6 years of age completed the CBCL (Achenbach & Rescorla, 2000), of which aggression is one of seven syndromes. Each syndrome scale has a criterion above which a behavior is considered clinically significant or severe enough to warrant intervention. Among this sample of children, 22.5% showed clinically significant levels of aggression.

Several studies have assessed rates of challenging behavior such as aggression in samples of individuals with ASD and ID. For example, in a large sample ($n = 3,065$) of adults with profound to mild ID, which in 68 cases was combined with autism, aggression was found in 29% of the subsample (i.e., cases with ID and autism) (Tyrer et al., 2006). In Kanne and Mazurek's (2011) study, 1,380 children between 4 and 17 years participated, all of whom had some type of ASD. Total IQ ranged between 13 and 167, and data were collected on ASD symptomatology, cognitive and adaptive functioning, and aggressive behavior. Results showed that 56% of the sample engaged in some form of aggressive behavior, ranging from mild (24%) to severe physical aggression or violence (32%), towards caregivers.

Matson and Rivet (2008b) have investigated prevalence rates of several forms of aggression in 298 adults with ASD and ID who lived in two residential facilities. It was found that among participants with autism, 7% engaged in throwing objects at others, 15% engaged in aggression towards people, and 14% engaged in property destruction.

Dominick, Ornstein Davis, Lainhart, Tager-Flusberg, and Folstein (2007) assessed various topographies of aggression (e.g., hitting, biting others) in a sample of 54 children with ASD and compared outcomes to 38 children with language impairment. Children in both groups were between 4 and 14 years old. Groups were matched on age and nonverbal IQ. Aggression occurred more frequently in children with ASD (i.e., 33%) than in those without ASD (i.e., 21%), but the difference was not statistically significant. Over half of the children had the onset of their aggressive behavior during the toddler years. However, the prevalence of temper tantrums was significantly higher in children with ASD (i.e., 71%) than in children with language impairment (i.e., 23%). A temper tantrum was operationally defined as crying, flailing, and yelling usually in response to some aversive stimulus, such as change in activity. For 60% of these children, temper tantrums occurred on a daily basis, and 20% of children with ASD had the onset of tantrums by 1 year of age.

Matson and Rivet (2008a) compared prevalence rates of various topographies of challenging behavior (including aggression/destruction) of adults with autism/ID ($n = 62$) to rates among individuals with PDD-NOS/ID ($n = 99$) and individuals with ID only (controls; $n = 159$) of whom most had profound ID. Data on aggression/destruction were collected using the ASD-BPA. Prevalence rates across various topographies of aggression/destruction ranged from 11% (ripping clothes) to 29% (yelling or shouting at others). Comparative analyses revealed that participants with autism had significantly higher rates of aggression/destruction than both the PDD-NOS group and the ID only group. These results indicate that among adults with profound ID who live in a facility aggression/destruction is associated with severity of ASD symptoms.

Elevated rates of aggression have been found in individuals with ID who also have genetic disorders, which are frequently associated with ASD symptomatology. For example, Arron, Oliver, Moss, Berg, and Burbridge (2011) have investigated prevalence rates of physical aggression in several syndrome groups. Physical aggression was most common in Smith-Magenis syndrome (74%) and in Angelman syndrome (73%) and, to a lesser extent, in Cri du Chat, Fragile X, and Prader–Willi syndrome (43%), with rates of 70, 52, and 43%, respectively. Compared to a control group (46%), aggression was significantly higher for Angelman and Smith-Magenis syndromes.

Risk Factors

Among 298 adults with ASD and severe to profound ID who were living in a residential facility, Matson and Rivet (2008b) found that aggression/destruction (as measured by the ASD-BPA) was not related to severity of ASD symptomatology. However, a closer look revealed that communication impairment was a significant predictor of aggression/destruction.

In Kanne and Mazurek's (2011) sample of children and youngsters (4–17 years old), a relationship was found between aggressive behavior and age, and social and communication deficits. The likelihood of aggression decreased with increasing age, while it increased with ASD-related social and communication skill deficits.

IQ and gender and severity of ASD symptoms were not related to aggression, while self-injurious behavior, ritualistic behaviors, and resistance to change were predictive of aggression.

Hartley et al. (2008) showed that among 169 young children with autism, severity of aggressive behavior was negatively correlated with nonverbal cognitive functioning, expressive language, and adaptive skills. No associations were found between externalizing behaviors and age, gender, or severity of autistic symptoms. These results were largely corroborated by those from a study by Dominick et al. (2007) who found that aggression in children with ASD was negatively correlated (albeit moderately) with cognitive and language measures such as verbal and nonverbal IQ, and level of receptive and expressive language. By contrast, in Hartley et al.'s study, severity of autistic symptoms was positively associated with challenging behavior. Aggression was also positively associated with self-injury and temper tantrums. Other studies have not found such a relationship. For example, Matson, Boisjoli, and Mahan (2009) investigated relationships between challenging behavior and expressive and receptive communication skills in 168 toddlers who met DSM-IV-TR (APA, 2000) criteria for ASD and who were enrolled in an early intervention program. Data on ASD symptoms and challenging behavior (e.g., aggression) were collected using the *Baby and Infant Screen for Children with aUtism Traits* (BISCUIT). A range of developmental skills were measured using the *Battelle Developmental Inventory-2nd edition* (BDI-2). Results showed that in this group of toddlers low levels of receptive and expressive communication were associated with low levels of aggression. These results suggest that communication deficits may not be a risk factor for aggression in infants and toddlers with ASD. Differences in sample characteristics and type of measurement may also account for the discrepancies in outcomes among the aforementioned studies.

Recent studies have shown that certain genetic disorders may also be a risk factor for aggression. For example, Arron et al. (2011) have compared prevalence rates of aggressive behavior (physical aggression) among several syndrome groups and one control group. Participants were between 4 and 52 years of age, and data were collected through a range of questionnaires. Results showed that aggressive behavior was significantly more common in Angelman syndrome and in Smith-Magenis syndrome. Across all syndrome groups, impulsivity and overactivity were positively correlated with aggression. Physical aggression was more likely in younger individuals with Cri du Chat, Fragile X, and Prader–Willi syndrome. Aggression was associated with being male in Prader–Willi syndrome and with being of lower ability in Prader–Willi and Cornelia de Lange syndromes. The latter results imply that there may be syndrome-specific associations between physical aggression and certain risk factors.

Adverse Consequences

Kanne and Mazurek (2011) have reviewed studies on adverse consequences of aggression in people with ID and/or ASD and concluded that aggression is one of the strongest predictors of crisis intervention re-referrals, admission to residential facilities, and use of psychotropic medication. It may lead to increased levels of stress among parents and out-of-home placements of children and it is associated with an increased risk of physical abuse from caregivers. Aggression in children with ASD and ID is significantly associated with burnout and emotional exhaustion among teachers and special education support staff. In this way, this behavior has negative effects on teachers' instructional efforts, and it interferes with instruction. Related to this, Tyrer et al. (2006) have found that almost half of carers of adults with ID who engaged in aggression reported that they were unable to cope with the aggressive behavior compared to 10% of those caring for adults without aggression.

Feeding Disorders

Definition

The APA (2000) defined Feeding Disorder of Infancy and Early Childhood (hereafter "Feeding Disorders") as

" … persistent failure to eat adequately, as reflected in persistent failure to gain weight or significant weight loss over at least one month (Criterion A) … " (p. 98) and this disorder is not better accounted for by other disorders such as general medical conditions (Criterion B), another mental disorder, including other disorders of eating such as Rumination Disorder or lack of food (Criterion C), and the disorder must onset before the age of 6 years (Criterion D.)

Feeding Disorders are difficult to diagnose for several reasons. Food refusal lies along a continuum in terms of both its severity and duration, and it may wax and wane in severity over time. The presence of medical problems, which is common, can also distract family members and professionals away from psychological aspects of food refusal, which may coexist with relevant medical problems and which may or may not be related to a Feeding disorder. Additionally, parental tolerance and societal norms for children's eating behavior have probably changed dramatically over time and vary tremendously over cultures. Thus, diagnosis of feeding disorders can be problematic.

Forms and Classification

Feeding disorders can take several forms. This can include food refusal and food selectivity. In food refusal, a child may refuse all or many foods such that the child does not consume sufficient calories and has other nutritional deficiencies and/or associated medical problems, such as malnutrition or chronic gastrointestinal feeding. Food selectivity refers to eating a very narrow range of foods and/or being very sensitive to apparently minor differences in foods presentation or other food-related stimuli. For example, a child may eat only milk from a preferred bottle and cream cheese, but refuse to drink milk from any other container, refuse to consume similar foods such as yogurt, and refuse to consume cream cheese on a cracker. Such children might also be highly sensitive to with whom and where they eat, refusing to eat with certain caretakers or only eating a limited range of foods in certain settings.

Although the APA (2000) requires failure to gain weight or low weight, some children do not meet this criterion, but still may have significant behavior management issues regarding food selectivity or refusal.

Prevalence

Recently, research has paid more attention to feeding disorders, especially in the context of early intervention for young children with ASD. Williams, Seiverling, and Field (in press) provided a partial review of the epidemiology of food refusal and concluded that the prevalence of food refusal was unclear. For example, Field, Garland, and Williams (2003) reported a prevalence of 34% of children with special needs rising to 69% of children with gastrointestinal reflux. Similarly, Fodstad and Matson (2008) reported that 25% of adults with disabilities in an institutional setting have some form of a feeding disorder as assessed by a psychometric screening measure. Both of these studies, however, were samples of convenience rather than random samples from some population of interest, and there are simply too few studies to make any strong conclusions regarding the prevalence of feeding disorders.

Even less is known about the prevalence of food selectivity (Williams & Seiverling, 2010). Recently, however, Raspa, Bailey, Bishop, Holiday, and Olmsted (2010) surveyed a sample of 1,075 children with Fragile X syndrome, a condition associated with ASD symptoms. Questions related to food selectivity included items related to selectivity by texture, color, smell, and type of food. Selectivity by texture was most common and ranged from 63% of boys aged 6–10 years to 19% of girls aged 11–15 years. Food selectivity was generally less prevalent in adults. For example, food selectivity was reported in only 39% of men and 19% of women. These results suggest that food selectivity is common in people with Fragile X syndrome; however, the validity of the data, which were reported by family members, is unclear.

Adverse Consequences

Food Refusal may be associated with various medical and social problems. These may include gastrointestinal reflux, esophagitis, vomiting and regurgitation, painful or otherwise difficult swallowing and chronic gastrointestinal tube feeding, etc. It is difficult to disentangle cause and effect here. Food refusal may begin after the occurrence of one or more painful or invasive medical or other procedures related to swallowing or food consumption. Chronic gastrointestinal feeding may begin as a feeding strategy but then contribute to the maintenance of food refusal by failing to provide opportunities to relearn how to eat or by providing an easy alternative to feeding a child who is difficult to feed.

Food selectivity can be associated with a number of adverse consequences. For example, food selectivity may make meal times difficult for families as meal consumption may take extensive lengths of time to complete and family members may need to engage in a range of behavior management strategies to persuade their child to eat. Sometimes the family members' behavior management strategies fail, provoking distressing and/or dangerous challenging behavior and perhaps even maintaining food refusal and inadvertently shaping even more difficult challenging behavior. Sometimes, children with high food selectivity also refuse to eat any new food for prolonged periods of time. This can be highly distressing to family members and perhaps place the child at risk for medical problems.

Risk Factors

Due to the limited epidemiology for food refusal and selectivity, it is difficult to identify risk factors with certainty. Children who display food refusal and selectivity often present with a history of medical problems that could function as classical and operant conditioning events that might result in the onset and maintenance of food refusal (Williams, Seiverling et al., 2010). It is easy to speculate as to how parental management strategies might inadvertently shape food refusal, especially in the case of children who have weak or absent adaptive feeding behavior. The function of food refusal may be that of escaping demands (i.e., food presented), while food selectivity may be maintained by access to preferred food items.

Some empirical evidence for risk factors comes from Field et al. (2003) who reported on risk factors for five feeding problems: food refusal, food selectivity by type, food selectivity by texture, oral motor delays, or dysphagia in children with autism, Down syndrome, and cerebral palsy. Esophageal reflux was the most common problem and predicted food refusal, whereas neuroanatomical abnormalities were associated with skill deficits. Although Raspa et al. (2010) reported age- and gender-related differences in the prevalence of food selectivity in people with Fragile X syndrome, these data do not shed any light on what the mechanisms might be that place certain demographic groups at greater or lesser risk. Thus, although there is a limited quantity of data on risk factors for feeding disorders, the data that are available suggest the notion of classical conditioning and difficulties in acquisition of adaptive feeding responses as plausible mechanisms for explaining the onset of some Feeding disorders.

Pica, Vomiting, and Rumination

Definition

Pica is the ingestion of nonnutritive or inedible objects (Matson, Belva, Hattier, & Matson, 2011). Pica can be food-based (e.g., eating rotten food, frozen food, or scavenging for food in the trash) or nonfood-based (e.g., ingesting cigarette butts, feces, hair, or paint). The individual who engages in pica seeks out inedible objects in their environment, places the object in their mouth, and then either chews the object or immediately swallows it. Some people will engage in pica with several different types of objects, and other people will only ingest one specific type of object (e.g., only cigarette butts) (Matson et al., 2011). When an individual ingests only a specific type of nonedible material, a more specific term may be used to describe the pica (Stiegler, 2005). In order to diagnose pica as a stand-alone disorder, the behavior (a) must persist for longer than 1 month,

(b) must be developmentally inappropriate, and (c) cannot be part of cultural or religious practice (APA [DSM-IV-TR], 2000). However, pica is not typically diagnosed separately in individuals with autism due to the prevalence of other problem behaviors within the autism population.

Rumination is the deliberate regurgitation, chewing, and swallowing of stomach contents, and vomiting (or emesis) is the expulsion of regurgitated stomach contents from the mouth (Lang et al., 2011; Starin & Fuqua, 1987). A combination of these regurgitation behaviors may be called ruminative vomiting (e.g., Mulick, Schroeder, & Rojahn, 1980). Individuals who engage in ruminative vomiting often obtain access to vomitus by tilting back their head, arching their torso, and creating suction with their tongue on the roof of the mouth or by thrusting their fingers down their throat (Tierney & Jackson, 1984). In order for these regurgitation behaviors to be considered ruminative vomiting, the regurgitation cannot be due to physiological issues, such as illness, drug side effects, or gastroesophageal abnormality (APA, 2000). Like pica, rumination may be diagnosed as a stand-alone disorder. However, this diagnosis is not typically made with individuals with autism due to the common association between the behavior and autism (i.e., other problem behaviors).

Prevalence

Estimates of the prevalence of pica among people with autism are rare (Myles, Simpson, & Hirsch, 1997). However, Kinnell (1985) found that 60% of a sample of 70 people with severe autism engaged in pica. Several studies have estimated the prevalence of pica among groups of people with ID, without, however, specifying how many of those people also had autism (c.f., Ashworth, Martin, & Hirdes, 2008). In these studies, prevalence estimates of pica among people living in institutions ranged from 9.2 to 25.8% (Matson, Sipes et al., 2011). Studies providing estimations of prevalence outside institutional settings are rare. Rojahn (1986) conducted a postal survey of over 25,000 people in Germany and estimated the prevalence of pica among individuals with ID living in the community to be 0.3%. This large discrepancy in prevalence data may be due to different estimation methods (e.g., direct observation vs. review of patient records) and the different definitions of pica used across the prevalence studies (Ali, 2001; Danford & Huber, 1982). For example, although all definitions of pica have included the ingestion of inedible objects, some studies have also included compulsive eating of food (e.g., Danford & Huber, 1982), mouthing but not swallowing of objects (e.g., McAlpine & Singh, 1986), and eating frozen foods that should be heated (e.g., Tewari, Krishnan, Valsalan, & Ashok, 1995). Danford and Huber compared case records to direct observations and found that pica was often not reported in patients' records. Therefore, studies relying solely on reviews of case records may underestimate prevalence (Danford & Huber, 1982).

Data on the prevalence of ruminative vomiting among individuals with autism is sparse and no large-scale studies have been published (Lang et al., 2011). However, the available data suggests that approximately 5–10% of individuals with ID may engage in these behaviors (Danford & Huber, 1981; Gravestock, 2000; Tewari et al., 1995). One potential reason for the lack of prevalence data for ruminative vomiting may be due to difficulties distinguishing between regurgitation caused by medical issues and psychogenic or operant regurgitation (i.e., regurgitation maintained by automatic and social reinforcement contingencies) (Lang et al., 2011). For example, Rogers, Stratton, Victor, Kennedy, and Andres (1992) found gastroesophageal abnormalities that could cause chronic regurgitation in 91% of the people identified by hospital staff as engaging in ruminative vomiting.

Adverse Consequences

Pica is associated with a variety of serious health risks including vomiting, malnutrition, poisoning, anemia, parasitic infection, gastroesophageal trauma, and death (e.g., Ali, 2001; Ashworth et al., 2008; Decker, 1993; Matson, Sipes, et al., 2011;

Matson & Bamburg, 1999; Stiegler, 2005). Decker (1993) reviewed the treatment history of 35 patients that engaged in pica at a community hospital over a period of 15 years and found that 75% of the patients had required surgery. For these individuals, the complication rate for surgery was 30%, and the death rate was 11% (Decker, 1993). Even in cases in which behavioral treatments are utilized, the ingestion of a single object (e.g., a safety pin) may result in life-threatening complications (e.g., Falcomata, Roane, & Pabico, 2007). For some people with autism, pica is also associated with aggressive behavior that occurs when their attempts to obtain specific inedible objects for the purpose of ingestion are impeded (Danford & Huber, 1982; Matson & Bamburg, 1999). However, other people with autism who engage in pica are not aggressive and may be notably withdrawn and submissive (Tewari et al., 1995).

Chronic ruminative vomiting may lead to serious health risks including malnutrition, weight loss, dehydration, increased susceptibility to disease, tooth decay, choking, gastrointestinal bleeding, and death (Fredericks, Carr, & Williams, 1998; Singh, 1981; Starin & Fuqua, 1987). Rumination is the primary cause of death in 5 to 10% of people who ruminate (Fredericks et al., 1998). In addition to adverse health effects, vomiting and rumination may also exacerbate the social deficits associated with autism. For example, frequent contact with vomitus may hinder a person's appearance and cause foul odors leading to social isolation and reduced educational or vocational opportunities (Starin & Fuqua, 1987).

Risk Factors

Dementia, pregnancy, and sickle cell anemia are risk factors for the development of pica in individuals with and without ID (Ali, 2001; Ashworth et al., 2008). For individuals with autism, pica appears to be more common among individuals with the most severe to profound ID, suggesting that pica is more common in individuals with autism than in people with Asperger's syndrome (Ashworth et al., 2008; Danford & Huber, 1982;

Matson, Sipes et al., 2011; McAlpine & Singh, 1986). Pica also appears to be more common in individuals with autism than in individuals with other developmental disabilities (Ashworth et al., 2008; Myles et al., 1997; Stiegler, 2005). For example, Kinnell (1985) compared an autism group to a Down syndrome group and found pica in 60% of the autism group and only 4% of the Down syndrome group. Several studies have reported that pica appears to decrease with age (e.g., Ali, 2001), and other studies have reported that pica persists over time (e.g., Matson & Bamburg, 1999). One reason for the reduced rates of pica in older groups of people with ID may be the shorter life expectancy of individuals with profound ID (Danford & Huber, 1981).

Ruminative vomiting can occur in typically developing children but is more common among people with autism and severe to profound ID (Gravestock, 2000; Tierney & Jackson, 1984). When rumination occurs in typically developing children, it often begins and ends early in life; however, in individuals with autism and ID, it often begins later in life and persists over time (Winton & Singh, 1983). For people with autism, the risk of developing ruminative vomiting may be equal across ages and level of intellectual functioning (Parry-Jones, 1994; Rastam, 2008). Lang et al. (2011) reviewed the intervention research targeting rumination and operant vomiting and found that many of the participants receiving treatment had a comorbid visual impairment suggesting that visual impairment may be a risk factor. Johnston and Greene (1992) reviewed data on 10 patients across 10 years and found that the quantity of food consumed during meals is related to frequency of rumination. Interventions in which more food is provided to people who ruminate often result in reductions in ruminative vomiting (Lang et al., 2011).

Conclusion

In this chapter, we have provided a selective review of studies on the nature, prevalence, and characteristics of challenging behaviors in individuals with ASD and/or ID. A relatively large number of studies have been published on the prevalence and associated factors of challenging behavior in children and adults with ASD and/or ID. Overall, these rates may vary as a result of differences in operational definitions, ASD diagnosis, measurement instrument, and sample characteristics. Despite this, it is now well established that individuals with ASD and/or ID are at risk for various types of challenging behavior and that these behaviors add to the "severity" of ASD condition (Matson & Rivet, 2008b).

An increasing number of studies have identified risk factors for challenging behavior in individuals with ASD and/or ID. Risk factors may be biological, for example, in case the challenging behavior is part of the behavioral phenotype of the genetic disorder. It should be noted, however, that results of studies on risk factors are correlational and it is often unclear to what extent a risk factor is also a cause of challenging behavior (Matson, Kozlowski et al., 2011). For example, several studies have shown that also phenotypic behaviors may be influenced by environmental events and that such behaviors may be reduced by procedures based on functional analysis (see, e.g., Radstaake, Didden, Oliver, Allen & Curfs, in press). Other risk factors are related to skill deficits, such as deficits in the area of communication and adaptive skills that may be targeted for intervention. For example, training of cognitive and adaptive skills has shown to result in improved functioning in children with ASD and/or ID (see results of a recent meta-analysis by Peters-Scheffer, Didden, Korzilius, & Sturmey, 2011).

References

Achenbach, T., & Rescorla, L. (2000). *Child Behavior Checklist*. Burlington: ASEBA.

American Psychiatric Association. (2000). *Diagnostic and statistical manual of mental disorders (Revised)* (4th ed.). Washington, DC: Author.

Ali, Z. (2001). Pica in people with intellectual disability: A literature review of aetiology, epidemiology and complications. *Journal of Intellectual & Developmental Disability, 26*, 205–215.

Arron, K., Oliver, C., Moss, J., Berg, K., & Burbidge, C. (2011). The prevalence and phenomenology of self-injurious and aggressive behaviour in genetic syndromes. *Journal of Intellectual Disability Research, 55*, 109–120.

Ashworth, M., Martin, L., & Hirdes, J. P. (2008). Prevalence and correlates of pica among adults with intellectual disability in institutions. *Journal of Mental Health Research in Intellectual Disabilities, 1*, 176–190.

Baghdadli, A., Pascal, C., Grisi, S., & Aussilloux, C. (2003). Risk factors for self-injurious behaviors among 222 children with autistic disorders. *Journal of Intellectual Disability Research, 47*, 622–627.

Bienstein, P., & Nussbeck, S. (2009). Reliability of a German version of the Questions About Behavioral Function (QABF) Scale for self-injurious behavior in individuals with intellectual disabilities. *Journal of Mental Health Research in Intellectual Disabilities, 2*, 249–260.

Bodfish, J. W., Crawford, T. W., Powell, S. B., Parker, D. E., Golden, R. N., & Lewis, M. H. (1995). Compulsion in adults with mental retardation: Prevalence, phenomenology, and comorbidity with stereotypy and self-injury. *American Journal on Mental Retardation, 100*, 183–192.

Danford, D. E., & Huber, A. M. (1981). Eating dysfunctions in an institutionalized mentally retarded population. *Appetite, 2*, 281–292.

Danford, D. E., & Huber, A. M. (1982). Pica among mentally retarded adults. *American Journal on Intellectual and Developmental Disabilities, 87*, 141–146.

Deb, S. (1998). Self-injurious behaviour as part of genetic syndromes. *British Journal of Psychiatry, 172*, 385–388.

Decker, C. J. (1993). Pica in the mentally handicapped: A 15 year surgical perspective. *Canadian Journal of Surgery, 36*, 551–554.

Dib, N., & Sturmey, P. (2007). Reducing student stereotypy by improving teachers' implementation of discrete-trial teaching. *Journal of Applied Behavior Analysis, 40*, 339–343.

Dominick, K., Ornstein Davis, N., Lainhart, J., Tager-Flusberg, H., & Folstein, S. (2007). Atypical behaviors in children with autism and children with a history of language impairment. *Research in Developmental Disabilities, 28*, 145–162.

Emerson, E. (2005). *Challenging behaviour: Analysis and intervention in people with severe intellectual disabilities*. Cambridge: Cambridge University Press.

Emerson, E., Kiernan, C., Alborz, A., Reeves, D., Mason, H., & Swarbrick, R., et al. (2001). The prevalence of challenging behaviors: A total population study. *Research in Developmental Disabilities, 22*, 77–93.

Falcomata, T., Roane, H., & Pabico, R. (2007). Unintentional stimulus control during the treatment of pica displayed by a young man with autism. *Research in Autism Spectrum Disorders, 1*, 350–359.

Falcomata, T. S., Roane, H. S., Feeney, B. J., & Stephenson, K. M. (2010). Assessment and treatment of elopement maintained by access to stereotypy. *Journal of Applied Behavior Analysis, 43*, 513–517.

Farmer, C., & Aman, M. (2011). Aggressive behavior in a sample of children with autism spectrum disorders. *Research in Autism Spectrum Disorders, 5*, 317–323.

Fee, V. E., & Matson, J. L. (1992). Definition, classification, and taxonomy. In J. K. Luiselli, J. L. Matson, & N. N. Singh (Eds.), *Self-injurious behavior: Analysis, assessment, and treatment* (pp. 3–20). New York: Springer.

Field, D., Garland, M., & Williams, K. (2003). Correlates of specific childhood feeding problems. *Journal of Pediatrics and Child Health, 39*, 299–304.

Fodstad, J. C., & Matson, J. L. (2008). A comparison of feeding and mealtime problems in adults with intellectual disabilities with and without autism. *Journal of Developmental and Physical Disabilities, 20*, 541–550.

Fredericks, D. W., Carr, J. E., & Williams, W. L. (1998). Overview of the treatment of rumination disorder for adults in a residential setting. *Journal of Behavior Therapy and Experimental Psychiatry, 29*, 31–40.

Goldman, S., Wang, C., Salgado, M., Greene, P., Kim, M., & Rapin, I. (2009). Motor stereotypies in children with autism and other developmental disorders. *Developmental Medicine and Child Neurology, 51*, 30–38.

Gravestock, S. (2000). Eating disorders in adults with intellectual disability. *Journal of Intellectual Disability Research, 44*, 625–637.

Guess, D., & Carr, E. (1991). Emergence and maintenance of stereotypy and self-injury. *American Journal on Mental Retardation, 96*, 299–319.

Hall, S. S., Lighthouse, A. A., & Reiss, A. L. (2008). Compulsive, self-injurious, and autistic behavior in children and adolescents with fragile X syndrome. *American Journal on Mental Retardation, 113*, 44–53.

Hartley, S., Sikora, D., & McCoy, R. (2008). Prevalence and risk factors of maladaptive behaviour in young children with autistic disorder. *Journal of Intellectual Disability Research, 52*, 819–829.

Holden, B., & Gitlesen, J. P. (2006). A total population study of challenging behavior in the county of Hedmark, Norway: Prevalence and risk markers. *Research in Developmental Disabilities, 27*, 456–465.

Iwata, B., Pace, G., Dorsey, M., Zarcone, J., Vollmer, T., Smith, R., et al. (1994). The functions of self-injurious behavior: An experimental-epidemiological analysis. *Journal of Applied Behavior Analysis, 27*, 215–240.

Johnston, J. M., & Greene, K. S. (1992). Relation between ruminating and quantity of food consumed. *Mental Retardation, 30*, 7–11.

Jones, R. S. (1987). The relationship between stereotyped and self-injurious behaviour. *British Journal of Medical Psychology, 60*, 287–289.

Kanne, S., & Mazurek, M. (2011). Aggression in children and adolescents with ASD: Prevalence and risk factors. *Journal of Autism and Developmental Disorders, 41*, 926–937.

Kinnell, H. G. (1985). Pica as a feature of autism. *British Journal of Psychiatry, 147*, 80–82.

Klonsky, E. D., & Meuhlenkamp, J. J. (2007). Self-injury: A research review for the practitioner. *Journal of Clinical Psychology: In Session, 63*, 1045–1056.

Lang, R., Mulloy, A., Giesbers, S., Pfeiffer, B., Delaune, E., Didden, R., et al. (2011). Behavioral interventions for rumination and operant vomiting in individuals with intellectual disabilities: A systematic review. *Research in Developmental Disabilities, 32*, 2193–2205.

Lord, C., Rutter, M., & Lecoutteur, A. (1994). Autism Diagnostic Interview Revised: A revised version of a diagnostic interview for caregivers of individuals with possible pervasive developmental disorders. *Journal of Autism and Developmental Disorders, 24*, 659–683.

Lowe, K., Allen, D., Jones, E., Brophy, S., Moore, K., & James, W. (2007). Challenging behaviours: Prevalence and topographies. *Journal of Intellectual Disability Research, 51*, 625–636.

Mandell, D. S. (2008). Psychiatric hospitalization among children with autism spectrum disorders. *Journal of Autism and Developmental Disorders, 38*, 1059–1065.

Matson, J. L., & Bamburg, J. W. (1999). A descriptive study of pica in persons with mental retardation. *Journal of Developmental and Physical Disabilities, 11*, 353–361.

Matson, J. L., Belva, B., Hattier, M. A., & Matson, M. L. (2011). Pica in persons with developmental disabilities: Characteristics, diagnosis, and assessment. *Research in Autism Spectrum Disorders, 5*, 1459–1464.

Matson, J. L., Boisjoli, J., & Mahan, S. (2009). The relation of communication and challenging behaviors in infants and toddlers with autism spectrum disorders. *Journal of Developmental and Physical Disabilities, 21*, 253–261.

Matson, J. L., Fostad, J. C., Mahan, S., & Rojahn, J. (2010). Cut-offs, norms and patterns of problem behaviours in children with developmental disabilities on the Baby and Infant Screen for Children with autism (BISCUIT-Part 3). *Developmental Neurorehabilitation, 13*, 3–9.

Matson, J. L., Kozlowski, A. M., Worley, J. A., Shoemaker, M. E., Sipes, M., & Horowitz, M. (2011). What is the evidence for environmental causes of challenging behaviors in persons with intellectual disabilities and autism spectrum disorders? *Research in Developmental Disabilities, 32*, 693–698.

Matson, J. L., & LoVullo, S. V. (2008). A review of behavioral treatments for self-injurious behaviors of persons with autism spectrum disorders. *Behavior Modification, 32*, 61–76.

Matson, J. L., & Rivet, T. T. (2008a). Characteristics of challenging behaviours in adults with autistic disorder, PDD-NOS, and intellectual disability. *Journal of Intellectual & Developmental Disability, 33*, 323–329.

Matson, J. L., & Rivet, T. T. (2008b). The effects of severity of autism and PDD-NOS symptoms on challenging behaviors in adults with intellectual disabilities. *Journal of Developmental and Physical Disabilities, 20*, 41–51.

Matson, J. L., Sipes, M., Horovitz, M., Worley, S., Shoemaker, M., & Kozlowski, A. M. (2011). Behaviors and corresponding functions addressed via functional assessment. *Research in Developmental Disabilities, 32*, 625–629.

Matson, J. L., Terlonge, C., & Gonzáles, M. L. (2006). *Autism Spectrum Disorders—Diagnosis—Adult Version*. Baton Rouge: Disability Consultants.

McAlpine, C., & Singh, N. N. (1986). Pica in institutionalized mentally retarded persons. *Journal of Mental Deficiency Research, 30*, 171–178.

McClintock, K., Hall, S., & Oliver, C. (2003). Risk markers associated with challenging behaviours in people with intellectual disabilities: A meta-analytic study. *Journal of Intellectual Disability Research, 47*, 405–416.

Ming, X., Brimacombe, M., Chaaban, J., Zimmerman-Bier, B., & Wagner, G. (2008). Autism spectrum disorders: Concurrent clinical disorders. *Journal of Child Neurology, 23*, 6–13.

Mulick, J. A., Schroeder, S. R., & Rojahn, J. (1980). Chronic ruminative vomiting: A comparison of four treatment procedures. *Journal of Autism and Developmental Disorders, 10*, 203–213.

Murphy, G. H., Oliver, C., Corbett, J., Crayton, L., Hales, J., Head, D., et al. (1993). Epidemiology of self-injury, characteristics of people with severe self-injury and initial treatment outcome. In C. Kiernan (Ed.), *Research to practice? Implications of research on challenging behaviour of people with learning disability* (pp. 1–35). Avon: British Institute of Learning Disabilities.

Murphy, G., Hall, S., Oliver, C., & Kissi-Debra, R. (1999). Identification of early self-injurious behaviour in young children with intellectual disability. *Journal of Intellectual Disability Research, 43*, 149–163.

Murphy, O., Healy, O., & Leader, G. (2009). Risk factors for challenging behaviors among 157 children with autism spectrum disorders in Ireland. *Research in Autism Spectrum Disorders, 3*, 474–482.

Myles, B. S., Simpson, R. L., & Hirsch, N. C. (1997). A review of literature on interventions to reduce pica in individuals with developmental disabilities. *Autism, 1*, 77–95.

National Institutes of Health. (1989). *Treatment of destructive behaviors in persons with developmental disabilities* (Consensus Development Conference Statement, Vol. 7, No. 9). Bethesda: Author.

O'Reilly, M. F., Rispoli, M., Davis, T., Machalicek, W., Lang, R., Sigafoos, J., et al. (2010). Functional analysis of challenging behavior in children with autism spectrum disorder: A summary of 10 cases. *Research in Autism Spectrum Disorders, 4*, 1–10.

Oliver, C., Murphy, G. H., & Corbett, J. A. (1987). Self-injurious behaviour in people with mental handicap:

A total population study. *Journal of Mental Deficiency Research, 31*, 147–162.

Oliver, C., Petty, J., Ruddick, L., & Bacarese-Hamilton, M. (2011). The association between repetitive, self-injurious and aggressive behavior in children with severe intellectual disability. *Journal of Autism and Developmental Disorders* [Epub ahead of print].

Parry-Jones, B. (1994). Merycism or rumination disorder: A historical investigation and current assessment. *British Journal of Psychiatry, 165*, 303–314.

Percy, M., Cheetham, T., Gitta, M., Morrison, B., Machalek, K., Bega, S., et al. (2007). Other syndromes and disorders associated with intellectual and developmental disabilities. In I. Brown & M. Percy (Eds.), *A comprehensive guide to intellectual and developmental disabilities* (pp. 229–267). Baltimore: Paul H. Brookes.

Peters-Scheffer, N., Didden, R., Korzilius, H., & Sturmey, P. (2011). A meta-analytic study on the effectiveness of comprehensive ABA-based early intervention programs for children with autism spectrum disorders. *Research in Autism Spectrum Disorders, 5*, 60–69.

Radstaake, M., Didden, R., Oliver, C., Allen, D., & Curfs, L. (In press). Functional analysis and functional communication training in individuals with Angelman syndrome. *Developmental Neurorehabilitation*.

Raspa, M., Bailey, D. B., Bishop, E., Holiday, D., & Olmsted, M. (2010). Obesity, food selectivity, and physical activity in individuals with fragile-X Syndrome. *American Journal on Mental Retardation, 115*, 482–495.

Rastam, M. (2008). Eating disturbances in autism spectrum disorders with focus on adolescent and adult years. *Clinical Neuropsychiatry, 5*, 31–42.

Rogers, B., Stratton, P., Victor, J., Kennedy, B., & Andres, M. (1992). Chronic regurgitation among persons with mental retardation: A need for combined medical and interdisciplinary strategies. *American Journal on Mental Retardation, 96*, 522–527.

Rojahn, J. (1986). Self-injurious stereotypic behavior of noninstitutionalized mentally retarded people: Prevalence and classification. *American Journal of mental Deficiency, 91*, 268–276.

Rojahn, J., Matson, J. L., Lott, D., Esbensen, A. J., & Smalls, Y. (2001). The Behavior Problems Inventory: An instrument for the assessment of self-injury, stereotyped behavior and aggression/destruction in individuals with developmental disabilities. *Journal of Autism and Developmental Disorders, 31*, 577–588.

Rojahn, J., Whittaker, K., Hoch, T. A., & Gonzáles, M. L. (2007). Assessment of self-injurious and aggressive behavior. In J. L. Matson (Ed.), *Handbook of assessment in persons with intellectual disability* (pp. 281–319). San Diego: Academic.

Sallustro, F., & Atwell, C. W. (1978). Body rocking, head banging, and head rolling in normal children. *The Journal of Pediatrics, 93*, 704–708.

Schloper, E., Reichler, R. J., & Rochen Renner, B. (1988). *The Childhood Autism Rating Scale*. Los Angeles: Western Psychological Services.

Schroeder, S. R., Mulick, J. A., & Rojahn, J. (1980). The definition, taxonomy, epidemiology and ecology of self-injurious behavior. *Journal of Autism and Developmental Disorders, 10,* 417–432.

Schroeder, S. R., Tessel, R. E., Loupe, P. S., & Stodgell, C. J. (1997). Severe behavior problems among people with developmental disabilities. In W. E. MacLean Jr. (Ed.), *Ellis' handbook of mental deficiency, psychological theory and research* (3rd ed., pp. 439–464). Mahwah: Lawrence Erlbaum.

Sigafoos, J., Arthur, M., & O'Reilly, M. (2003). *Challenging behavior and developmental disability.* Baltimore: Paul H. Brookes.

Sigafoos, J., Reichle, J., & Light Shriner, C. (1994). Distinguishing between socially and nonsocially motivated challenging behavior: Implications for the selection of intervention strategies. In M. F. Hayden & B. H. Abery (Eds.), *Challenges for a service system in transition: Ensuring quality community experiences for persons with developmental disabilities* (pp. 147–169). Baltimore: Paul H. Brookes.

Singh, N. N. (1981). Rumination. In N. R. Ellis (Ed.), *International review of research in mental retardation* (Vol. 10, pp. 139–182). New York: Academic.

Smith, R. T., Vollmer, T. R., & St. Peter Pipkin, C. (2007). Functional approaches to assessment and treatment of problem behavior in persons with autism and related disabilities. In P. Sturmey & A. Fitzer (Eds.), *Autism spectrum disorders: Applied behavior analysis, evidence, and practice* (pp. 187–234). Austin: Pro-Ed.

Sparrow, S. S., Balla, D. A., & Cicchetti, D. V. (1984). *Vineland Adaptive Behavior Scales* (Interviewth ed.). Circle Pines: American Guidance Service.

Starin, S. P., & Fuqua, W. (1987). Rumination and vomiting in the developmentally disabled: A critical review of the behavioral, medical, and psychiatric treatment research. *Research in Developmental Disabilities, 8,* 575–605.

Stiegler, L. N. (2005). Understanding pica behavior: A review for clinical and educational professionals. *Focus on Autism and Other Developmental Disabilities, 20,* 27–38.

Tate, B. G., & Baroff, G. S. (1966). Aversive control of self-injurious behavior in a psychotic boy. *Behavior Research and Therapy, 4,* 281–287.

Tewari, S., Krishnan, V. H. R., Valsalan, V. C., & Ashok, R. (1995). Pica in learning disability hospital: A critical survey. *British Journal of Developmental Disabilities, 41,* 13–22.

Thelen, E. (1981). Rhythmical behavior in infancy: An ethological perspective. *Developmental Psychology, 17,* 237–257.

Tierney, D., & Jackson, H. J. (1984). Psychosocial treatments of rumination disorder: A review of the literature. *Australia and New Zealand Journal of Developmental Disabilities, 10,* 81–112.

Tyrer, F., McGrother, C., Thorp, C., Donaldson, M., Bhaumik, S., Watson, J., et al. (2006). Physical aggression towards others in adults with learning disabilities: Prevalence and associated factors. *Journal of Intellectual Disability Research, 50,* 295–304.

Van Ingen, D. J., Moore, L. L., Zaja, R. H., & Rojahn, J. (2010). The Behavior Problems Inventory (BPI-01) in community-based adults with intellectual disabilities: Reliability and concurrent validity vis-à-vis the Inventory for Client and Agency Planning (ICAP). *Research in Developmental Disabilities, 31,* 97–107.

Vitiello, B., & Stoff, D. M. (1997). Subtypes of aggression and their relevance to child psychiatry. *Journal of the American Academy of Child and Adolescent Psychiatry, 36,* 307–315.

Weiss, J. (2003). Self-injurious behaviours in autism: A literature review. *Journal on Developmental Disabilities, 9,* 129–143.

Williams, K. E., & Seiverling, L. J. (2010). Eating problems in children with autism spectrum disorders. *Topics in Clinical Nutrition, 25,* 27–37.

Williams, K.E., Seiverling, L.J., & Field, D.G. (in press). Feeding problems. In P. Sturmey & R. Didden (Eds.), *Evidence-base practice in intellectual disabilities.* Chichester: Wiley UK.

Winchel, R. M., & Stanley, M. (1991). Self-injurious behavior: A review of the behavior and biology of self-mutilation. *American Journal of Psychiatry, 148,* 306–317.

Winton, A., & Singh, N. (1983). Rumination in pediatric populations: A behavioral analysis. *Journal of the American Academy of Child and Adolescent Psychiatry, 22,* 269–275.

World Health Organization. (1992). *The ICD-10 classification of mental and behavioural disorders: Clinical descriptions and diagnostic guidelines.* Geneva: Author.

Function of Challenging Behaviors

Giulio E. Lancioni, Nirbhay N. Singh, Mark F. O'Reilly, Jeff Sigafoos, and Robert Didden

Introduction

Challenging behavior is a label/definition normally used to identify a variety of performance expressions that (a) can be dangerous to the person's physical safety or to the safety of others sharing the person's context, and/or (b) can seriously interfere with the person's access to the typical community facilities (Carr, Dozier, Patel, Adams, & Martin, 2002; Emerson, 1995;

G.E. Lancioni (✉)
Department of Psychology, University of Bari,
Via QuintinoSella 268, Bary 70100, Italy
e-mail: g.lancioni@psico.uniba.it

N.N. Singh
American Health and Wellness Institute,
P.O. Box 80466, Raleigh, NC 27623, USA
e-mail: nirbsingh52@aol.com

M.F. O'Reilly
Department of Special Education, College of Education,
The University of Texas at Austin, Austin,
TX 78712, USA
e-mail: markoreilly@mail.utexas.edu

J. Sigafoos
School of Educational Psychology and Pedagogy,
Victoria University of Wellington, Karori Campus,
PO Box 17-310, Wellington, New Zealand
e-mail: jeff.sigafoos@vuw.ac.nz

R. Didden
Behavioural Science Institute, Radboud University
Nijmegen, P.O. Box 9104, Nijmegen 6500 HE,
The Netherlands
e-mail: r.didden@pwo.ru.nl

McLaughlin et al., 2003; Stewart & Alderman, 2010; Wood, Blair, & Ferro, 2009). In particular, challenging behaviors include a variety of self-injurious stereotypies (e.g., hitting, scratching, biting one's own body parts), other apparently nonself-injurious stereotypies (e.g., flapping own hands, body rocking, and repeated verbalizations), aggression toward others, and property destruction (Lancioni, Singh, O'Reilly, & Sigafoos, 2009; Matson & LoVullo, 2008; Neidert, Dozier, Iwata, & Hafen, 2010; Stokes & Luiselli, 2009; Watson & Watson, 2009; Wilder, Kellum, & Carr, 2000).

Challenging behaviors are highly likely among persons with general developmental disorders, autism, severe and profound intellectual disabilities, and multiple disabilities (Kurtz et al., 2003; Lancioni et al., 2009). The first consideration about challenging behaviors is that they have a definitely negative impact on the person's developmental and adaptive opportunities and on his or her context and therefore their occurrence needs to be reduced through appropriate intervention strategies (Singh et al., 2009; Tarbox et al., 2009). The second consideration is that challenging behaviors may have their emergence and continuous occurrence justified by the functions (consequences) that they have for the person. In other words, they may have an important role for the person (e.g., in terms of stimulation and reinforcement), irrespective of whether an external observer could attribute them an immediate/obvious meaning or not

J.L. Matson (ed.), *Functional Assessment for Challenging Behaviors*,
Autism and Child Psychopathology Series, DOI 10.1007/978-1-4614-3037-7_4,
© Springer Science+Business Media, LLC 2012

(LaBelle & Charlop-Christy, 2002; Najdowski, Wallace, Ellsworth, MacAleese, & Cleveland, 2008; Noell & Gansle, 2009). The third consideration is that any attempt to intervene to reduce the occurrence of challenging behaviors should rely on (a) an understanding of the possible functions of such behaviors and (b) intervention strategies that are matched to those functions (Matson & Minshawi, 2007; Neidert et al., 2010; Singh et al., 2009; Tarbox et al., 2009).

These three considerations have over time become a widely agreed way of thinking and the common approach is that an assessment of the person's challenging behavior is a preliminary condition for the development of the intervention strategy. Assessment can occur in different ways. The three most common forms may involve the use of rating scales, observational descriptive strategies, and functional analysis procedures (Borrero & Borrero, 2008; Harvey, Luiselli, & Wong, 2009; Kates-McElrath, Agnew, Axelrod, & Bloh, 2007; Pence, Roscoe, Bourret, & Ahearn, 2009).

Assessment Strategies

Rating Scales

The use of rating scales relies on the notion that staff/caregivers, who know the person with challenging behavior, can provide relevant information when faced with structured questions about the behavior and its possible functions within a reasonably short amount of time (Carter, Devlin, Doggett, Harber, & Barr, 2004; Singh et al., 2009; Watson & Watson, 2009). Two of the rating scales may be considered particularly useful and practical, that is, the Motivation Assessment Scale (MAS) (Durand & Crimmins, 1988) and the Questions about Behavioral Function (QABF) (Matson et al., 2005; Matson & Wilkins, 2009; Singh et al., 2009). The MAS includes 16 questions, through which it attempts to identify the functions of the person's challenging behavior. The specificity of the questions with the clear definition of the challenging behavior are supposed to increase the probability of providing useful information as to when the behavior is

more likely to occur (e.g., in situations in which the person is alone, in difficult task situations, in situations where attention is diverted or when environmental events not scheduled are likely to occur). In essence, the scale is provided with many of the questions that functional analysis procedures pose and attempt to resolve through manipulation of the situations. Through those questions, the scale attempts to evaluate four different functions as potentially responsible for the challenging behavior, that is, access to specific items/activities, attention, escape from demands, and sensory or automatic consequences.

The QABF was originally conceived as a 25-item questionnaire and evaluated over a large number of participants with highly encouraging results in terms of its ability to identify the function of the challenging behavior for a large percentage of participants (Matson, Bamburg, Cherry, & Paclawskyj, 1999; Paclawskyj, Matson, Rush, Smalls, & Vollmer, 2000). Recently, research has shown that a 15-item version may preserve the same potential as the longer version (Singh et al., 2009). One possible difference of this scale compared to the MAS is that the questions are even more explicit as to the target of their inquiry (e.g., engages in the behavior to get attention, engages in the behavior as a form of self-stimulation, and engages in the behavior when he/she does not want to do something). Through those questions, the scale attempts to evaluate five different functions, which add physical discomfort to those already contemplated in the MAS.

Descriptive Methods

The use of observational, descriptive strategies involves direct observation and recording of the challenging behavior as well as of the environmental variables that might be relevant for such behavior. The most common form of descriptive strategy consists of recording the antecedent event and the consequence for each occurrence of the target behavior (Noell & Gansle, 2009; Tarbox et al., 2009). This strategy, which is also known as the ABC (antecedent–behavior–consequence) approach, requires the person's behavior to be recorded in combination with what occurs immediately before its emission and what follows it. For example, one may record that a student's screaming and self-hitting behavior in the classroom is generally preceded by the teacher asking him or her specific (task-related) questions and followed by the teacher's silence or gentle physical interaction directed at calming the student. In that case, one could hypothesize that the student's challenging behavior has the function of avoiding task-related questions and possibly obtaining attention and physical contact (Borrero & Borrero, 2008; Harvey et al., 2009; Pence et al., 2009).

Another direct observation strategy involves the use of time charts, the most popular of which is the scatter plot (Noell & Gansle, 2009; Touchette, MacDonald, & Langer, 1985). The first step in this type of strategies is to develop a grid that divides the time of observation into specific periods (e.g., half hours, quarter hours or any other time unit that might seem appropriate). Each time unit is then filled with the frequencies of the behavior under observation. After several observation days, a pattern may emerge with the problem behavior concentrated in certain periods of the day and virtually absent in others. The differences in the occurrence of the behavior might then be correlated to the presence or absence of certain staff/caregivers, the presence or absence of certain activities, the presence or absence of task-related demands, the presence or absence of certain groups of stimuli and reinforcers, as well as the presence or absence of other recognizable variables. This type of picture/evidence may not be sufficient to identify the function of the behavior and its controlling variables. Nonetheless, it may facilitate the efforts to discover the relationship between the challenging behavior and one or more environmental variables. The manipulation of some of those variables may then help reduce or eliminate the problem (Touchette et al., 1985).

Functional Analysis

The functional analysis is an experimental method that involves the manipulation of antecedents and consequences of the challenging behavior in order to identify or exclude functional relations between the behavior and the specific environmental variables being manipulated. The standard functional analysis approach described by Iwata, Dorsey, Slifer, Bauman, and Richman (1982/1994) involves four specific assessment conditions across which the challenging behavior is measured and compared, that is, attention, demand, play, and alone. These conditions are presented several times non-consecutively, according to a multielement baseline design. The attention condition involves the use of some forms of reprimand or concern (e.g., Don't do that or you should not hurt yourself) delivered contingent on the occurrence of the challenging behavior. The demand condition involves the presentation of fairly difficult tasks (e.g., educational or occupational tasks, such as coloring or arranging objects, that are considered demanding for the participant) or of questions waiting to be answered. The task or questions would be momentarily interrupted/halted by the occurrence of the challenging behavior. The play condition involves the availability of preferred material and activities and the positive interaction of the therapist in charge of the session, who delivers attention with overall regularity except when the challenging behavior occurs. The alone condition involves the request that the participant stays in a room with no stimuli or persons present.

To establish whether attention is playing a role in maintaining the challenging behavior, the data obtained in this condition are compared with the data resulting from the play and alone conditions. Relatively high levels of challenging behavior during the attention condition and low levels of the behavior during the latter two conditions would strongly suggest that the behavior is directed at obtaining environmental attention (i.e., social positive reinforcement). Relatively high levels of challenging behavior in the demand condition and lower levels in the other conditions would suggest that the behavior is directed at escaping difficult demand situations (i.e., tasks or questions), thus obtaining negative reinforcement. Relatively high levels of challenging behavior during the alone situation, as compared to the other situations, may suggest that the behavior provides a form of reinforcement not mediated by environmental variables (i.e., automatic reinforcement).

Functional Analysis and Possible (Desirable or Necessary) Adaptations

There is broad consensus as to the fact that functional analysis represents the best, more powerful approach to determine the functions of challenging behaviors. Indeed, most of the functional analysis studies published in scientific journals apparently reported interpretable data as to the possible behavioral function with important practical implications for intervention (Hanley, Iwata, & McCord, 2003; Hanley, Piazza, Fisher, & Maglieri, 2005). Notwithstanding the positive results and utility of functional analysis, a number of issues have been raised that call for possible adaptations/changes of the classical Iwata et al.'s (1982/1994) model or conventional versions following the original model (e.g., Buchanan & Fisher, 2002; Carter et al., 2004; Tarbox et al., 2009). Those issues, which may also present some level of contradiction with one another, concern (a) the occasional need of extending the number of assessment conditions available so that the analysis becomes more representative of complex daily environments and ultimately more reliable, (b) the practical importance of designing short versions of the assessment procedure, (c) the opportunity of drawing different assessment sequences in cases of inconclusive data, and (d) the importance of carrying out the assessment within the same educational/rehabilitation context in which the person spends his or her time (and of maintaining a number of basic elements of that context) (Carter et al., 2004; LaBelle & Charlop-Christy, 2002; Lang et al., 2008; 2009; Wallace & Knights, 2003; White et al., 2011).

Extending the Range (Number) of Assessment Conditions

The desirability (need) of extending the assessment range has frequently been addressed and a

number of studies have reported additional conditions compared to those included in the classical model. For example, a number of studies have added the tangible condition, that is, a condition within which a toy or a food item is visible but out of reach and its delivery is arranged contingent on the occurrence of the challenging behavior (e.g., Asmus, Franzese, Conroy, & Dozier, 2003; Kuhn, Hardesty, & Sweeney, 2009; Kurtz, Chin, Rush, & Dixon, 2008; Lancioni, Walraven, O'Reilly, & Singh, 2002; Tarbox et al., 2009). Some studies have divided attention into social and physical attention components so as to determine whether one or the other of these components could be motivating for the challenging behavior (e.g., Britton, Carr, Kellum, Dozier, & Weil, 2000). Other studies have replaced or supplemented some of the traditional conditions with new ones such as response blocking and response blocking with attention so as to represent daily program arrangements available for the participants (Hagopian & Toole, 2009).

Designing Short Versions of Functional Analysis

While the utility of functional analysis procedures is not in discussion, their practicality (affordability) in terms of time costs may raise some questions (Matson & Minshawi, 2007; Moore, Fisher, & Pennington, 2004; Northup et al., 1991; Perrin, Perrin, Hill, & DiNovi, 2008; Wallace & Knights, 2003). Iwata et al. (1982/1994) reported that the mean number of sessions included in early functional analysis studies was 26 with an average time cost of about 6.5 h (seemingly high in many daily contexts). In response to this question, various attempts were made to design and evaluate shorter, more affordable procedures. For example, Northup et al. (1991) successfully designed a functional analysis procedure that lasted a 90-min period (i.e., a period typically reserved for outpatient psychological evaluations) and was carried out within a single day. Kahng and Iwata (1999) compared a full-length functional analysis with a one-session-per-condition functional analysis with 50 participants with developmental disabilities and self-injurious or aggressive behavior and found that the outcomes corresponded in 66% of the cases. Wallace and Knights (2003) reported comparable results with brief and extended functional analysis procedures applied with three adults with developmental disabilities and disruptive behavior. The brief analysis was based on 2-min sessions and the extended analysis on 10-min sessions. The time durations of the two were 36 min and 310 min, respectively. Perrin et al. (2008) carried out a brief functional analysis of elopement with two 3-year-old children with a diagnosis of autism. The functional analysis included five conditions each of which was presented over four 5-min sessions. The results of the functional analysis were differentiated and the intervention strategies based on the identified behavioral functions were effective.

Drawing Different (Special) Assessment Conditions or Sequences

The results of the functional analysis can occasionally be largely undifferentiated. This outcome may be an indication that (a) the challenging behavior is idiosyncratic and requires very specific assessment conditions (different from those usually included in the functional assessment procedure) or (b) the multielement methodology used to alternate the conditions is less than optimal to differentiate those conditions and help clarify among them (DeLeon, Kahng, Rodriguez-Catter, Sveinsdóttir, & Sadler, 2003; Hausman, Kahng, Farrell, & Mongeon, 2009; Healey, Ahearn, Graff, & Libby, 2001; Ringdahl, Christensen, & Boelter, 2009). For example, DeLeon et al. (2003) reported that the level of challenging behavior was undifferentiated in conventional conditions but clearly dominant in a specially designed condition called "contingent wheelchair movement." Hausman et al. (2009) reported low levels of self-injurious and aggressive behavior in a 9-year-old girl under conventional conditions. Yet, her challenging behavior increased quite drastically when the assessment allowed the girl to access a ritualistic behavior

(i.e., change the position of the door). Healey et al. (2001) suggested that lack of response differentiation under multielement designs (with quickly alternating conditions) may advise the use of blocked phases, that is, phases in which the conditions are repeated for some time rather than being regularly rotated.

Carrying Out the Assessment within the Educational/Rehabilitation Context (or Maintaining Similar Task or Attention Condition)

The fact that functional analysis can be arranged in different settings and carried out by different persons can be considered a practical advantage, but can also present serious risks in terms of outcome dependability (Lang et al., 2008; 2009; McAdam, DiCesare, Murphy, & Marshall, 2004; Tiger, Fisher, Toussaint, & Kodak, 2009). For example, Lang et al. (2008) showed that the results of the functional analysis carried out with two children of 12 and 7 years of age with autism and related communication and behavioral disorders corresponded across settings (i.e., a therapy room and a classroom) only for one of the children. Lang et al. (2009) replicated the earlier findings with a 4-year-old child whose challenging behaviors included screaming and aggression. Indeed, the functional analysis carried out in the playground seemed to indicate that the child's behaviors were mainly maintained by adult attention. The functional analysis carried out in the classroom, however, seemed to indicate that the behaviors were maintained prevalently by access to toys. Intervention procedures based on non-contingent use of attention and toys indicated that the former was more effective in the playground and the latter more effective in the classroom. Tiger et al. (2009) found discrepancies between the problems identified in the daily program and the outcome of their early functional analyses. For example, the early functional analysis carried out with a 10-year-old child with intellectual disability, hydrocephalus, and mild visual impairment did not evidence the high rates of aggressive behavior for which the child had been referred. In an attempt to extend the assessment and understand the reasons of the discrepancies, it was discovered that the therapist in charge of the functional analysis used a graduated-prompting procedure to help the child during academic tasks while the classroom teacher did not apparently do so and resorted to repeating the verbal instructions multiple times. This difference was finally found to be responsible for the discrepancies.

Selected Studies of Functional Analysis Divided by Identified Functions

The number of studies reported on functional analysis is quite vast and involves a wide range of participants, behaviors, environments, and assessment conditions. The aim of this section is to present a small selection of studies (see list in Table 4.1) serving as descriptive examples of procedural approaches and of outcomes, that is, of identified functions. These examples may serve as guidelines for setting up the assessment and using its results for designing a matching intervention. The first group of studies presented below concerns research reports, which identified attention either alone or in combination with other variables as the behavioral function (e.g., Lancaster et al., 2004; Roane & Kelly, 2008; Stokes & Luiselli, 2009). The second group of studies concerns research reports, which identified tangible items as the behavioral function (e.g., Ingvarsson, Kahng, & Hausman, 2008; Lang et al., 2010). The third group of studies concerns research reports, which pointed out escape from demand as the behavioral function (e.g., O'Reilly & Lancioni, 2000; Rooker & Roscoe, 2005). The fourth group of studies concerns research reports, which suggested automatic reinforcement as the behavioral function (e.g., Falcomata, Roane, Hovanetz, Kettering, & Keeney, 2004; Piazza, Adelinis, Hanley, Goh, & Delia, 2000; Wilder, Register, Register, Bajagic, & Neidert, 2009). The final group of studies includes research reports, which pointed out idiosyncratic events such as door manipulation as the behavioral function (e.g., DeLeon et al., 2003; Hausman et al., 2009).

Attention Alone or in Combination

Lindauer, Zarcone, Richman, and Schroeder (2002) carried out a functional analysis with a 25-year-old man who had a diagnosis of profound intellectual disability, Lennox Gastaut syndrome, and autism. The man presented self-injurious behaviors, such as hitting his head, biting his hands, and banging his head, as well as aggression. The functional analysis assessment was based on 10-min sessions carried out in the man's bedroom and included five conditions, that is, attention, demands, ignore, tangible items, and free play. During the attention condition, the therapist intervened following the instances of self-injurious behavior for about 5 s. During the tangible items condition, the man had access to a preferred item (a tape recorder) for 30 s contingent on the occurrence of challenging behavior. Similarly, in the demands condition, the occurrence of the behavior interrupted any demand for 30 s. The man displayed relatively high rates of challenging behavior in the attention condition suggesting that this was the main function of the behavior. In a subsequent intervention program, the authors combined a functional communication training (FCT) program and extinction for the challenging behavior with highly satisfactory results.

Fyffe, Kahng, Fittro, and Russell (2004) conducted a functional analysis with a 9-year-old boy who had a diagnosis of traumatic brain injury and seizure disorder. The boy presented inappropriate sexual behavior, which consisted of touching or attempting to touch others in the area of the groin, buttocks, or breast. The functional analysis procedure was carried out in a therapy room through 20-min sessions and included three assessment conditions, that is, demand, social attention, and toy play. During the demand condition, there was a 30-s break in the task contingent on the challenging behavior while praise was scheduled for compliance. In the social attention condition, the boy received a 5-s reprimand at the occurrence of the behavior. In the toy play condition, the boy had access to preferred items and received attention at 30-s intervals. The task analysis showed that the behavior was exhibited only in the social attention condition. Based on these

Table 4.1 List of studies divided by identified functions

Functions/authors	Participants (No.)	Age	Challenging behaviors
Attention			
Lindauer et al. (2002)	1	25	Self-injurious behavior
Fyffe et al. (2004)	1	9	Inappropriate sexual behavior
Lancaster et al. (2004)	4	34–56	Bizarre speech
Borrero et al. (2005)	3	7–12	Aggression and disruption
Dwyer-Moore and Dixon (2007)	3	70–90	Disruptive vocalizations or wandering and attempts to exit place
Roane and Kelley (2008)	1	16	Self-injurious behavior
Stokes and Luiselli (2009)	1	4	Elopement
Tangible items			
Hagopian et al. (2001)	1	6	Aggression/disruption and self-injurious behavior
Tarbox et al. (2003)	3	6–39	Elopement
Ingvarsson et al. (2008)	1	8	Aggression/disruption and self-injurious behavior
Reed et al. (2009)	1	16	Destruction and self-injurious behavior
Lang et al. (2010)	1	3	Elopement
Demand escape			
O'Reilly and Lancioni (2000)	1	4	Aggression and self-injurious behaviors
Peyton et al. (2005)	1	10	Noncompliant vocal behavior
Rooker and Roscoe (2005)	1	5	Self-injurious behavior
Wilder et al. (2005)	1	40	Self-injurious behavior
Butler and Luiselli (2007)	1	13	Aggression, tantrums, and self-injurious behavior
Alone (automatic reinforcement)			
Richman et al. (1998)	1	27	Disruption and self-injurious behavior
Roscoe et al. (1998)	3	20–38	Self-injurious behavior
Kuhn et al. (1999)	1	35	Self-injurious behavior
Piazza et al. (2000)	3	6–17	Disruption and self-injurious behavior
Wilder et al. (2000)	1	30	Head rocking
Tang et al. (2003)	6	4–17	Disruption, stereotypies, and self-injurious behaviors
Falcomata et al. (2004)	1	18	Inappropriate verbalizations
Moore et al. (2004)	1	12	Self-injurious behavior
Wilder et al. (2009)	1	37	Rumination
Idiosyncratic events			
DeLeon et al. (2003)	1	14	Aggression
Ringdahl et al. (2009)	1	18	Aggression and attempts to leave the room

data, an intervention strategy was implemented that involved FCT (i.e., the boy was taught to request for attention via a card) and momentary blocking followed by extinction/ignoring for the challenging behavior. The intervention impact was positive and the availability of the communication card was gradually reduced.

Lancaster et al. (2004) studied four adults of 34–56 years of age, who had dual (i.e., intellectual and psychiatric) diagnoses and presented with bizarre speech. The assessment was carried out in a therapy room over 10-min sessions and included the standard four conditions suggested by Iwata et al. (1982/1994) for one of the participants and several condition and design variations for the other participants. The outcome of the assessment showed that the bizarre speech of two of the participants was clearly higher in the attention condition. In relation to this outcome, noncontingent attention was subsequently scheduled for both these participants with encouraging results. Both participants had clear declines (but not the elimination) of the challenging behavior. For one of them, the decline in bizarre speech was accompanied by an increase in appropriate speech.

Borrero, Vollmer, Borrero, and Bourret (2005) reported the evaluation of three children of 12, 8, and 7 years of age who presented with mild intellectual disability, autism and moderate intellectual disability, and mild intellectual disability and seizure disorder, respectively. The participants' challenging behaviors consisted of aggression towards other persons and disruption. The functional analysis procedure was based on sessions of 10 or 5 min and included four conditions, that is, attention, demands (instructions), tangible, and play. During the attention condition, the participants received a brief reprimand in relation to the challenging behavior. During the demand condition (which included task instructions presented at intervals of about 10 s and supplemented with prompts), the occurrence of the challenging behavior caused a 30-s interruption of all instructions and prompts. During the tangible condition, the behavior ensured a 30-s access to preferred items. During the play condition, the participants had free access to preferred items and received attention from the therapist at 30-s intervals. The first participant showed a clear increase in disruptive behavior during the attention condition (suggesting that attention was the specific variable that maintained the behavior). The third participant had an increase in aggression and disruptive behavior during attention, demand, and tangible conditions. The second participant, to the contrary, showed a behavior increase only in the tangible condition.

Dwyer-Moore and Dixon (2007) studied three elderly persons of 70–90 years of age who were affected by dementia and resided in a care facility. Their challenging behaviors consisted of disruptive vocalizations or wandering and attempting to exit the locked facility. The functional analysis procedure was carried out in a room of the care facility and consisted of the rapid alternation of four standard conditions (i.e., attention, demand, alone, and leisure/play). The conditions were implemented over sessions of 10 min separated by intervals of 5 min. In the attention condition,

the therapist sat far from the patient and intervened with 5–10 s of attention (i.e., a number of sentences frequently used within the facility) only in relation to the problematic behaviors. In the demand condition, the therapist required the patients to perform simple motor activities or computation tasks, which were involved in the patients' exercise programs. Compliance resulted in praise. No response or incorrect responding resulted in prompting. Challenging behavior resulted in interruption of any demands for 30 s. In the leisure/play condition, leisure items such as magazines and television were available and the therapist provided social attention at intervals of about 30 s. In the alone condition, the patients were alone in the assessment room and had no leisure items available while the therapist watched them unobtrusively from outside the room. The results of the functional analysis showed that the disruptive verbalizations of one of the two patients with such a challenging behavior and the wandering of the third patient were clearly higher during the attention condition. The disruptive verbalization of the other patient seemed to be higher during the demand condition. In order to determine the dependability of the assessment data, intervention conditions matching these data were organized. Attention contingent on appropriate verbalizations was used for the first person. Noncontingent attention was arranged for the patient with the wandering problem, and FCT and extinction were used for the last participant. The results of the intervention supported the findings of the functional analysis with all three patients and improved their general performance.

Roane and Kelley (2008) investigated the case of a 16-year-old girl who had a diagnosis of moderate intellectual disability, generalized anxiety disorder, and cerebral degenerative chorea. The girl's challenging behavior consisted of hitting herself with her hands and banging her head. The functional analysis was conducted in a fully padded room over sessions of 10 min. The two assessment conditions consisted of continuous and contingent physical attention. In the first of these conditions (continuous attention), a therapist sat next to the girl on the floor so that the girl could wrap her arms around the therapist or the therapist held hands with the girl throughout the length of the session. During the second (contingent attention) condition, the two forms of physical contact/attention were the same as those mentioned above. They were applied only in connection with the occurrence of the challenging behavior when the therapist moved close to the girl for 20 s. The levels of challenging behavior seemed definitely higher in the contingent condition suggesting that this form of attention was responsible for it. Based on these data, the authors applied continuous physical attention as the intervention variable to reduce foot withdrawal and promote correct step performance during walking sessions. Consistent with the results of the functional analysis, the walking data showed that continuous physical attention reduced foot withdrawal and increased step performance. By contrast, attention contingent on foot withdrawal increased this behavior and reduced step performance.

Stokes and Luiselli (2009) reported the assessment and treatment of a 26-year-old man with Prader–Willi syndrome who attended a community-based vocational training program and lived in a supervised group-home. The man's main challenging behavior consisted of rectal picking, which had a long history and was health threatening. He also presented with skin picking, which consisted of excoriating the skin around his fingernails, arms, and lips. Following the application of functional assessment scales such as the MAS and the Functional Analysis Screening Tool (Iwata & DeLeon, 1996), the authors also conducted a specific functional analysis assessment using skin picking as target behavior (rather than rectal picking as they wanted to avoid undue risks in relation to this particular behavior). The functional analysis was based on four standard conditions (i.e., attention, demand/escape, play, and alone) implemented in a small room at the vocational training context. Each condition was implemented over three 5-min sessions that were carried out by a specific staff person (i.e., different from the persons involved in the other sessions/conditions). The results of the assessment showed that the behavior had high frequency in the attention and alone conditions suggesting that it could be motivated by staff attention as

well as by sensory consequences (i.e., automatic reinforcement; Lancioni et al., 2009). Although, the man did not show the skin picking behavior during the demand condition, staff hypothesized that rectal picking could also be motivated by task escape (as it often resulted in the interruption of all he was doing and visits to the hospital). The intervention program, which was matched to the assessment, included reduced toilet times, FCT, and differential social reinforcement of positive toilet behavior. The program outcome showed a successful elimination of rectal picking and the maintenance of the positive effects over time.

Access to Tangible Items

Hagopian, Wilson, and Wilder (2001) followed the case of a 6-year-old boy with autism and mild intellectual disability who presented with aggression, disruption, and self-injurious behaviors. The functional analysis was eventually concentrated on social attention, task demand, social demand, and tangible conditions through 10-min sessions. The social demand condition involved the therapist talking to the boy and commenting on his play. This stopped for 30 s in connection with the boy's challenging behavior. Similarly, the challenging behavior allowed 30-s access to a preferred toy in the tangible condition. The assessment results indicated that the boy had high levels of challenging behavior in the tangible and social demand conditions. In the subsequent intervention, the use of FCT (to require objects) was effective to reduce the challenging behavior to virtually zero levels.

Tarbox, Wallace, and Williams (2003) carried out an investigation with three participants of 6, 28, and 39 years of age who had diagnoses of Asperger's syndrome, profound intellectual disability and seizure disorder, and severe intellectual disability, respectively. The challenging behavior of each of the participants was elopement. The functional analysis was carried out by regular caregivers in situations that resembled the participants' typical settings (i.e., those in which the challenging behaviors occurred). The conditions implemented over 10-min sessions included attention, tangible, demand, and play. The results of the functional analysis showed that the first two participants had high levels of elopement responses during the tangible condition (i.e., when they could reach a toy store and obtain a potato chip, respectively). In the subsequent, matched intervention, the use of FCT to enable the two participants to formulate item requests combined with elopement blocking produced largely satisfactory results.

Ingvarsson et al. (2008) reported the case of an 8-year-old girl who had been diagnosed with autism, mild cerebral palsy, moderate intellectual disability, and obsessive–compulsive disorders. She also presented aggression, disruption and self-injurious behaviors. The assessment was carried out by a therapist in a bedroom of the facility in which the girl had been admitted through 10-min sessions. The conditions included attention, demand, toy play, ignore, and tangible items. In the tangible condition, the girl obtained her preferred food contingent on her challenging behavior. High rates of challenging behavior were consistently observed only in the tangible condition. A subsequent intervention provided preferred food items noncontingently within a task-like condition with positive results, irrespective of the density of the delivery.

Reed, Pace, and Luiselli (2009) studied a 16-year-old boy with a diagnosis of pervasive developmental disorder with seizure and mood problems, and a possible hemispheric brain lesion. The boy attended a school for students with brain injury and showed multiple forms of self-injury and destructive behaviors. The functional analysis was carried out within a special (assessment) room over 10-min sessions. The procedure involved three common conditions (i.e., demand, attention, and play), which were carried out according to standard rules. The only specificities were (a) the use of educational tasks of the participant's individualized program for the demand condition, (b) the availability of five preferred stimuli relevant for the participant engagement during the play condition, and (c) the use of different staff persons for the implementation of the diverse conditions. The tangible condition involved a new (fourth) staff person for

its implementation. Moreover, two condition variations were realized. One of these new conditions was preceded by the participant's choice of the tangible item that he would have during the sessions (i.e., contingent on the occurrence of the challenging behaviors). The other condition involved the same item across all sessions. The results showed that the frequency of the challenging behaviors was high only in the tangible condition, in which the participant was allowed to choose the preferred item to use.

Lang et al. (2010) conducted an assessment with a 4-year-old boy who had a diagnosis of Asperger's syndrome and presented the problem of elopement. Separate functional analyses were carried out in the boy's typical classroom and in a resource room in which the boy received individual instruction. The analyses were based on 5-min sessions covering attention, demand, play, and tangible conditions. In the tangible condition, a television and a DVD player were available. The child was shown his preferred DVD for 10 s prior to the session and contingent on each elopement episode during the session. The results of the two analyses differed. The rates of elopement were higher during the attention condition in the resource room and during the tangible condition in the classroom. Intervention strategies based on the noncontingent use of attention and tangible items validated the results of the functional analyses. In fact, the attention-based intervention was effective in the resource room while the tangible-based intervention was effective in the classroom.

Demand Escape

O'Reilly and Lancioni (2000) examined the situation of a 4-year-old girl with moderate level of intellectual disability who presented with self-injurious and aggressive behavior. The girl was residing at home with her family and the functional analysis and intervention were conducted in that context with the mother acting as therapist. The functional analysis included the standard attention, demand, play, and alone conditions and was implemented through 15-min sessions.

During the demand condition, the girl was presented with two tasks that she had difficulty carrying out. Both tasks were available within each session and the therapist/mother maintained her requests on them expect in case of challenging behaviors. Contingent on these behaviors, the task was removed and the mother stepped away for a minimum of 10 s starting from the cessation of those behaviors. The results showed high levels of challenging behaviors during the demand condition and virtually no challenging behaviors during the other conditions. The authors also found out that the level of challenging behaviors co-varied with the level of sleep deprivation. That is, more severe sleep deprivation tended to increase the challenging behavior.

Peyton, Lindauer, and Richman (2005) reported a study with a 10-year-old girl who had a diagnosis of autism and developmental delays. The girl's challenging behavior consisted of noncompliant vocal behavior (e.g., the girl declaring her inability to do what she was asked to do). The assessment was carried out at home with the girl's mother acting as therapist and video-recording the sessions for subsequent expert scoring. The functional analysis included the attention, demand, play, and alone conditions. During the demand condition, the mother prompted her to complete tasks dealing with number, letter, and picture identifications. Compliance led her to receive praise and to be presented with additional instructions/prompts. Noncompliance led to task interruption and material removal for about 20 s. Data showed high levels of noncompliant vocal behavior only in the demand condition with the suggestion that the behavior served to escape the demand situation. Subsequent investigations in which the instructions were provided in an indirect way demonstrated that the noncompliant vocal behavior decreased to virtually zero levels (thus suggesting that the instruction mode rather than the task demand was responsible for the challenging behavior) while task performance was very high.

Rooker and Roscoe (2005) carried out an assessment with a 5-year-old boy with a diagnosis of autism and a serious self-injurious behavior consisting of chin-to-shoulder hitting. The initial functional analysis was carried out in a special room through 10-min sessions covering the four standard (i.e., attention, demand, play, and alone) conditions. During the demand condition, a difficult task was used and the challenging behavior allowed a 15-s interruption of such a task. The results of the analysis indicated that the boy exhibited clearly higher levels of the challenging behavior in the demand condition and suggested that such behavior served to escape the difficult task situation. Repetitions of functional analysis with noncontingent access to forms of self-restraint or contingent access to self-restraint indicated that the challenging behavior occurred only when self-restraint was contingent. This latter data would seem to modify the early suggestion that challenging behavior served as escape.

Wilder, Normand, and Atwell (2005) reported the evaluation of a 40-year-old woman with a diagnosis of autism, gastro-esophageal reflux and food allergies. She presented with food refusal and exhibited various forms of severe self-injurious behavior. The functional analysis was carried out in a therapy room through 10-min sessions that covered the four standard conditions. During the attention condition, the therapist followed every instance of challenging behavior with a verbal reprimand and a brief physical touch. During the play condition, the woman had free access to preferred items and activities and received the therapist's attention every 30 s, while no consequences were available for her challenging behavior. During the demand condition, the therapist presented a bite of food on a spoon every 30 s. Brief praise was used if the woman accepted the bite. If the woman did not accept the bite but did not show the challenging behavior, the spoon remained at her lips for 30 s at which time a new bite was presented. In case of challenging behavior, the spoon was removed and the therapist took a distance from the woman for about 15 s. The woman was reported to show the challenging behavior almost exclusively during the demand condition and it was suggested that such behavior served to escape the feeding situation. In a subsequent intervention effort, the authors tested the effects of continuous stimulation (children's video), which was briefly interrupted (i.e., for 15 s) only in connection with the occurrence of the challenging behavior. Data showed that the level of challenging behavior dropped drastically and the level of bite acceptance increased to about 90% of the total.

Butler and Luiselli (2007) reported an elaborate three-phase functional analysis with a 13-year-old girl who had a diagnosis of autism and presented with self-injurious behavior as well as aggression and tantrums. The analysis was carried out within the girl's daily educational context through 10-min sessions. The first phase of the functional analysis involved the four standard (attention, demand, play, and alone) conditions. During the demand condition, the therapist presented academic tasks that were part of the girl's educational plan. For each task, the initial instruction would be followed by prompting if the girl failed to respond. Every correct response was followed by praise. Challenging behavior led to the removal of the task and distancing of the therapist for 30 s. The second phase of the functional analysis was directed at assessing different demand conditions. One of these conditions involved the same requests/tasks used during the first phase of the functional analysis. Another condition involved requests concerning the simple manipulation of objects such as puzzles, beads, clay, and sensory toys already familiar to the girl. The final condition involved requests concerning basic motor activities such as sitting down and putting something away. The third phase of the functional analysis served to assess the impact of five different therapists within a demand condition that matched the one used during the first phase of the analysis. The five therapists were known to the girl and included the one responsible for the first two phases of the analysis, the classroom teacher, and three classroom assistants.

The results of the first phase of the analysis showed that the girl had low or zero levels of challenging behavior except in the demand condition, in which those levels were very high. The results of the second phase of the analysis indicated that the levels of challenging behavior were highest in the first demand condition, in which the educational (most demanding/difficult) tasks were presented and lowest in the third demand

condition, in which basic motor activities (least demanding forms of engagement) were used. The results of the third phase of the analysis showed that the highest levels of challenging behavior occurred with the therapist in charge of the previous assessment phases and the classroom teacher (i.e., the two persons with whom the girl had a longer learning history, that is, the longest practice time for consolidating the relationship between demands, challenging behavior, and escape opportunities). Based on the aforementioned results, the intervention program was directed at (a) smoothing (attenuating the aversiveness/difficulties of) the instructions so as to reduce the motivation to engage in challenging behavior to escape them, (b) implementing noncontingent escape occasions to allow the girl multiple break (reinforcement) occasions, and (c) avoiding task removal and therapist distancing in relation to challenging behavior. Those basic principles were combined with fading strategies concerning the number of instructions presented within each session and the interval between the occasions of noncontingent reinforcement. This intervention package seemed to be very effective with an increased number of instructions available and a virtual disappearance of the challenging behavior.

Alone (Automatic Reinforcement)

Richman, Wacker, Asmus, and Casey (1998) carried out an assessment with a 27-year-old woman who had a diagnosis of profound intellectual disability and autism, and presented with disruptive behavior as well as finger picking. Functional analysis, which included the standard four conditions applied over 5-min sessions, showed a different picture for the two forms of challenging behavior. In essence, disruptive behavior seemed to occur (almost) exclusively within the demand condition, while finger picking was consistently present through all conditions. Based on these data, the hypothesis was that disruptive behavior was maintained by escape and finger picking was due to the sensory input it produced (i.e., was maintained by automatic reinforcement; see Kenzer & Wallace, 2007; Lyons,

Rue, Luiselli, & DiGennaro, 2007; Vollmer, 1994). The intervention program for finger picking consisted of (a) a combination of response blocking applied to prevent its occurrence and effects and prompting aimed at directing the woman's hand to a toy, and (b) praise contingent on independent toy play. The positive effects of this package, which were maintained over time, could not be replicated through the use of the reinforcement (praise) alone.

Roscoe, Iwata, and Goh (1998) studied three adults of 20–38 years of age who were diagnosed with profound or moderate intellectual disability and displayed self-injurious behaviors such as arm rubbing, object hitting, hand mouthing, and body picking and rubbing. The functional analysis included the four standard conditions, which were implemented by four different therapists over four different rooms through 15-min sessions. One participant showed high levels of challenging behavior in the demand, play and alone conditions, and somewhat lower levels in the attention condition. The second participant had comparably high levels across all conditions. The third participant had high levels only in the alone condition. Based on these data, the view was that the challenging behaviors did not have a social function and were probably maintained by automatic reinforcement. In line with this hypothesis, the intervention strategies carried out with the participants consisted of stimulation and sensory extinction. The two strategies were compared through 10-min sessions implemented alternatively. The stimulation condition consisted of providing the participants with preferred objects (e.g., a dumbbell massager or a plastic ring) that they could manipulate without incurring the challenging behaviors. The sensory extinction consisted of using devices (e.g., foam sleeves or latex gloves) that would mask the sensory effects of the challenging behaviors. The results were eventually positive with both intervention strategies. However, the effects of stimulation were apparently more rapid and accompanied by participants' object engagement.

Kuhn, DeLeon, Fisher, and Wilke (1999) reported the study of a 35-year-old man who had a diagnosis of autism, severe intellectual disability,

and obsessive–compulsive disorder and displayed severe face hitting and head banging. The functional analysis was carried out through 10-min sessions and included the four standard conditions. Given the severity of the challenging behaviors, the therapist tried to block their occurrence throughout the sessions. The behavior levels seemed to be highest in the alone and demand conditions, suggesting that automatic reinforcement, escape or both could be responsible for the outcome. To determine which hypothesis was more realistic, intervention strategies involving sensory extinction, escape extinction or both were arranged. The intervention effects were highly positive when the two forms of extinction together and when sensory extinction alone were used and largely unsatisfactory when escape extinction was applied. On this basis, it was concluded that the challenging behaviors were maintained by sensory reinforcement.

Piazza et al. (2000) conducted their investigations with three participants of 6–17 years of age who had a diagnosis of severe to profound intellectual disability and multiple challenging behaviors. Dangerous behavior (e.g., climbing on furniture), saliva play, and hand mouthing were exposed to functional analysis, which included the four standard conditions for one participant and a fifth (tangible) condition for the other two. Sessions were 10-min long and were carried out in a specially equipped context. The outcome of the analysis indicated that the dangerous behavior occurred at the highest level in the alone condition. The other two behaviors had high frequencies in all conditions, including the alone condition. Therefore, the hypothesis was that the behaviors were maintained by their sensory consequences (automatic reinforcement). On this basis, objects were selected that could produce sensory consequences similar to those related to the challenging behaviors, and the hope was that the participants could play with these objects and, thereby, produce sufficient sensory input to replace the need for the challenging behaviors. The intervention data comparing the effects of those objects with those of unmatched ones (i.e., producing stimulation unrelated to the challenging behaviors) supported the aforementioned anticipation.

All three participants had drastic reductions of their challenging behaviors when allowed to engage in activity with matched material.

Wilder et al. (2000) carried out a study with a 30-year-old woman who had a diagnosis of profound intellectual disability and visual impairment and presented with persistent bilateral head rocking. The functional analysis involving the four standard conditions, which were implemented over 10-min sessions, showed that the behavior was present at very high levels across all conditions. This outcome seemed to indicate that the behavior did not have any social function, but was rather maintained by automatic reinforcement. Intervention strategies based on this notion were subsequently examined to determine the reliability of the functional analysis conclusions. An assessment comparing the use of various forms of stimulation intervention through the sessions showed that a vibrating massage reduced the rocking behavior drastically, while illumination changes and increased noise inputs did not produce effects. A subsequent assessment involved the comparison of two environmental enrichment strategies, which included multiple stimuli, and varied from one another for the presence or absence of vibratory stimuli in the package. In line with the previous data, the package including vibratory stimuli was more effective in reducing head rocking.

Tang, Patterson, and Kennedy (2003) carried out functional analyses with six participants of 4–17 years of age who were diagnosed with profound intellectual or multiple disabilities and presented with one or two challenging behaviors such as hand mouthing and head shaking. The functional analyses involved the four standard conditions, which were applied over 5-min sessions. The results of the analyses indicated that the challenging behaviors were showing high levels of occurrence across all conditions or during the alone condition, therefore suggesting that automatic reinforcement was largely (or totally) responsible for their maintenance. In a related intervention assessment, masking (sensory-attenuation) strategies were implemented with five of the original participants. Auditory masking occurred through the use of safety plugs or headphones;

visual masking occurred through goggles or a dark screen; tactile masking occurred through gloves. Preliminary findings indicated some effects of one form of masking or another with three of the participants. In a subsequent effort to investigate masking and competing (substitutive) sensory stimulation, the authors reported encouraging results with at least two of the three participants involved. One of these two responded equally positively (with near zero levels of challenging behavior) to the masking and the competing stimulation and the other showing a very obvious reduction of the challenging behavior during the competing sensory stimulation.

Falcomata et al. (2004) examined an 18-year-old man who had a diagnosis of autism and presented with problem behaviors including inappropriate verbalizations. The first phase of the functional analysis involved five conditions, namely, the four standard ones plus a tangible condition. The second phase involved only the alone condition. Sessions lasted 10 min. Inappropriate verbalizations were consistently present during the alone, attention and demand conditions of the first assessment phase and remained very high during the second phase. The suggestion was therefore that they were maintained by automatic reinforcement. In a related treatment evaluation, two intervention strategies were compared. One included the use of noncontingent reinforcement, that is, the participant had continuous access to a radio and no consequences occurred for the inappropriate verbalizations. The other strategy differed from the previous one only in that the radio was removed for 5 s at the occurrence of inappropriate verbalizations. The first intervention strategy succeeded in reducing the inappropriate verbalizations to about 50% of the baseline level. The second intervention strategy reduced them to a virtually zero level.

Moore et al. (2004) conducted a study with a 12-year-old girl who had a diagnosis of autism and presented with a multitude of severe challenging behaviors, which included hand, head, shoulder, foot and leg. The study was organized into two different phases. The first phase was directed at assessing the occurrence or absence of the specific behaviors in relation to the presence or absence of protective equipment. The participant was alone within a padded room through all the assessment sessions. The results showed that the behaviors were at a virtually zero level when protective equipment was present on all relevant parts of the body. Shoulder-related behaviors occurred when this body part was freed from protective material. A similar outcome occurred with hand-related behaviors, but not with foot/leg-related behaviors. The second phase of the study was a functional analysis (with the four standard conditions) applied to the hand-related behaviors. The outcome of this phase showed that the occurrence of these behaviors increased drastically in each of the assessment conditions when the protective equipment was removed. On the basis of both sets of data, the authors' conclusion was that the participant's challenging behaviors were maintained by automatic reinforcement.

Wilder et al. (2009) conducted a study with a 37-year-old man who had a diagnosis of profound intellectual disability and autism and presented with rumination (i.e., regurgitation, chewing and re-swallowing of food previously ingested). The functional analysis involved the four standard conditions, which were presented by four different therapists wearing shirts of different colors. Each condition involved two sessions per day, one prior to the meal and one after the meal. Sessions were 10-min long. The participant showed no rumination during the sessions occurring prior to the meal. By contrast, he had high levels of rumination during all sessions carried out after the meal, irrespective of the conditions under which they occurred. In light of these findings, the suggestion was that the behavior did not have a social function, but was maintained by automatic reinforcement. Although the source of this reinforcement was not known, it was assumed that it would be related to oral stimulation. On this basis, an intervention strategy involving the use of preferred oral stimulation on a noncontingent schedule was implemented. The oral stimulation consisted of applying pie spray (i.e., a form of stimulation which was considered easy to use and advantageous on the long term because calorie-free). The rate of rumination during the baseline phases varied between 2.8 and 3.7 per min. During the

intervention phases, the rates decreased to around 1 per min. Eventually, the participant was able to maintain such a level by self-administering the spray at intervals of about 10 s.

Access to Idiosyncratic Events

DeLeon et al. (2003) reported the case of a 14-year-old boy who was diagnosed with profound intellectual disabilities, cerebral palsy, and visual impairment, and showed a multitude of challenging behaviors including aggression (e.g., hitting, pinching, and grabbing others). The functional analysis, which was carried out through 10-min sessions, included seven conditions. Three of them (i.e., attention, play, and alone) represented standard conditions. The other four (i.e., task demand, daily living activities, social demand, and contingent wheelchair movement) were arranged according to the participant's general characteristics/peculiarities. During task demand, the therapist required the performance of academic tasks but supplemented the requests with guidance/orientation toward the material and adapted prompting sequences. During daily living activities, the therapist performed hygiene activities for the boy and interrupted those activities for 30 s in concomitance with the challenging behaviors. During the social demand, the therapist provided continuous verbal and physical attention and interrupted it all for 30 s following challenging behaviors. Finally, during the contingent wheelchair movement, the therapist resumed wheelchair pushing for 30 s after each instance of challenging behavior. The findings showed that challenging behavior was highest within the last assessment condition. Based on these findings, the intervention included FCT (i.e., technology-assisted request of wheelchair movement), which allowed him 30 s of wheelchair pushing, and extinction for the challenging behavior. The boy increased his requests and reduced the challenging behavior to near zero levels.

Ringdahl et al. (2009) studied an 18-year-old woman who had a diagnosis of severe to profound intellectual disability and presented with challenging behaviors, which consisted of aggression and attempts to leave the room. The initial functional analysis included fairly standard conditions concerning attention, demand, and play. The outcome of this analysis showed that the challenging behaviors were largely distributed across all conditions and thus no conclusions could be drawn as to their possible social function. The subsequent functional analysis compared two conditions involving walking in the hallway. In one condition, the woman had continuous access to walking in the hallway with the therapist providing regular attention. In the other condition, the woman had continuous access to leisure items as well as attention from the therapist. Her access to walking (i.e., 30-s walking periods), however, was contingent on the occurrence of aggression. The woman showed aggression only in the latter condition. On the basis of this outcome, intervention strategies were successfully implemented, which involved FCT (to request walks), use of walks as reinforcement of simple activities, and use of walks on a noncontingent schedule.

Conclusion

Challenging behaviors are fairly common among persons with developmental disorders, autism, severe and profound intellectual disabilities, and multiple disabilities (Lancioni et al., 2009; Rehfeldt & Chambers, 2003; Stewart & Alderman, 2010). The fact that these behaviors have a negative impact on the person's developmental and adaptive opportunities calls for the application of appropriate intervention strategies (Singh et al., 2009; Tarbox et al., 2009). Intervention is more likely to succeed if it is matched to the function of the person's challenging behavior (Borrero & Borrero, 2008; Matson & Minshawi, 2007; Neidert et al., 2010). In this chapter, five groups of studies were reviewed to illustrate different outcomes of the functional analysis, that is, the identification of five different functions for challenging behaviors. The first group of studies identified attention (e.g., Fyffe et al., 2004; Roane & Kelley, 2008). The second group of studies identified access to tangible items (e.g., Hagopian et al., 2001; Reed et al., 2009).

The third group of studies identified demand escape (e.g., O'Reilly & Lancioni, 2000; Rooker & Roscoe, 2005). The fourth group of studies identified automatic reinforcement (e.g., Piazza et al., 2000; Wilder et al., 2009). The fifth group of studies identified idiosyncratic events (e.g., Ringdahl et al., 2009).

The intervention strategies developed on the basis of the results of the functional analyses were generally satisfactory thus providing support for the reliability of those results and the notion that the intervention should be planned in accordance with the function of the challenging behaviors. Three questions would seem to be open to additional research in this area. The first question pertains to the functional analysis' model, implementation procedures, and time requirements/costs. With regard to the model, suggestions were made about the occasional necessity of contemplating additional or alternative conditions compared to those available in the standard format, that is, the one provided by Iwata et al. (1982/1994) and followed by most of the studies in the field. With regard to the implementation procedures, evidence was presented about the possible relevance of (a) carrying out the assessment in the same contexts in which the person normally is and shows his or her challenging behavior and (b) involving in the assessment the personnel responsible of the daily programs. With regard to the assessment duration (time costs), the point was made that the length of many of the published analyses might be excessive (too costly) for several daily contexts. Indications also exist that shorter versions of those analyses might be sufficient to provide usable information (e.g., Northup et al., 1991; Perrin et al., 2008; Wallace & Knights, 2003).

The second question concerns the fact that intervention may need to reconcile the elimination of the challenging behavior with the establishment of adaptive skills, which are essential to foster development (Lancioni et al., 2009). For example, the effectiveness of a noncontingent strategy to reduce challenging behaviors maintained by access to attention or tangible items would need to be combined with efforts to develop useful skills, through which the participant can have new opportunities of engagement and stimulation (Kazdin, 2001; Lancioni et al., 2009).

The third question concerns the notion of idiosyncratic situations and functions. In essence, one could argue that idiosyncrasy concerned the forms of reinforcement that worked for the persons involved in the studies, which differed from the attention and tangible conditions/reinforcers generally proposed within standard functional analyses (e.g., DeLeon et al., 2003; Ringdahl et al., 2009). The evidence available suggests that one cannot design a functional analysis assessment independent of the participants' daily experience and possible reinforcement sources.

In conclusion, the vast literature on functional analysis of challenging behaviors has produced a large body of evidence on the possibility of identifying the functions of those behaviors and therefore of designing more respondent treatment programs. At present, there is wide agreement on the need of carrying out the functional analysis of challenging behaviors and of using the results of such analysis to design the intervention. There is also a clear understanding that future research would need to concentrate on and clarify several aspects of both the functional analysis and the subsequent intervention processes (e.g., Healey et al., 2001; Lang et al., 2010; Perrin et al., 2008; Wilder et al., 2009).

References

Asmus, J. M., Franzese, J. C., Conroy, M. A., & Dozier, C. L. (2003). Clarifying functional analysis outcomes for disruptive behaviors by controlling consequence delivery for stereotypy. *School Psychology Review, 32,* 624–630.

Borrero, C. S. W., & Borrero, J. C. (2008). Descriptive and experimental analyses of potential precursors to problem behavior. *Journal of Applied Behavior Analysis, 41,* 83–96.

Borrero, C. S. W., Vollmer, T. R., Borrero, J. C., & Bourret, J. (2005). A method for evaluating parameters of reinforcement during parent-child interactions. *Research in Developmental Disabilities, 26,* 577–592.

Britton, L. N., Carr, J. E., Kellum, K. K., Dozier, C. L., & Weil, T. M. (2000). A variation of noncontingent reinforcement in the treatment of aberrant behavior. *Research in Developmental Disabilities, 21,* 425–435.

Buchanan, J. A., & Fisher, J. E. (2002). Functional assessment and noncontingent reinforcement in the treatment

of disruptive vocalization in elderly dementia patients. *Journal of Applied Behavior Analysis, 35,* 99–103.

Butler, L. R., & Luiselli, J. K. (2007). Escape-maintained problem behavior in a child with autism. *Journal of Positive Behavior Interventions, 9,* 195–202.

Carr, J. E., Dozier, C. L., Patel, M. R., Adams, A. N., & Martin, N. (2002). Treatment of automatically reinforced object mouthing with noncontingent reinforcement and response blocking: Experimental analysis and social validation. *Research in Developmental Disabilities, 23,* 37–44.

Carter, S. L., Devlin, S., Doggett, R. A., Harber, M. M., & Barr, C. (2004). Determining the influence of tangible items on screaming and handmouthing following an inconclusive functional analysis. *Behavioral Interventions, 19,* 51–58.

DeLeon, I. G., Kahng, S. W., Rodriguez-Catter, V., Sveinsdóttir, I., & Sadler, C. (2003). Assessment of aberrant behavior maintained by wheelchair movement in a child with developmental disabilities. *Research in Developmental Disabilities, 24,* 381–390.

Durand, V. M., & Crimmins, D. B. (1988). Identifying the variables maintaining self-injurious behavior. *Journal of Autism and Developmental Disorders, 18,* 99–117.

Dwyer-Moore, K. J., & Dixon, M. R. (2007). Functional analysis and treatment of problem behavior of elderly adults in long-term care. *Journal of Applied Behavior Analysis, 40,* 679–683.

Emerson, E. (1995). *Challenging behaviour: Analysis and intervention with people with learning difficulties.* Cambridge: Cambridge University Press.

Falcomata, T. S., Roane, H. S., Hovanetz, A. N., Kettering, T. L., & Keeney, K. M. (2004). An evaluation of response cost in the treatment of inappropriate vocalizations maintained by automatic reinforcement. *Journal of Applied Behavior Analysis, 37,* 83–87.

Fyffe, C. E., Kahng, S. W., Fittro, E., & Russell, D. (2004). Functional analysis and treatment of inappropriate sexual behavior. *Journal of Applied Behavior Analysis, 37,* 401–404.

Hagopian, L. P., & Toole, L. M. (2009). Effects of response blocking and competing stimuli on stereotypic behavior. *Behavioral Interventions, 24,* 117–125.

Hagopian, L. P., Wilson, D. M., & Wilder, D. A. (2001). Assessment and treatment of problem behavior maintained by escape from attention and access to tangible items. *Journal of Applied Behavior Analysis, 34,* 229–232.

Hanley, G. P., Iwata, B. A., & McCord, B. E. (2003). Functional analysis of problem behavior: A review. *Journal of Applied Behavior Analysis, 36,* 147–185.

Hanley, G. P., Piazza, C. C., Fisher, W. W., & Maglieri, K. A. (2005). On the effectiveness of and preference for punishment and extinction components of function-based interventions. *Journal of Applied Behavior Analysis, 38,* 51–65.

Harvey, M. T., Luiselli, J. K., & Wong, S. E. (2009). Application of applied behavior analysis to mental health issues. *Psychological Services, 6,* 212–222.

Hausman, N., Kahng, S. W., Farrell, E., & Mongeon, C. (2009). Idiosyncratic functions: Severe problem behavior maintained by access to ritualistic behaviors. *Education and Treatment of Children, 32*, 77–87.

Healey, J. J., Ahearn, W. H., Graff, R. B., & Libby, M. E. (2001). Extended analysis and treatment of self-injurious behavior. *Behavioral Interventions, 16*, 181–195.

Ingvarsson, E. T., Kahng, S. W., & Hausman, N. L. (2008). Some effects of noncontingent positive reinforcement on multiply controlled problem behavior and compliance in a demand context. *Journal of Applied Behavior Analysis, 41*, 435–440.

Iwata, B. A., & DeLeon, I. G. (1996). *Functional analysis screening tool (FAST)*. Gainesville: The Florida Center on Self-Injury, University of Florida.

Iwata, B. A., Dorsey, M. F., Slifer, K. J., Bauman, K. E., & Richman, G. S. (1994). Toward a functional analysis of self-injury. *Journal of Applied Behavior Analysis, 27*, 197–209 (Reprinted from *Analysis and Intervention in Developmental Disabilities, 2*, 3–20, 1982).

Kahng, S. W., & Iwata, B. A. (1999). Correspondence between outcomes of brief and extended functional analyses. *Journal of Applied Behavior Analysis, 32*, 149–159.

Kazdin, A. E. (2001). *Behavior modification in applied settings* (6th ed.). Belmont: Wadsworth.

Kates-McElrath, K., Agnew, M., Axelrod, S., & Bloh, C. L. (2007). Identification of behavioral function in public schools and clarification of terms. *Behavioral Interventions, 22*, 47–56.

Kenzer, A. L., & Wallace, M. D. (2007). Treatment of rumination maintained by automatic reinforcement: A comparison of extra portions during a meal and supplemental post-meal feedings. *Behavioral Interventions, 22*, 297–304.

Kuhn, D. E., DeLeon, I. G., Fisher, W. W., & Wilke, A. E. (1999). Clarifying an ambiguous functional analysis with matched and mismatched extinction procedures. *Journal of Applied Behavior Analysis, 32*, 99–102.

Kuhn, D. E., Hardesty, S. L., & Sweeney, N. M. (2009). Assessment and treatment of excessive straightening and destructive behavior in an adolescent diagnosed with autism. *Journal of Applied Behavior Analysis, 42*, 355–360.

Kurtz, P. F., Chin, M. D., Huete, J. M., Tarbox, R. S. F., O'Connor, J. T., Paclawskyj, T. R., et al. (2003). Functional analysis and treatment of self-injurious behavior in young children: A summary of 30 cases. *Journal of Applied Behavior Analysis, 36*, 205–219.

Kurtz, P. F., Chin, M. D., Rush, K. S., & Dixon, D. R. (2008). Treatment of challenging behavior exhibited by children with prenatal drug exposure. *Research in Developmental Disabilities, 29*, 582–594.

LaBelle, C. A., & Charlop-Christy, M. H. (2002). Individualizing functional analysis to assess multiple and changing functions of severe behavior problems in children with autism. *Journal of Positive Behavior Interventions, 4*, 231–241.

Lancaster, B. M., LeBlanc, L. A., Carr, J. E., Brenske, S., Peet, M. M., & Culver, S. J. (2004). Functional analysis and treatment of the bizarre speech of dually diagnosed adults. *Journal of Applied Behavior Analysis, 37*, 395–399.

Lancioni, G. E., Singh, N. N., O'Reilly, M. F., & Sigafoos, J. (2009). An overview of behavioral strategies for reducing hand-related stereotypies of persons with severe to profound intellectual and multiple disabilities: 1995-2007. *Research in Developmental Disabilities, 30*, 20–43.

Lancioni, G. E., Walraven, M., O'Reilly, M. F., & Singh, N. N. (2002). Persistent humming by a man with multiple disabilities: Evaluating function and treatment opportunities. *European Journal of Behavior Analysis, 3*, 75–80.

Lang, R., Davis, T., O'Reilly, M., Machalicek, W., Rispoli, M., Sigafoos, J., et al. (2010). Functional analysis and treatment of elopement across two school settings. *Journal of Applied Behavior Analysis, 43*, 113–118.

Lang, R., O'Reilly, M., Lancioni, G., Rispoli, M., Machalicek, W., Chan, J. M., et al. (2009). Discrepancy in functional analysis results across two applied settings: Implications for intervention design. *Journal of Applied Behavior Analysis, 42*, 393–398.

Lang, R., O'Reilly, M., Machalicek, W., Lancioni, G., Rispoli, M., & Chan, J. M. (2008). A preliminary comparison of functional analysis results when conducted in contrived versus natural settings. *Journal of Applied Behavior Analysis, 41*, 441–445.

Lindauer, S. E., Zarcone, J. R., Richman, D. M., & Schroeder, S. R. (2002). A comparison of multiple reinforcer assessments to identify the function of maladaptive behavior. *Journal of Applied Behavior Analysis, 35*, 299–303.

Lyons, E. A., Rue, H. C., Luiselli, J. K., & DiGennaro, F. D. (2007). Brief functional analysis and supplemental feeding for postmeal rumination in children with developmental disabilities. *Journal of Applied Behavior Analysis, 40*, 743–747.

Matson, J. L., Bamburg, J. W., Cherry, K. E., & Paclawskyj, T. R. (1999). A validity study on the Questions About Behavior Function (QABF) scale: Predicting treatment success for self-injury, aggression, and stereotypies. *Research in Developmental Disabilities, 20*, 163–175.

Matson, J. L., & LoVullo, S. V. (2008). A review of behavioral treatments for self-injurious behaviors of persons with autism spectrum disorders. *Behavior Modification, 32*, 61–76.

Matson, J. L., Mayville, S. B., Kuhn, D. E., Sturmey, P., Laud, R., & Cooper, C. (2005). The behavioral function of feeding problems as assessed by the questions about behavioral function (QABF). *Research in Developmental Disabilities, 26*, 399–408.

Matson, J. L., & Minshawi, N. F. (2007). Functional assessment of challenging behavior: Toward a strategy for applied settings. *Research in Developmental Disabilities, 28*, 353–361.

Matson, J. L., & Wilkins, J. (2009). Factors associated with the questions about behavior function for functional assessment of low and high rate challenging behaviors in adults with intellectual disability. *Behavior Modification, 33,* 207–219.

McAdam, D. B., DiCesare, A., Murphy, S., & Marshall, B. (2004). The influence of different therapists on functional analysis outcomes. *Behavioral Interventions, 19,* 39–44.

McLaughlin, T. F., Derby, K. M., Gwinn, M., Taitch, H., Bolich, B., Weber, K., et al. (2003). The effects of active and violent play activities on brief functional analysis outcomes. *Journal of Developmental and Physical Disabilities, 15,* 93–99.

Moore, J. W., Fisher, W. W., & Pennington, A. (2004). Systematic application and removal of protective equipment in the assessment of multiple topographies of self-injury. *Journal of Applied Behavior Analysis, 37,* 73–77.

Najdowski, A. C., Wallace, M. D., Ellsworth, C. L., MacAleese, A. N., & Cleveland, J. M. (2008). Functional analyses and treatment of precursor behavior. *Journal of Applied Behavior Analysis, 41,* 97–105.

Neidert, P. L., Dozier, C. L., Iwata, B. A., & Hafen, M. (2010). Behavior analysis in intellectual and developmental disabilities. *Psychological Services, 7,* 103–113.

Noell, G. H., & Gansle, K. A. (2009). Introduction to functional assessment. In A. Akin-Little, S. G. Little, M. A. Bray, & T. J. Kehle (Eds.), *Behavioral interventions in schools: Evidence-based positive strategies* (pp. 43–58). Washington, DC: American Psychological Association.

Northup, J., Wacker, D., Sasso, G., Steege, M., Cigrand, K., Cook, J., et al. (1991). A brief functional analysis of aggressive and alternative behavior in an outclinic setting. *Journal of Applied Behavior Analysis, 24,* 509–522.

O'Reilly, M. F., & Lancioni, G. (2000). Response covariation of escape-maintained aberrant behavior correlated with sleep deprivation. *Research in Developmental Disabilities, 21,* 125–136.

Paclawskyj, T. R., Matson, J. L., Rush, K. S., Smalls, Y., & Vollmer, T. R. (2000). Questions about behavioral functions (QABF): A behavioral checklist for functional assessment of aberrant behavior. *Research in Developmental Disabilities, 21,* 223–229.

Pence, S. T., Roscoe, E. M., Bourret, J. C., & Ahearn, W. H. (2009). Relative contributions of three descriptive methods: Implications for behavioral assessment. *Journal of Applied Behavior Analysis, 42,* 425–446.

Perrin, C. J., Perrin, S. H., Hill, E. A., & DiNovi, K. (2008). Brief functional analysis and treatment of elopement in preschoolers with autism. *Behavioral Interventions, 23,* 87–95.

Peyton, R. T., Lindauer, S. E., & Richman, D. M. (2005). The effects of directive and nondirective prompts on noncompliant vocal behavior exhibited by a child with autism. *Journal of Applied Behavior Analysis, 38,* 251–255.

Piazza, C. C., Adelinis, J. D., Hanley, G. P., Goh, H. L., & Delia, M. D. (2000). An evaluation of the effects of matched stimuli on behaviors maintained by automatic reinforcement. *Journal of Applied Behavior Analysis, 33,* 13–27.

Reed, D. D., Pace, G. M., & Luiselli, J. K. (2009). An investigation into the provision of choice in tangible conditions of a functional analysis. *Journal of Developmental and Physical Disabilities, 21,* 485–491.

Rehfeldt, R. A., & Chambers, M. R. (2003). Functional analysis and treatment of verbal perseverations displayed by an adult with autism. *Journal of Applied Behavior Analysis, 36,* 259–261.

Richman, D. M., Wacker, D. P., Asmus, J. M., & Casey, S. D. (1998). Functional analysis and extinction of different behavior problems exhibited by the same individual. *Journal of Applied Behavior Analysis, 31,* 475–478.

Ringdahl, J. E., Christensen, T. J., & Boelter, E. W. (2009). Further evaluation of idiosyncratic functions for severe problem behavior: Aggression maintained by access to walks. *Behavioral Interventions, 24,* 275–283.

Roane, H. S., & Kelley, M. E. (2008). Decreasing problem behavior associated with a walking program for an individual with developmental and physical disabilities. *Journal of Applied Behavior Analysis, 41,* 423–428.

Rooker, G. W., & Roscoe, E. M. (2005). Functional analysis of self-injurious behavior and its relation to self-restraint. *Journal of Applied Behavior Analysis, 38,* 537–542.

Roscoe, E. M., Iwata, B. A., & Goh, H. L. (1998). A comparison of noncontingent reinforcement and sensory extinction as treatments for self-injurious behavior. *Journal of Applied Behavior Analysis, 31,* 635–646.

Singh, A. N., Matson, J. L., Mouttapa, M., Pella, R. D., Hill, B. D., & Thorson, R. (2009). A critical item analysis of the QABF: Development of a short form assessment instrument. *Research in Developmental Disabilities, 30,* 782–792.

Stewart, I., & Alderman, N. (2010). Active versus passive management of post-acquired brain injury challenging behaviour: A case study analysis of multiple operant procedures in the treatment of challenging behaviour maintained by negative reinforcement. *Brain Injury, 24,* 1616–1627.

Stokes, J. V., & Luiselli, J. K. (2009). Applied behavior analysis assessment and intervention for health: Threatening self-injury (rectal picking) in an adult with Prader-Willi syndrome. *Clinical Case Studies, 8,* 38–47.

Tang, J.-C., Patterson, T. G., & Kennedy, C. H. (2003). Identifying specific sensory modalities maintaining the stereotypy of students with multiple profound disabilities. *Research in Developmental Disabilities, 24,* 433–451.

Tarbox, R. S. F., Wallace, M. D., & Williams, L. (2003). Assessment and treatment of elopement: A replication and extension. *Journal of Applied Behavior Analysis, 36,* 239–244.

Tarbox, J., Wilke, A. E., Najdowski, A. C., Findel-Pyles, R. S., Balasanyan, S., Caveney, A. C., et al. (2009). Comparing indirect, descriptive, and experimental functional assessments of challenging behavior in

64

children with autism. *Journal of Developmental and Physical Disabilities, 21*, 493–514.

Tiger, J. H., Fisher, W. W., Toussaint, K. A., & Kodak, T. (2009). Progressing from initially ambiguous functional analyses: Three case examples. *Research in Developmental Disabilities, 30*, 910–926.

Touchette, P. E., MacDonald, R. F., & Langer, S. N. (1985). A scatter plot for identifying stimulus control of problem behavior. *Journal of Applied Behavior Analysis, 18*, 343–351.

Vollmer, T. R. (1994). The concept of automatic reinforcement: Implications for behavioral research in developmental disabilities. *Research in Developmental Disabilities, 15*, 187–207.

Wallace, M. D., & Knights, D. J. (2003). An evaluation of a brief functional analysis format within a vocational setting. *Journal of Applied Behavior Analysis, 36*, 125–128.

Watson, T. S., & Watson, T. S. (2009). Behavioral assessment in the schools. In A. Akin-Little, S. G. Little, M. A. Bray, & T. J. Kehle (Eds.), *Behavioral interventions in schools: Evidence-based positive strategies* (pp. 27–41). Washington, DC: American Psychological Association.

White, P., O'Reilly, M., Fragale, C., Kang, S., Muhich, K., & Falcomata, T. (2011). An extended functional analysis protocol assesses the role of stereotypy in aggression in two young children with autism spectrum disorder. *Research in Autism Spectrum Disorders, 5*, 784–789.

Wilder, D. A., Kellum, K. K., & Carr, J. E. (2000). Evaluation of satiation-resistant head rocking. *Behavioral Interventions, 15*, 71–78.

Wilder, D. A., Normand, M., & Atwell, J. (2005). Noncontingent reinforcement as treatment for food refusal and associated self-injury. *Journal of Applied Behavior Analysis, 38*, 549–553.

Wilder, D. A., Register, M., Register, S., Bajagic, V., & Neidert, P. L. (2009). Functional analysis and treatment of rumination using fixed-time delivery of a flavor spray. *Journal of Applied Behavior Analysis, 42*, 877–882.

Wood, B. K., Blair, K.-S. C., & Ferro, J. B. (2009). Young children with challenging behavior: Function-based assessment and intervention. *Topics in Early Childhood Special Education, 29*, 68–78.

Populations and Problems Evaluated with Functional Assessment

5

John M. Huete, Patricia F. Kurtz, and R. Justin Boyd

B.F. Skinner (1953) first emphasized that a scientific analysis of behavior requires an understanding of the cause–effect relationship between behavior and the environmental conditions that are associated with its occurrence. Skinner termed the understanding of this cause–effect relationship "a functional analysis of behavior." As methods for examining these relationships have expanded, the analyses of behavioral contingencies have come to be known more generally as functional assessment. The terms functional assessment and functional analysis are frequently used interchangeably; however, it is useful to distinguish between these two terms, as they often connote different meanings. Functional assessment typically is conceptualized as a broad category of procedures used to assess the function of behavior. These include indirect methods and direct methods (Miltenberger, 1999). Indirect methods assess the function of behavior without requiring any direct observation or experimental manipulation of the behavior, such as structured interviews (O'Neill, Horner, Sprague, Storey, & Newton, 1997) and questionnaires/checklists (Paclawskyj, Matson, Rush, Smalls, & Vollmer,

2000; Singh, Donatelli, Best, & Williams, 1993). Direct methods of functional assessment are procedures that utilize direct observation or experimental manipulation for assessing the function of behavior (Miltenberger, 1999). Included in direct observational methods are assessment techniques that result in correlational outcomes, such as gathering Antecedent–Behavior–Consequence (A–B–C) data (Bijou, Peterson, & Ault, 1968) and structured descriptive assessments (Anderson & Long, 2002), but also include experimental methods that result in the demonstration of cause–effect relationships (Iwata, Dorsey, Slifer, Bauman, & Richman, 1982/1994). The term functional analysis often is used to refer to more direct and experimental assessment procedures. The selection of procedures often is dependent on a number of factors, including the individual being assessed, the behavior of interest, resources available for assessment, context of the assessment, and the cost–benefit analysis of conducting the assessment (Johnston & O'Neill, 2001; Scott, Anderson, Mancil, & Alter, 2009). Vollmer, Marcus, Ringdahl, and Roane (1995) have provided practical guidance on making decisions about and progressing through functional assessment procedures, suggesting that practitioners begin with more brief assessment procedures and proceed to more time-consuming, costly extended assessments as needed.

Importantly, functional assessment should be understood not as a specific tool, but rather as a broad approach to understanding the relationship

J.M. Huete (✉) • P.F. Kurtz • R.J. Boyd
Department of Behavioral Psychology, Kennedy Krieger Institute and The Johns Hopkins University School of Medicine, 707 N. Broadway, Baltimore, MD 21205, USA
e-mail: Huete@kennedykrieger.org;
Kurtz@kennedykrieger.org; boydj@kennedykrieger.org

J.L. Matson (ed.), *Functional Assessment for Challenging Behaviors*,
Autism and Child Psychopathology Series, DOI 10.1007/978-1-4614-3037-7_5,
© Springer Science+Business Media, LLC 2012

of behavior to the factors associated with its occurrence. As such, the numerous functional assessment procedures that have been developed, ranging from caregiver interviews (O'Neill et al., 1997) to direct experimental testing of functional hypotheses (Iwata et al., 1982/1994), are a testament to the flexibility and applicability of the approach to understanding a growing list of behaviors. Therefore, no specific procedure has ownership over the term functional assessment nor is necessarily a better approach to understanding the function of behavior. Optimally, information from a variety of functional assessment procedures (e.g., interview, questionnaires, and direct observation) is combined to best understand the function of behavior (Vollmer et al., 1995).

While Skinner's initial emphasis was to understand all behaviors of the organism in terms of a functional analysis, specific technologies of functional assessment have evolved and grown mostly in an attempt to understand problem and challenging behaviors. Indeed, the flexibility of functional assessment procedures has spurred its application to the assessment and understanding of a variety of problems, including the treatment of substance use disorders (Budney & Higgins, 1998; Tuten, Jones, Ertel, Jakubowski, & Sperlein, 2006), depression (Dougher & Hackbert, 1994; Martell, 2008), and anxiety disorders (Kearney, Cook, Wechsler, Haight, & Stowman, 2008; Virues-Ortega & Haynes, 2005). The hallmark of functional assessment, and what has separated it from other assessment approaches, is its ability to lead to more effective interventions for behavior as a result of identifying the function of the behavior more precisely (Carr et al., 1999; Didden, Duker, & Korzilius, 1997; Scotti, Evans, Meyer, & Walker, 1991).

Even though functional assessment has demonstrated broad applications to a variety of problems, its history is most associated with challenging behaviors of individuals with intellectual and developmental disabilities (IDD). From its beginnings as a conceptual framework to understand the function of self-injurious behavior (Carr, 1977), functional assessment has become the benchmark approach to assessment of challenging behavior for persons with IDD. Initially,

functional assessment procedures were confined to research study or specialized settings, such as hospitals or residential homes. However, over the past 25 years, interest in and use of functional assessment has grown exponentially (Hanley, Iwata, & McCord, 2003). As a result, numerous functional assessment procedures have been utilized with a variety of challenging behaviors demonstrated by individuals with IDD and Autism Spectrum Disorders (ASD). The purpose of this chapter is to succinctly describe the range of challenging behaviors and populations for whom functional assessment has been used. The primary focus will be on the application of functional assessment to individuals diagnosed with ASD and IDD. The first part of this chapter briefly will review the variety of populations diagnosed with ASD or IDD with whom functional assessments have been used. Then, research on the use of functional assessment with common challenging behaviors most associated with individuals diagnosed with ASD and IDD will be reviewed.

Populations Evaluated with Functional Assessment

The specific populations of persons diagnosed with ASD and IDD for whom functional assessment has been used are numerous and varied, and the groups themselves are not necessarily mutually exclusive of one another (Sturmey, 1996). A comprehensive review of each IDD population evaluated with functional assessment is beyond the scope of this chapter. Therefore, the populations discussed will be delineated based primarily on the most common developmental diagnostic categories for which functional assessments have been used.

At first glance, it may appear that functional assessment procedures are utilized almost exclusively with individuals diagnosed with intellectual disability or mental retardation. This group certainly is well represented in the functional assessment literature likely because they are at higher risk for exhibiting more severe challenging behaviors (Matson & Rivet, 2008; McClintock, Hall, & Oliver, 2003). Previous epidemiological studies have supported that increased severity of intellectual disability, such as a diagnosis of severe and profound mental retardation, is correlated with a higher incidence of certain severe challenging behaviors (Berkson, 1983; McClintock et al., 2003). However, not all individuals diagnosed with ASD have a diagnosis of intellectual disability (Edelson, 2006; Hurley & Levitas, 2007; Matson & Rivet, 2008). Furthermore, functional assessments are commonly used to assess challenging behaviors of individuals with mild to moderate intellectual disabilities (Crockett & Hagopian, 2006; Hanley et al., 2003), as well as typically developing individuals, such as children diagnosed with Attention-Deficit/Hyperactivity Disorder (Northup & Gulley, 2001; Stahr, Cushing, Lane, & Fox, 2006) or Emotional or Behavioral Disorders (EBD: Nahgahgwon, Umbreit, Liaupsin, & Turton, 2010; Rasmussen & O'Neill, 2006; Restori, Gresham, Chang, Lee, & Laija-Rodriquez, 2007).

In terms of specific developmental diagnoses, Pervasive Developmental Disorder (PDD) represents one of the larger diagnostic groupings of individuals for whom functional assessments are conducted. This is due largely to the various challenging behaviors which are observed in many individuals diagnosed with PDD (Weiss, Fiske, & Ferraioli, 2009). PDD, however, is a broad diagnostic category and includes specific diagnoses of Autistic Disorder, Rett's Disorder, Childhood Disintegrative Disorder, Asperger's Disorder, and PDD Not Otherwise Specified (American Psychiatric Association, 2000). Much of the functional assessment literature has been devoted to the challenging behaviors of individuals with autism that interfere with adaptive and daily living skills (LaBelle & Charlop-Christy, 2002; Tarbox et al., 2009; Weiss et al., 2009). Specifically, severe challenging behaviors often are the primary targets of these assessments (O'Reilly et al., 2010). Many challenging behaviors of individuals diagnosed with autism, such as inappropriate vocalizations, stereotyped movements, and self-injury, are thought to be maintained by automatic reinforcement. Functional assessments of these behaviors often support this conclusion (O'Reilly et al., 2010). It would be

erroneous, though, to conclude that all challenging behaviors of autistic individuals are nonsocially maintained or the result of automatic reinforcement. Functional assessment procedures have been integral in demonstrating social operant functions for challenging behaviors of autistic individuals often dismissed as nonsocial behaviors (Franco et al., 2009; Hausman, Kahng, Farrell, & Mongeon, 2009; Kuhn, Hardesty, & Sweeney, 2009). For example, Franco et al. (2009) identified escape and access to tangible functions for vocal stereotypy of a 7-year-old boy diagnosed with autism. Recent studies have further demonstrated social operant functions for challenging behaviors that are associated with nonsocial behaviors, such as self-injurious behavior or aggression functioning to allow access to ritualistic behaviors (Hausman et al., 2009; Murphy, Macdonald, Hall, & Oliver, 2000). These studies highlight the important contributions that functional assessment has made to the understanding of behavior in autism.

While there are several reported examples of functional assessment with persons diagnosed with autism, there are considerably fewer with other PDDs. Only a handful of published reports exist where functional assessment procedures are used to evaluate challenging behaviors of individuals diagnosed with Asperger's Disorder (Clarke, Dunlap, & Vaughn, 1999; Tarbox, Wallace, & William, 2003; Arvans & LeBlanc, 2009; Lang, Didden et al., 2009; Lang, Didden et al., 2010), Rett's Disorder (Oliver, Murphy, Crayton, & Corbett, 1993), and Childhood Disintegrative Disorder (Carter & Wheeler, 2007). It may be that there are fewer reports of functional assessments with these disorders due to their smaller prevalence compared to autism. However, to the extent that individuals diagnosed with PDDs share similar challenging behaviors (e.g., stereotypies, self-injurious behaviors, aggression, elopement), there is a robust literature supporting the efficacy of functional assessment of these challenging behaviors.

Down's Syndrome is the most common chromosomal disorder associated with intellectual disability (Deitz & Repp, 1989). While challenging behaviors are not a necessary characteristic of

Down's Syndrome, recent evidence suggests a behavioral phenotype associated with avoidance behavior that increases the likelihood of challenging behaviors (Feeley & Jones, 2006; Patti & Tsiouris, 2006). Several studies have documented the utility of functional assessments for individuals with Down's Syndrome, addressing such challenging behaviors as self-injurious behavior (O'Reilly, Murray, Lancioni, Sigafoos, & Lacey, 2003), aggression (McComas, Thompson, & Johnson, 2003), and vocal stereotypy (Athens, Vollmer, Sloman, & Pipkin, 2008). In one unique application of functional assessment, Millichap et al. (2003) utilized descriptive assessments to demonstrate that certain behavioral excesses exhibited by elderly persons diagnosed with Down's Syndrome and dementia were functionally associated with environmental events, rather than randomly occurring. Using A–B–C data collection techniques, the authors examined the relationship of certain behavioral excesses (e.g., crying, shouting, stereotypies, inappropriate vocalizations, self-injury) to environmental events for four adults ages 42 to 56 years living in group or nursing homes. The behavioral excesses observed of these participants were significantly correlated with increases in social contact from peers and staff.

In addition to PDDs and Down's syndrome, there are several genetic disorders that are associated with challenging behaviors for which functional assessment has proved useful. Some of the most notable disorders include Fragile X, Cornelia de Lange, Lesch–Nyhan, Prader–Willi, Smith–Magenis, and Angelman syndromes. Although as a whole these genetic disorders are relatively rare, it is surprising that few published reports exist regarding the use of functional assessments for these populations. This is unfortunate given the relationship of these genetic disorders to challenging behaviors. As previously stated, it may be falsely assumed that challenging behaviors in these populations are inherently associated with the syndrome. However, several functional assessment studies have demonstrated that many of these challenging behaviors are sensitive to and vary as a function of environmental changes. For example, Hall, DeBernardis, and

Reiss (2006) used experimental functional analyses to demonstrate social escape as a function for several challenging behaviors of 114 children diagnosed with Fragile X. Likewise, several studies have examined operant mechanisms for challenging behaviors using functional analysis technology in persons diagnosed with Cornelia de Lange syndrome (Kern, Mauk, Marder, & Mace, 1995; Moss et al., 2005; Oliver et al., 2006). Oliver et al. (2006) conducted experimental functional analyses with 18 children ages 1 to 16 years diagnosed with Cornelia de Lange, where the influence of varying adult interaction on subject social avoidance and self-injury was evaluated. For six participants, level of adult attention was associated with social initiation and termination behaviors, while for three others, self-injury was associated with adult attention. Collectively, these studies have demonstrated that challenging behaviors thought to be part of the syndrome's behavioral phenotype, including self-injurious behavior, were sensitive to social contingencies particularly attention from others.

Lesch–Nyhan syndrome is a genetic disorder of purine metabolism in which severe self-injurious self-biting is a hallmark characteristic (Nyhan, 2002). Research using functional assessment has demonstrated social attention functions for self-injurious behaviors in individuals diagnosed with Lesch–Nyhan syndrome (Bergen, Holbern, & Scott-Huyghebaert, 2002; Hall, Oliver, & Murphy, 2001). These findings have been further supported with evidence that interventions using manipulations of social attention, such as extinction and differential attention, have decreased the occurrence of self-injury in individuals diagnosed with Lesch–Nyhan syndrome (Olson & Houlihan, 2000).

Prader–Willi syndrome (PWS) is a congenital disorder in which obsession with food is one key behavioral characteristic, as well as several other challenging behaviors, including skin picking and temper tantrums (Dykens, Cassidy, & DeVries, 2011). Research examining skin picking in PWS using functional assessments has shown that the behavior is associated with self-stimulation (Didden, Korzilius, Curfs, 2007; Lang et al., 2010; Radstaake et al., 2011; Slifer, Iwata, &

Dorsey, 1984), arousal reduction (Radstaake et al., 2011), as well as attention from others and escape from work (Stokes & Luiselli, 2009). Woodcock, Oliver, and Humphreys (2009) used interviews and questionnaires to assess the function of temper tantrums in persons diagnosed with PWS. Temper tantrums were more likely to occur following a change in routine.

Finally, functional assessments have been used to evaluate self-injurious and aggressive behaviors of individuals diagnosed with Smith–Magenis syndrome (SMS) and Angelman syndrome (Bass & Speak, 2005; Strachan et al., 2009; Taylor & Oliver, 2008). In each of these studies, functional assessments identified social operants for the challenging behaviors, including attention from others and escape from demands.

In summary, functional assessment is applicable to a broad range of individuals diagnosed with ASD and IDD. The key feature of functional assessment is that the results more directly suggest intervention for specific target challenging behaviors (Carr et al., 1999; Didden et al., 1997; Scotti et al., 1991). One important and prominent theme from the functional assessment literature with ASD and IDD populations is that social operant functions have been demonstrated for certain challenging behaviors, when perhaps previously they were dismissed as nonsocial or nonfunctional. As a result of identifying social functions for these challenging behaviors, more acceptable, reinforcement-based interventions, rather than punishment-based interventions, tend to be selected (Pelios, Morren, Tesch, & Axelrod, 1999).

Challenging Behaviors Evaluated with Functional Assessment

Self-Injurious Behavior

Perhaps no other challenging behavior was more responsible for ushering in the use of functional assessment than self-injurious behavior (SIB). SIB is defined as any behavior directed towards self that results in tissue damage or injury to the person (Tate & Baroff, 1966). SIB is observed in non-IDD populations, usually individuals with severe psychiatric disorder, such as Borderline Personality Disorder (Andover & Gibb, 2010; Kerr & Muehlenkamp, 2010). However, SIB is most notable as a challenging behavior for persons with IDD, where prevalence recently has been estimated at 4.9% in adults (Cooper et al., 2009), but likely is higher for individuals diagnosed with ASD (Oliver & Richards, 2010). Baghdadli, Pascal, Grisi, and Aussiloux (2003) found a SIB prevalence rate of 53% in a sample of 222 children under the age of 7 years diagnosed with autism.

SIB often is discussed as a class of behaviors, which may falsely suggest homogeneity of these behaviors. The topographies of SIB in individuals with IDD, and ultimately their behavioral functions, actually are varied and include head banging, head hitting, body hitting, self-scratching, self-biting, eye poking, and hair pulling. These individual topography categories can be delineated even further by identifying specific behaviors within a category. For example, head hitting can be defined as face slapping with an open hand, head punching with a closed fist, or head hitting with an object.

The personal and societal costs of SIB in individuals with IDD prompted researchers in the 1960s and 1970s to develop better interventions and treatments (Carr, 1977). An outgrowth of this push was an emphasis on identifying the function of SIB, which would suggest and lead to better interventions. Carr (1977) initially summarized several functional hypotheses for SIB, noting that more effective interventions were needed and dependent on understanding the motivational aspects of SIB. These hypotheses included SIB as a learned operant, maintained by positive social reinforcement or negative reinforcement; a means of providing sensory stimulation; or the product of aberrant physiological processes (Carr, 1977).

Drawing from these hypotheses, Iwata and colleagues (1982/1994) described the first experimental procedure for evaluating the operant functions of self-injury, demonstrating that for six of the nine participants, SIB was associated with a specific stimulus condition. The initial formulation of functional assessment for SIB

(Iwata et al., 1982/1994) consisted of using analog conditions to experimentally evaluate the effects of contingent delivery of attention, escape from academic demands, and being alone on the occurrence of SIB. These conditions separately tested if SIB was functionally related to social positive reinforcement, social negative reinforcement, or automatic reinforcement, respectively. Specifically, rates of SIB which were consistently elevated when compared to the other conditions in the assessment were considered to be demonstrations of a causal, functional relationship between SIB and that consequence. For example, if SIB occurred at higher rates in the social disapproval, or attention, condition, then a conclusion of the functional analysis would be that SIB was associated with periods of low attention and reinforced by attention from others as a consequence.

Functional assessment has broadened the understanding of SIB by demonstrating that many forms of the behavior were maintained entirely, or in part, by social consequences. To illustrate this, Iwata, Pace, Dorsey, and Zarcone (1994) conducted experimental functional analyses with 152 subjects exhibiting SIB in order to understand the epidemiology of SIB functions. Results showed that SIB was maintained by social positive reinforcement for 26.3% of cases, social negative reinforcement for 38.1% of cases, automatic reinforcement for 25.7% of cases, and multiple factors (e.g., social positive and social negative reinforcement) for 5.3% of cases; results were undifferentiated for the remaining 4.6% of cases. While the Iwata et al. (1994) sample was heterogeneous with respect to age and diagnoses, additional similar epidemiological evaluations provide valuable information about the distribution of SIB functions for specific populations (Didden et al., 2007; Kurtz et al., 2003). For example, Kurtz et al. (2003) reviewed functional analysis results for 30 children under the age of 5 years who exhibited SIB and found a considerably lower percentage of cases where SIB was maintained by social negative reinforcement (3.4%) and a higher percentage where SIB was maintained by social positive reinforcement (37.9%). The authors reasoned that for very young children, there likely is not as much opportunity for a history of SIB to be established in demand or instructional situations, because these situations are not as prevalent for this age group. Similarly, Didden et al. (2007) found that self-injurious skin picking in persons diagnosed with PWS is predominantly maintained by automatic reinforcement and likely associated with the compulsive behaviors typical of Prader–Willi.

The single-subject, multielement experimental design used by Iwata et al. (1982/1994) is one of the more common methods for assessment of SIB, but is just one of many approaches to functional assessment. Additionally, this method tests more general hypotheses regarding maintaining variables for SIB. The methods and sophistication with which the function of SIB is assessed have greatly expanded over the past 25 years. In particular, functional assessments are not confined to evaluating general hypotheses regarding the function of challenging behavior (i.e., attention, escape, tangible objects) and are increasingly guided by more specific hypotheses, which provide improved information regarding the function of challenging behavior and thus appropriate intervention. For example, following initial inconclusive functional analysis results, Hausman et al. (2009) utilized an A-B-A-B reversal design to demonstrate that a child's SIB and other challenging behaviors were maintained by access to rituals, specifically opening and closing cabinet doors. Similarly, Hagopian, Wilson, and Wilder (2001), after observing that SIB and other challenging behaviors for a 6-year-old child with autism occurred at highest rates during the toy play control condition, included an escape from attention condition during subsequent functional analysis. The function of the child's challenging behavior was maintained, in part, by social avoidance. In a couple of other examples, additional modified functional analyses have demonstrated SIB to be maintained by increased compliance with an individual's demands, or requests (Bowman, Fisher, Thompson, & Piazza, 1997), as well as by a specific quality of attention, such as physical contact (Richman & Hagopian, 1999). In each of these cases, evaluating more specific hypotheses about SIB resulted in improved assessment outcomes and better interventions.

One issue that often arises in the functional assessment of SIB is the time and cost of conducting experimental functional analyses (Axelrod, 1987; Oswald, Ellis, Singh, & Singh, 1994). In many settings, such as schools, resources may not be readily available to conduct these analyses. Increasingly, indirect functional assessment measures are used in these settings to offset the time and cost of conducting direct functional assessment. Several instruments, including the Functional Assessment Interview (FAI: O'Neill et al., 1997) and Questions About Behavioral Function questionnaire (QABF: Paclawskyj et al., 2000), have been used extensively and possess good psychometric properties (Freeman, Walker, & Kaufman, 2007; Nicholson, Konstantinidi, & Furniss, 2006; Paclawskyj, Matson, Rush, Smalls, & Vollmer, 2001; Stage et al., 2006). However, indirect functional assessment measures do not always correlate with the results of experimental functional analyses. As such, some researchers have concluded that indirect functional assessment measures should be used as a preliminary step to direct functional analysis procedures (Alter, Conroy, Mancil, & Haydon, 2008; Paclawskyj et al., 2001; Stage et al., 2006).

Brief functional analysis methods also are available (Kahng & Iwata, 1999; Northup, Wacker, Sasso, & Steege, 1991), but still require some time and expertise to conduct. Additionally, non-experimental functional assessments have been used, particularly structured descriptive assessments, which generally produce similar results as analog functional analyses (Anderson & Long, 2002; Sasso, Reimers, Cooper, & Wacker, 1992). However, similar to indirect functional assessment methods, brief functional assessment results do not always correlate with the results of extended experimental analyses and may tend to overestimate attention as a function of challenging behavior (Kahng & Iwata, 1999; Lerman & Iwata, 1993; Thompson & Iwata, 2007).

Another related issue in the functional assessment of SIB is how to ethically and safely conduct assessment, particularly experimental analyses. Although there is little disagreement regarding the utility of functional assessments in identifying the most effective interventions for SIB (Carr et al., 1999; Didden et al., 1997; Scotti et al., 1991), there continues to be concern regarding the use of procedures that evoke SIB (Hastings & Noone, 2005). Direct functional assessment of SIB, whether from observation or experimental manipulation, involves allowing a potentially harmful behavior to occur and in the case of structured descriptive and experimental analyses, purposely introducing conditions that set the occasion for SIB. Iwata et al. (1982/1994) set a standard for ethically conducting direct functional analysis of SIB by stipulating termination criteria for the assessment and having medical personnel involved, examining each subject prior to and during each assessment. The authors' focus was to ensure that each subject was not exposed to any greater risk than would occur in the natural environment.

One method to reduce the risk of injury while conducting direct functional assessment of SIB is to utilize protective equipment, such as padded helmets or arm splints, in the assessment. However, protective equipment itself can either inhibit the occurrence of SIB or reduce its occurrence, thus resulting in inconclusive functional analysis results and inhibiting evaluation of the operant function of SIB (Borrero, Vollmer, Wright, Lerman, & Kelley, 2002; Le & Smith, 2002). Another method for conducting functional analyses of SIB safely involves the assessment of precursor behaviors (Bergen et al., 2002; Langdon, Carr, & Owen-DeSchryver, 2008; Najdowski, Wallace, Ellsworth, MacAleese, & Cleveland, 2008). Specifically, precursor behaviors are behaviors that reliably precede and serve the same function as the challenging behavior, such as SIB. For example, a less severe behavior such as screaming or stomping of a foot may typically precede head banging. In this scenario, the dependent variable is screaming or foot stomping rather than head banging. Functional analyses that make precursor behaviors the dependent variable can assess the function of SIB without observing its occurrence by instead assessing the function of the precursor behavior. In this way, the functional analysis may be conducted more safely for the individual; however, limitations of this approach exist as identifying reliable precursors that are in the same response class as SIB can be difficult.

In summary, SIB is common and one of the more severe challenging behaviors exhibited by individuals diagnosed with ASD and IDD. Functional assessment procedures have aided in the understanding of SIB, which has lead to improved interventions. While direct functional assessment, particularly experimental functional analyses, provides the most valid assessment results for SIB, there are several factors that should be considered in determining an assessment approach. Ultimately, practitioners should make decisions based on a cost–benefit analysis, which includes weighing the advantages of conducting direct assessment of SIB function (i.e., more accurate and thorough assessment of function) with the cost of conducting the assessment (i.e., safety concerns, staff time). If direct functional assessment is likely to result in improved intervention that can reduce or eliminate SIB, the short-term costs of the procedures may be outweighed by the longer-term benefits for the individual.

Stereotyped Behaviors

Stereotyped behaviors, or stereotypies, are defined as repetitive, rhythmic, and seemingly purposeless behaviors that tend to be inappropriate (Goldman et al., 2009; Turner, 1999). Stereotyped movements and interests are a core diagnostic feature of ASD (American Psychiatric Association, 2000), as well as a common behavioral feature of many IDDs (Dominick, Davis, Lainhart, Tager-Flusberg, & Folstein, 2007; Hill & Furniss, 2006). Prevalence estimates vary, but suggest that as many as two-thirds of individuals diagnosed with IDDs exhibit some form of stereotypy, with estimates for individuals diagnosed with ASD perhaps higher (Berkson, 1983; Bodfish, Symons, Parker, & Lewis, 2000; Goldman et al., 2009; Matson, Dempsey, & Fodstad, 2009; Matson & Rivet, 2008). Some common stereotypies include body rocking, head shaking, hand and arm flapping, finger tapping, clapping, spinning objects, shaking

objects, jumping, and inappropriate vocalizations (Cunningham & Schreibman, 2008; Goldman et al., 2009). Although most stereotypies are considered innocuous, in many instances, stereotypy can significantly interfere with skill development, can be self-directed and classified as self-injurious, and can result in negative social consequences for the individual, such as social avoidance and isolation (Jones, 1991; Matson et al., 2009; Matson, Kiely, & Bamburg, 1997; Matson & Rivet, 2008). As a result, stereotypies often have been targets of functional assessments (Kennedy, 2007; Patel, Carr, Kim, Robles, & Eastridge, 2000; Vollmer et al., 1995).

The initial and prevailing conceptualization of stereotyped movements is that these behaviors serve an automatic function for the individual, usually in the form of sensory stimulation (Lovaas, Newsom, & Hickman, 1987; Rapp & Vollmer, 2005). There exists a considerable research literature utilizing functional assessments with stereotypies that supports the theory that stereotypies are maintained by sensory consequences or self-stimulation (Dawson, Matson, & Cherry, 1998; Piazza, Adelinis, Hanley, Goh, & Delia, 2000; Rapp, 2006). The sensory function of stereotypy often is demonstrated by providing the individual with items or activities that produce a similar sensory consequence as the stereotypy, which results in reductions in stereotypy (Piazza et al., 2000). Additionally, research has shown that other severe challenging behaviors are maintained by an individual's access to stereotypy, suggesting that stereotypy is a reinforcer itself (Falcomata, Roane, Feeney, & Stephenson, 2010; Hanley, Iwata, Thompson, & Lindberg, 2000; Hausman et al., 2009).

However, it should be noted that there are several examples of stereotypies being multiply maintained and varying as a function of socially mediated consequences (Ahearn, Clark, Gardener, Chung, & Dube, 2003; Durand & Carr, 1987). Durand and Carr (1987) examined the relationship of stereotypies (i.e., hand flapping and body rocking) to instructional situations in three children diagnosed with PDDs. Stereotypy increased with the presentation of difficult tasks and decreased with the termination of these tasks.

These results demonstrated that stereotyped movements, in part, functioned as a means of escape from non-preferred tasks. In these examples, stereotypy originally may have served a self-stimulatory function, but obtained socially mediated functions after a history was established of the behavior resulting in social consequences, such as escape from non-preferred situations or attention from others (Durand & Carr, 1987). For example, Goh, Iwata, Shore, and DeLeon (1995) conducted experimental functional analyses with 12 adults diagnosed with developmental disabilities who engaged in stereotypic hand mouthing. For 2 of the participants, hand mouthing was maintained by social positive reinforcement in the form of attention and access to preferred items.

Aggression

Aggressive behaviors include inappropriate physical contact directed towards another person that may result in harm or injury (Luiselli, 2009). Common aggressive behaviors observed in ASD and IDD populations include hitting, kicking, biting, pinching, scratching, hair pulling, grabbing, and choking (Luiselli, 2009). Aggression is estimated to occur in up to 22% of individuals diagnosed with IDD (Gardner & Cole, 1990; Jacobson, 1982) and can have significant adverse consequences for individuals with ASD and IDD, often interfering with learning and skill acquisition, increasing the likelihood of social isolation, and often leading to more restrictive school and home placements (Luiselli, 2009). Because of the serious consequences of aggression, it is not surprising that much of the functional assessment literature has been devoted to this challenging behavior. In a review of 277 studies using functional analysis methodology to evaluate challenging behavior, Hanley et al. (2003) found that aggression was second only to SIB as the most evaluated challenging behavior, occurring in 40.8% of the sample.

Unlike SIB, functional assessments of aggressive behaviors primarily have identified social factors mediating their occurrence (Hanley et al., 2003; Marcus, Vollmer, Swanson, Roane, &

Ringdahl, 2001). Dawson et al. (1998) examined the functions of various challenging behaviors via QABF (Paclawskyj et al., 2000) in a sample of 36 adults diagnosed with autism, PDD-NOS, or mental retardation. Results showed that aggression was primarily endorsed as maintained by social consequences, such as access to attention or tangibles. Marcus et al. (2001), using experimental functional analyses in a sample of 8 children and adolescents diagnosed with developmental disabilities, found aggression to be maintained by social positive and social negative consequences for each individual.

Much of the recent functional assessment literature on aggression has focused on idiosyncratic variables associated with its occurrence. For example, aggression has been demonstrated to be maintained by such specific consequences as access to certain conversation topics (Roscoe, Kindle, & Pence, 2010), access to walks (Ringdahl, Christensen, & Boelter, 2009), and wheelchair movement (DeLeon, Kahng, Rodriguez-Catter, Sveinsdóttir, & Sadler, 2003). Adelinis and Hagopian (1999) conducted a functional analysis with a 27-year-old male diagnosed with autism and moderate mental retardation and found that his aggressive behaviors were associated with the use of "don't" instructions, especially those that interrupted preferred activities. Kahng, Leak, Vu, and Mishler (2008) demonstrated that the aggression of a 16-year-old boy occurred when mechanical arm splints, which were an intervention for SIB, were removed. Functional analysis indicated that the participant's aggression was maintained by access to his arm splints. Similarly, aggression has been shown to follow blocking of and be maintained by access to stereotyped movements (Hagopian & Toole, 2009).

While most functional assessments of aggressive behaviors identify social operant functions for the behaviors, there have been examples of aggression maintained by automatic reinforcement (Luiselli, 2009; Thompson, Fisher, Piazza, & Kuhn, 1998). Thompson et al. (1998) described the functional analysis of a 7-year-old boy diagnosed with pervasive developmental disorder and severe mental retardation, whose aggressive chin pressing was maintained independent of social consequences. Subsequent assessment of this behavior suggested that it was maintained by tactile stimulation (i.e., the sensation of rubbing his chin).

Property Destruction

Property destruction generally is defined as any behavior that results in damage to or destruction of the physical environment and includes such behaviors as throwing objects, hitting or kicking objects, ripping or tearing paper/books, slamming doors, and banging on furniture, to name a few (Ebanks & Fisher, 2003; Fisher, Lindauer, Alterson, & Thompson, 1998; Petursdottir, Esch, Sautter, & Stewart, 2010; Schieltz et al., 2010). Property destruction is a noted common challenging behavior of persons diagnosed with ASD and IDD (Smith & Matson, 2010). Although it has been evaluated in numerous functional assessment studies (Hanley et al., 2003), property destruction seldom has been the sole subject of assessment and more often is included with other severe challenging behaviors often under the general category of destructive behaviors (Harding et al., 2001; Schieltz et al., 2010; Tarbox, Wallace, Tarbox, Landaburu, & Williams, 2004) and occasionally under the category of disruptions (Kuhn et al., 2009). This is likely due to the presumption that property destruction is in the same response class or is part of a similar response chain as other challenging behaviors (Fisher et al., 1998; Harding et al., 2001).

In general, results of functional assessments with property destruction have identified social operant functions for the behavior, including escape from aversive tasks (Ebanks & Fisher, 2003), access to preferred items (Reed, Pace, & Luiselli, 2009), and attention (Harding et al., 2001). Some unique findings, though, regarding property destruction have been made via functional assessment. For example, Bowman et al. (1997) found that property destruction, along with other challenging behaviors, was associated with increased compliance with the demands of two children diagnosed with developmental disabilities. Additionally, Fisher et al. (1998)

demonstrated that property destruction was part of a response chain that produced broken object pieces with which subjects engaged in automatically maintained stereotypy (i.e., tapping the broken pieces). Intervention that provided the subjects with already broken materials or preferred toys resulted in significant reductions in property destruction.

Tantrums

Tantrum behaviors can diminish the positive interactions between children and their parents (Vollmer, Northup, Ringdahl, LeBlanc, & Chauvin, 1996). Such behaviors can place a strain on parents and caregivers by causing them to avoid community or other social outings and activities with their child (Patterson, Chamberlain, & Reid, 1982). Although tantrum behavior may include a constellation of disruptive and destructive behaviors, it usually is operationally defined as periods of screaming and/or crying with or without other problem behaviors. Current literature on tantrum behavior suggests that tantrums most commonly co-occur with other disruptive or destructive behaviors in children with ASD (Baghdadli et al., 2003; Fox, Keller, Grede, & Bartosz, 2007; Petursdottir et al., 2010) and that a particularly strong relation exists between aggressive behavior and tantrums (Matson, 2009). This point is evident in the literature as few studies have focused on tantrum behavior alone, but in conjunction with other destructive or socially disruptive behaviors (e.g., Campbell & Lutzker, 1993; Luiselli & Murbach, 2002).

In terms of assessment, variations of functional analysis procedures have been used to evaluate tantrums. For example, Wilder, Chen, Atwell, Pritchard, and Weinstein (2006) evaluated tantrums associated with transitions. In addition, descriptive functional assessments of tantrum behaviors (Campbell & Lutzker, 1993; Luiselli & Murbach, 2002) and discrete screaming behavior (Graff, Lineman, Libby, & Ahearn, 1999) in naturalistic settings have been described in the literature. Campbell and Lutzker (1993) utilized descriptive functional assessment procedures to evaluate the environmental determinants of severe tantrum behaviors which often co-occurred with property destruction for an 8-year-old boy with ASD who was reported to have no existing functional communication skills. Given that the participant's challenging behaviors were most problematic at home, the researchers trained the child's mother to collect A–B–C data and subsequently developed functional hypotheses from those data. For this participant, tantrum behavior was hypothesized to be maintained by both negative reinforcement (i.e., escape from demand situations) and positive reinforcement (i.e., access to tangible items). Following functional communication training and an activity planning component, significant reductions in both the frequency and duration of this child's tantrum behavior were achieved.

In addressing discrete screaming behavior, Graff et al. (1999) used descriptive functional assessment procedures with a young girl with ASD and IDD in her school setting. After examining A–B–C data collected by the participant's teacher and determining that no positive correlation existed between screaming and any specific antecedent, the researchers hypothesized that screaming was maintained by automatic reinforcement. This information was also consistent with informal functional assessment interviews conducted with the participant's mother. Upon conclusion of these methods and a functional analysis which corroborated the descriptive assessment hypothesis, the researchers implemented a function-based intervention which was effective in reducing screaming for this participant.

Pica

Although the majority of studies using functional assessment methods have targeted severe challenging behaviors such as self-injury, aggression, and disruptive behavior (Hanley et al., 2003), the procedures have been modified or refined in various ways to assess other challenging behaviors. For example, pica, the ingestion of inedible objects such as rocks, paper, glass, cigarette butts,

clothing, etc., occurs in up to 25% of individuals with IDD (Danford & Huber, 1982), but is one of the most difficult problem behaviors to assess and effectively treat (Favell, McGimsey, & Schell, 1982; Madden, Russo, & Cataldo, 1980). Pica places the individual at risk of illness, medical complications, or injury due to choking, intestinal obstruction, bowel perforation, or parasitic infection (Fisher et al., 1994; Foxx & Martin, 1975). Pica presents significant challenges for caregivers and service providers, often necessitating the provision of continuous supervision, use of protective equipment and/or punishment procedures, and a more secure residential placement (Mace & Knight, 1986).

The application of functional analysis methods to this serious problem has led to new approaches to both assessment and treatment. In an early study, Mace and Knight (1986) examined both the amount of social interaction provided and the types of protective equipment used with an adult with severe pica (i.e., ingestion of ripped/shredded clothing or other materials), who resided in an institution and was prescribed a helmet with face shield to prevent pica. In the first analysis, three levels of staff–client social interaction during vocational work were assessed: frequent interaction (close, continuous staff supervision), limited interaction (staff physically distant, attention provided on fixed time, 3-min schedule), and no interaction (staff distant, turned away, no contact). In the second analysis, three forms of protective equipment were assessed: helmet with face shield, helmet without face shield, and no helmet. The two sets of assessment results were used to develop a comprehensive intervention that surprisingly involved limited levels of staff interaction and no protective helmet; this intervention was effective in achieving substantial reductions in pica.

Functional analysis procedures have been modified to permit safe occurrence and direct observation of pica (Piazza, Hanley & Fisher, 1996; Piazza, Fisher, Hanley, & Lindauer, 1998; Piazza, Roane, Keeney, Boney, & Abt, 2002). For example, Piazza et al. (1998) conducted functional analyses of pica for 4 children admitted to an inpatient unit. Sessions were conducted in experimental rooms where the individual was permitted to engage in pica within a "baited" environment; that is, the session room was baited with pica items deemed medically safe and/or items that simulated pica items (e.g., bits of flour tortilla to simulate paint chips) that the individual would typically seek to ingest in home or community settings. Then, analog functional analysis conditions as described by Iwata et al. (1982/1994) were conducted. As expected, pica was maintained by automatic reinforcement for two of four participants. Interestingly, for two participants, pica was maintained at least in part by social consequences, specifically access to adult attention and tangibles.

The baited environment approach has also been utilized with individuals displaying cigarette butt pica (Piazza et al., 1996; Goh, Iwata, & Kahng, 1999). In most of these cases, functional analysis outcomes indicated pica was maintained by automatic reinforcement, and reinforcement-based treatments were effective in reducing pica. However, Goh et al. (1999) noted that in one case, despite clear functional assessment findings, multiple attempts at intervention were unsuccessful, necessitating use of preventive measures for pica. More recently, blocking the individual's attempts at pica has been assessed within the baited environment (Hagopian & Adelinis, 2001; McCord, Grosser, Iwata, & Powers, 2005). Thus, assessment of pica via functional analysis has been critical in moving researchers and practitioners away from use of protective equipment and punishment to development of reinforcement-based, less restrictive treatments, such as provision of stimuli matched to reinforcing properties of pica items, or provision of noncontingent reinforcement, for both automatically and socially maintained pica.

Elopement

Functional analysis procedures have also been successfully applied to elopement, i.e., leaving an area without supervision or caregiver consent (Tarbox et al., 2003). Although prevalence estimates are lacking, this behavior is frequently reported in individuals with IDDs (Jacobson, 1982; Lowe et al., 2007). Elopement not only may interfere with participation in educational, social, or vocational activities but may place the individual at great risk for injury (e.g., running into traffic) (Piazza et al., 1997). In cases where elopement persists or is dangerous to the individual, additional staff support or restrictive residential care may be required to minimize risk. Similar to the assessment of pica, research in this area has been limited. It is difficult to assess and understand the contextual variables surrounding the occurrence of elopement (i.e., what is the individual running to or from), and there are significant challenges in safely assessing the behavior as permitting even one occurrence can be dangerous. In the first application of functional analysis procedures to this problem, Piazza et al. (1997) assessed elopement in three children with intellectual disabilities admitted to an inpatient unit. Functional analysis procedures (Iwata et al., 1982/1994) were modified such that attention, tangible, and demand sessions were conducted in the hospital, in settings which simulated the natural environment where elopement was likely to occur for each participant, but were safe for repeated sessions. For example, elopement for two participants was assessed in a restricted two-room area, where the participant could leave one room and enter the other to access consequences specified for that condition. For a third participant, elopement was assessed in a large common area where exit was not available, as he reportedly engaged in elopement in open spaces. Across all conditions, elopement was allowed to occur, corresponding contingencies were applied, and the individual was then brought back to the starting location with minimal attention. In cases where functional analysis results were unclear, reinforcer assessments were conducted to clarify behavioral function. Assessment results indicated that for two children, elopement was maintained by access to tangible items, and for a third participant, elopement was maintained by access to adult attention. While effective treatments were developed for these participants, generality of results was limited, as assessment and treatment were conducted in an inpatient setting.

In an effort to improve external validity of this assessment, more recent studies have focused on conducting functional analyses of elopement in natural settings while maintaining a high level of safety and experimental control. For example, Tarbox et al. (2003) replicated Piazza et al.'s (1997) procedures but conducted all sessions in an enclosed mall and in a vocational day program, using a confederate to monitor the participant and maintain safety. Additionally, to further simulate conditions in the natural environment, parents were trained to serve as therapists during all assessment and treatment sessions. Results of the three functional analyses indicated that elopement was maintained by positive reinforcement in the form of access to a toy store, access to tangible items, and access to adult attention for the three respective participants. Similarly, Kodak, Grow, and Northup (2004) conducted a functional analysis of elopement outdoors on a kickball field with a 5-year-old girl diagnosed with ADHD. The participant's elopement was shown to be sensitive to adult attention and was treated effectively with noncontingent reinforcement and time-out. Most recently, Lang, Davis et al., (2010) assessed a student's elopement in two school settings, the student's classroom and a resource room where discrete trial training was conducted, using procedures similar to those described by Piazza et al. (1997) and Tarbox et al. (2003). Interestingly, the two functional analyses identified different maintaining variables for elopement across the two settings: elopement within the classroom was maintained by access to a preferred activity (watching videos), while elopement from the resource room was maintained by access to adult attention.

Taken together, the above studies illustrate the utility and flexibility of functional analysis procedures in identifying behavioral function for different forms of problem behavior, Indeed, in a recent review of the treatment literature on elopement, Lang, Rispoli et al., (2009) noted that not only was elopement usually maintained by operant contingencies but that function-based interventions (i.e., those based on functional analysis results) were most effective in reducing elopement.

Feeding Problems

Functional analyses have also been successfully applied to the assessment of feeding problems. Feeding difficulties can take a variety of forms, including food refusal (refusal to eat all or most foods presented), food selectivity (consumption of select foods or food groups and refusal of others), and mealtime problem behaviors (turning head away from spoon, crying, throwing food, vomiting) (Piazza & Roane, 2009). The prevalence of feeding problems among children with intellectual and developmental disabilities is estimated at 35% (Dahl & Sundelin, 1986); however, a very high prevalence, as high as 90%, is reported in children with autism (Kodak & Piazza, 2008). It is important to note that for many children exhibiting food refusal, there is a comorbid medical condition such as gastroesophageal reflux, cardiopulmonary condition, neurological condition, food allergy, or anatomical anomaly (Williams, Field, & Sieverling, 2010). Feeding problems can have a serious impact on child health; typically reported complications include malnourishment, lack of growth, failure to thrive, and reliance on supplemental feeding via gastrostomy tube (Williams et al., 2010).

One focus of the research on feeding problems in children with intellectual disabilities has been on functional analysis of inappropriate mealtime behaviors. In the first such study, Piazza et al. (2003) initially conducted descriptive assessments at home with six parents and their children to identify potential reinforcers for inappropriate mealtime behaviors such as head turning, batting at the spoon, throwing food/utensils, crying, expelling food, vomiting, self-injury, and aggression. Descriptive assessment results indicated that all parents provided attention, escape, and/or tangibles contingent upon food refusal behaviors. Additionally, following inappropriate behavior, all parents provided attention and removed food, and half of the parents provided access to a tangible item. Based on these data, modified functional analysis procedures described by Iwata et al. (1982/1994) were used to assess food refusal behaviors for 15 children. Brief meal sessions were conducted in experimental rooms by behavior therapists wherein a bite of food and the instruction "Take a bite" were presented. Inappropriate mealtime behaviors resulted in one of three types of consequences: removal of the spoon of food (escape condition), provision of verbal coaxing or statements of concern (attention condition), or provision of preferred toy, food, or drink (tangible condition). A play/control condition was also conducted. Functional analysis results indicated that for 12 children, inappropriate mealtime behaviors were sensitive to social consequences (three children displayed few problem behaviors during the assessment). Indeed, 60% of children exhibited problem behavior sensitive to negative reinforcement, suggesting that escape plays a primary role in maintenance of mealtime behavior problems. Also, more than 50% of children exhibited mealtime problem behaviors maintained by positive reinforcement. Importantly, as seen with studies of SIB and other challenging behaviors exhibited by children with intellectual disabilities, effective function-based interventions were derived from functional analysis results.

More recent studies have replicated and extended Piazza et al.'s (2003) research identifying social contingencies responsible for maintenance of mealtime behavior problems. For example, Borrero, Woods, Borrero, Masler, and Lesser (2010) conducted descriptive analyses of feeding problems with 25 children and their parents. They found that social reinforcement, primarily in the form of attention and escape, was most commonly provided by parents following mealtime problem behavior, which supports the validity of a functional analysis approach to assessment of feeding problems. In another study, Wilder, Normand, and Atwell (2005) assessed the food selectivity and SIB of a 3-year-old girl diagnosed with autism. They utilized a brief functional analysis methodology described by Northup et al. (1991) where each test and control condition consisted of single data points within a reversal design. This modified assessment was effective in identifying escape as a maintaining variable for the child's meal-related problem behaviors and in guiding development of an effective reinforcement-based intervention.

Research on functional assessment and treatment of feeding difficulties has expanded to include such topics as mealtime behavior problems that are maintained by multiple sources of reinforcement (Bachmeyer et al., 2009), feeding problems specific to children with autism (cf. review by Volkert & Vaz, 2010), and parent-conducted functional analyses of inappropriate mealtime behaviors displayed by children with autism spectrum disorders (Najdowski, Wallace, Penrod et al., 2008). Finally, modifications to functional analysis methodology have also been useful in assessing the feeding-related, post-meal problem behavior of rumination. Rumination is the regurgitation, chewing, and re-swallowing of previously ingested food; this behavior can produce esophagitis, dehydration, and other medical problems. Two studies (Lyons, Rue, Luiselli, & DiGennaro, 2007; Wilder, Register, Register, Bajacic, & Neidert, 2009) have reported on functional analyses with children with developmental delay or autism who displayed rumination; in all cases, rumination was maintained by automatic reinforcement, and effective treatments were identified for all participants. Thus, as demonstrated by research on self-injury and other behavior problems, functional analysis results have been useful in guiding development of highly specific and effective interventions (i.e., those based on the function of the behavior) for a range of inappropriate mealtime or food-related behaviors.

Noncompliance

Noncompliant behavior can be observed in many different forms and may often co-occur with other topographies of challenging behavior (e.g., aggressive and disruptive tantrum behavior). Among childhood problems, noncompliance has been noted as one of the most concerning problems for parents and teachers (Miles & Wilder, 2009). For children with ASD and IDD who often benefit from highly specialized academic programming and instruction, compliance with instructions may be essential in order to produce meaningful gains in academic and social skills.

For observational or data collection purposes, noncompliant behavior often is operationally defined by defining its inverse (i.e., compliance). For example, when providing discrete trial-based instruction using a least-to-most prompting sequence, compliance may be defined as "beginning or completing the request within 5 s of the verbal or gestural prompt." Noncompliance usually is defined as the child doing anything other than complying.

Not unlike other topographies of challenging behavior, researchers have utilized functional assessment methodologies to identify putative discriminative stimuli and establishing operations associated with noncompliance (Rortvedt & Miltenberger, 1994; Roscoe, Rooker, Pence, & Longworth, 2009), as well as the consequent environmental events maintaining these behaviors (Peyton, Lindauer, & Richman, 2005; Rodriguez, Thompson, & Baynham, 2010). Specifically, task features such as degree of difficulty or task presentation style (e.g., type of prompting or rate of prompt delivery) have been found to be particularly relevant.

McComas, Hoch, Paone, and El-Roy (2000) utilized multiple methods of functional assessment to identify idiosyncratic establishing conditions which contributed to the occurrence of problematic behaviors (i.e., aggression, disruption, and noncompliance) reported to occur during academic times for three children with ASD attending a small private school. Following functional analyses procedures (Iwata et al., 1982/1994) for each participant, it was hypothesized that problem behaviors and noncompliance were maintained by negative reinforcement in the form of escape from task demands. Following the functional analyses, descriptive assessments comprised of informal teacher interviews and A–B–C observations were conducted during academic work times in each participant's classroom. From these observations, different task features specific to each participant were hypothesized to be idiosyncratic establishing operations, such as difficult tasks, adult-selected task sequences, and repetitive tasks, and were associated with problem behavior and noncompliance. Finally, upon examining levels of problem behavior and compliance given the presence or absence of individually designed antecedent interventions (e.g., participant choice of task sequence), interventions were implemented which produced near-zero levels of problem behavior.

In a second study conducted by Peyton et al. (2005), the type of prompting used, independent of the task type, was found to set the occasion for challenging behaviors associated with noncompliant vocal behavior (NVB), but not *actual* noncompliance. In their study, modified functional analysis procedures were employed to examine the NVB of a 15-year-old girl with ASD who was referred for the assessment and treatment of disruptive and inappropriate vocalizations. For this individual, NVB was defined as "any vocal behavior involving a refusal to comply with a request" (e.g., "I can't ever do that," "I won't do it"). Interestingly, researchers found that although high levels of NVB were observed during demand conditions conducted as part of a standard functional analysis (i.e., Iwata et al., 1982/1994), only moderate levels of noncompliance were observed, causing them to question the validity of a negative reinforcement hypothesis. Next, a follow-up functional analysis comparing two demand conditions where NVB resulted in either task removal (i.e., escape) or no task removal demonstrated that NVB was not sensitive to escape, but was consistently occasioned by directive prompts. Finally, an intervention analysis comparing the use of directive (e.g., "show me the circle") versus nondirective prompts (e.g., "I wonder where the circle is") was conducted which demonstrated that nondirective prompts reduced NVB to near zero.

Although noncompliant behavior may be common during demand contexts and particularly when aversive stimuli, such as difficult tasks, are present, some functional assessments have also found noncompliance to be sensitive to positive reinforcement. Based on teacher concerns and reports of noncompliant behavior, Rodriguez et al. (2010) examined the noncompliant behavior of three preschool-aged children who attended a university-affiliated early childhood program. During their functional analysis procedures, the degree to which noncompliant behavior was maintained by either escape or attention was examined by alternating attention and escape conditions in a multielement design where the antecedent conditions in each test remained constant, yet the contingencies for compliance or noncompliance were programmed based on a contingency reversal strategy. That is, during the escape condition, noncompliance resulted in escape, while compliant behavior resulted in attention, and during the attention condition, the contingencies were reversed. Noncompliance was highest for all three participants when noncompliant behavior resulted in positive reinforcement in the form of attention (e.g., "come on, you know you can do this") but not escape, as may have been indicated by more naturalistic or descriptive methods.

Problems with Transitions

A transition can be defined as changing from one activity to a different activity which may or may not include a change in physical location (e.g., transitioning from recess to the classroom). Some authors have estimated that up to 35% of a child's waking hours may include transitions (Sainato, Strain, Lefebvre, & Rapp, 1987). For individuals with ASD and IDD, transitions may prove uniquely problematic for a number of reasons and have long been associated with occasioning problem behavior within this population (American Psychiatric Association, 2000). While intervention research has suggested the role of environmental predictability as being a particularly relevant variable when considering aberrant behaviors associated with transitions (Flannery & Horner, 1994), the application of functional assessment methodologies to evaluate challenging behaviors associated with transitions remains limited.

In natural settings, transitions often involve multiple stimulus changes, such as the removal or loss of multiple types of preferred stimuli, and functional assessment methods have been applied to examine these events (McCord, Thomson, & Iwata, 2001). In particular, examination of the following types of transitions has been suggested: from a high

preferred activity to a low preferred activity, from low to high, from low to low, and from high to high (McCord et al., 2001; Wilder et al., 2006).

McCord et al. (2001) conducted a functional analysis to examine the self-injurious behavior of two adults with ID by arranging activity initiation transitions (i.e., changes from no activity to a low or high preferred activity) as well as activity termination transitions (i.e., changes from an ongoing high or low preferred activity to no activity). Furthermore, each condition was evaluated when participants either were or were not required to make a physical change in location. The results of their analysis suggested that for both individuals, SIB was maintained by negative reinforcement in the form of avoiding physical location changes and that one of the participant's SIB was also maintained by escape from ongoing tasks and avoidance of task initiations.

Wilder, Harris, Reagan, and Rasey (2007) utilized methods similar to those used by McCord et al. (2001) to examine the tantrum behavior of typically developing children in preschool and identified different maintaining consequences for each. For one participant, problem behaviors were maintained by positive reinforcement in the form of gaining access to the previously interrupted activity. For the second participant, problem behaviors were maintained by negative reinforcement in the form of task avoidance. The use of a DRO plus extinction procedure resulted in reducing tantrum behaviors to near zero for both of these participants.

Although these examples provide evidence for the utility of functional analysis methodology to evaluate challenging behaviors associated with transitions, when transitions occur in the home, school, or community, they may involve multiple contextual variables which are difficult to replicate using analog arrangements (Kern & Vorndran, 2000). Furthermore, the use of descriptive assessments in naturalistic settings may enhance the treatment utility of the assessment (English & Anderson, 2006).

Kern and Vorndran (2000) provide an example of a less intensive functional assessment methods used to evaluate problems associated with transitions. These researchers examined the "flopping" behavior (i.e., dropping to the ground and refusing to move during transitions) of an 11-year-old girl diagnosed with IDD, ADHD, and moderate obesity in her school setting. Specifically, data were collected by coupling informal functional assessment interviews with naturalistic A–B–C observations conducted during transitions (e.g., from recess to the classroom) throughout the child's school day. After examining their functional assessment information, it was hypothesized that challenging behaviors were maintained by avoidance of low preferred environments or activities, such as activities involving high rates of demands.

School Refusal

As the preceding examples have demonstrated, noncompliance with immediate academic, daily living, or other tasks can be evaluated using functional assessment methods successfully. However, a related concern with respect to noncompliance is school refusal behavior (SRB). SRB has been defined as "child-motivated refusal to attend school and/or problems with remaining in classes for an entire day" and should be distinguished from absenteeism which is generally used to refer to child absences from school that are not due to their overt refusal (Kearney, 2008). SRB in typically developing children has been estimated to occur in 1–10% of the school-age population (Kearney, 2008; Kearney & Silverman, 1999; King & Bernstein, 2001), and others have suggested that the prevalence of this behavior in children with ASD and IDD may be comparable (Kurita, 1991).

To better understand the function of SRB, Kearney and Silverman (1993) developed the School Refusal Assessment Scale (SRAS), which is designed to identify one of the following four forms of hypothesized reinforcement for school refusal: avoidance of stimuli provoking negative affectivity, escape from aversive social or evaluative situations, attention seeking, or positive tangible reinforcement. However, while the treatment

validity of this measure is promising for use with typically developing children (Kearney & Silverman, 1999), the SRAS has not been evaluated with children with ASD or IDD. Fortunately, although scarce, examples of individualized functional assessments of SRB within this population are available and have shown promise (Meyer, Hagopian, & Paclawsky, 1999; Arvans & LeBlanc, 2009).

Meyer et al. (1999) used functional assessment methods to examine the SRB of an 18-year-old male diagnosed with moderate mental retardation, mild cerebral palsy, and Anxiety Disorder NOS who also engaged in physical and verbal aggression and disruptive behaviors. Although multiple phases of assessment and treatment were conducted as part of their study, the use of teacher and school attendance reports, informal interviews with the participant's teachers and parent, and unstructured descriptive observations during parent–child interactions allowed the researchers to hypothesize that school refusal was maintained by positive reinforcement in the form of access to preferred activities and social attention from his mother. Upon implementing a function-based intervention, an increase in school attendance and decreases in SRB and other noncompliant behaviors were observed.

In a second study, Arvans and LeBlanc (2009) evaluated the relation between migraine reports and SRB for a 15-year-old boy diagnosed with Asperger's Disorder. In this case, the authors used the Functional Assessment Interview (FAI; O'Neill et al., 1997) and the Functional Assessment Screening Tool (FAST; Iwata & DeLeon, 1995) to examine the antecedents and consequences associated with the boy's migraine reports. Upon conclusion, the maintaining consequence most reliably following migraine reports was determined to be escape from school or individual class periods during school. Subsequently, rather than treating migraines via medication, a function-based intervention consisting of a token economy and escape extinction were found to decrease migraine reports and increase school and class attendance.

Summary

Functional assessment is comprised of a broad range of indirect and direct procedures for examining the function, or purpose, of challenging behaviors. Functional assessment procedures have been applied to a variety of populations, but are most notably used with individuals diagnosed with IDD and ASD, likely due to the increased prevalence of challenging behaviors in these populations. While SIB has been most associated with the evolution of functional assessment and functional analysis methods, adaptations to procedures have allowed for successful assessment of numerous challenging behaviors, including stereotypies, aggression, property destruction, and feeding problems, to name a few. The most important element of functional assessment is that the results typically inform regarding intervention. For example, identification of SIB maintained by attention from others can be addressed with interventions such as noncontingent delivery of attention on a fixed-time schedule or differential reinforcement procedures. As a result of this link between functional assessment results and treatment, interventions have progressively become less punitive and more reinforcement-based and have resulted in less restrictive placements for numerous individuals with IDD or ASD. One other related and prominent effect of the increased use of functional assessments is a better understanding of the behavioral presentations for numerous populations of individuals with IDDs. Specifically, functional assessments have demonstrated that challenging behaviors once thought to be an inherent characteristic of particular diagnoses, and thus automatically maintained, may actually be regulated by, or at least sensitive to, social or environmental factors. This has allowed practitioners to develop interventions for challenging behaviors of individuals where it was once thought interventions would not be effective. As more research is conducted, and as more practitioners adopt functional assessment procedures, the already growing body of support for functional assessment as the most effective means of assessing challenging behaviors should expand greatly.

This will lead to the development and refinement of more effective and efficient functional assessment procedures and to the expansion and adaptation of procedures to more populations and challenging behaviors.

References

Adelinis, J. D., & Hagopian, L. P. (1999). The use of symmetrical 'do' and 'don't' requests to interrupt ongoing activities. *Journal of Applied Behavior Analysis, 32*, 519–523.

Ahearn, W. H., Clark, K. M., Gardener, N. C., Chung, B. I., & Dube, W. V. (2003). Persistence of stereotypic behavior: Examining the effects of external reinforcers. *Journal of Applied Behavior Analysis, 36*, 439–448.

Alter, P. J., Conroy, M. A., Mancil, G., & Haydon, T. (2008). A comparison of functional behavior assessment methodologies with young children: Descriptive methods and functional analysis. *Journal of Behavioral Education, 17*, 200–219.

American Psychiatric Association. (2000). *Diagnostic and statistical manual of mental disorders (DSM-IV-TR)*. Washington, DC: Author.

Anderson, C. M., & Long, E. S. (2002). Use of a structured descriptive assessment methodology to identify variables affecting problem behavior. *Journal of Applied Behavior Analysis, 35*, 137–154.

Andover, M. S., & Gibb, B. E. (2010). Non-suicidal self-injury, attempted suicide, and suicidal intent among psychiatric inpatients. *Psychiatry Research, 178*, 101–105.

Athens, E. S., Vollmer, T. R., Sloman, K. N., & Pipkin, C. (2008). An analysis of vocal stereotypy and therapist fading. *Journal of Applied Behavior Analysis, 41*, 291–297.

Arvans, R. K., & LeBlanc, L. A. (2009). Functional assessment and treatment of migraine reports and school absences in an adolescent with Asperger's disorder. *Education & Treatment of Children, 32*, 151–166.

Axelrod, S. (1987). Functional and structural analyses of behavior: Approaches leading to reduced use of punishment procedures. *Research in Developmental Disabilities, 8*, 165–178.

Bachmeyer, M. H., Piazza, C. C., Fredrick, L. D., Reed, G. K., Rivas, K. D., & Kadey, H. J. (2009). Functional analysis and treatment of multiply controlled inappropriate mealtime behavior. *Journal of Applied Behavior Analysis, 42*, 641–658.

Baghdadli, A., Pascal, C., Grisi, S., & Aussilloux, C. (2003). Risk factors for self-injurious behaviours among 222 young children with autistic disorders. *Journal of Intellectual Disability Research, 47*, 622–627.

Bass, M. N., & Speak, B. L. (2005). A behavioral approach to the assessment and treatment of severe self-injury in a woman with Smith-Magenis syndrome: A single case study. *Behavioural and Cognitive Psychotherapy, 33*(3), 361–368. doi:10.1017/S1352465805002110.

Bergen, A. E., Holbern, S. W., & Scott-Huyghebaert, V. C. (2002). Functional analysis of self-injurious behavior in an adult with Lesch-Nyhan syndrome. *Behavior Modification, 26*, 187–204.

Berkson, G. (1983). Repetitive stereotyped behaviors. *American Journal of Mental Deficiency, 88*, 239–246.

Bijou, S. W., Peterson, R. F., & Ault, M. H. (1968). A method to integrate descriptive and experimental field studies at the level of data and empirical concepts. *Journal of Applied Behavior Analysis, 1*, 175–191.

Bodfish, J. W., Symons, F. J., Parker, D. E., & Lewis, M. H. (2000). Varieties of repetitive behavior in autism: Comparisons to mental retardation. *Journal of Autism and Developmental Disorders, 30*, 237–243.

Borrero, J. C., Vollmer, T. R., Wright, C. S., Lerman, D. C., & Kelley, M. E. (2002). Further evaluation of the role of protective equipment in the functional analysis of self-injurious behavior. *Journal of Applied Behavior Analysis, 35*, 69–72.

Borrero, C. S., Woods, J. N., Borrero, J. C., Masler, E. A., & Lesser, A. D. (2010). Descriptive analyses of pediatric food refusal and acceptance. *Journal of Applied Behavior Analysis, 43*, 71–88.

Bowman, L. G., Fisher, W. W., Thompson, R. H., & Piazza, C. C. (1997). On the relation of mands and the function of destructive behavior. *Journal of Applied Behavior Analysis, 30*, 251–265.

Budney, A. J., & Higgins, S. T. (1998). *Community reinforcement plus vouchers approach: Manual 2: National Institute on Drug Abuse. Therapy manuals for drug addiction.* (NIH Publication Number 98-4309). Rockville: National Institute on Drug Abuse.

Campbell, R. V., & Lutzker, J. R. (1993). Using functional equivalence training to reduce severe challenging behavior: A case study. *Journal of Developmental and Physical Disabilities, 5*, 203–216.

Carr, E. G. (1977). The motivation of self-injurious behavior: A review of some hypotheses. *Psychological Bulletin, 84*, 800–816.

Carr, E. G., Horner, R. H., Turnbull, A. P., Marquis, J. G., McLaughlin, D., McAtee, M. L., et al. (Eds.). (1999). *Positive behavior support for people with developmental disabilities: A research synthesis.* Washington, DC: American Association on Mental Retardation.

Carter, S. L., & Wheeler, J. J. (2007). Analysis of behavioural responding across multiple instructional conditions for a child with childhood disintegrative disorder. *Journal of Research in Special Educational Needs, 7*, 137–141.

Clarke, S., Dunlap, G., & Vaughn, B. (1999). Family-centered, assessment-based intervention to improve behavior during an early morning routine. *Journal of Positive Behavior Interventions, 1*, 235–241.

Cooper, S. A., Smiley, E. E., Allan, L. M., Jackson, A. A., Finlayson, J. J., Mantry, D. D., et al. (2009). Adults with intellectual disabilities: Prevalence, incidence and remission of self-injurious behaviour, and related factors. *Journal of Intellectual Disability Research, 53*, 200–216.

Crockett, J. L., & Hagopian, L. P. (2006). Prompting procedures as establishing operations for escape-maintained behavior. *Behavioral Interventions, 21*, 65–71.

Cunningham, A. B., & Schreibman, L. (2008). Stereotypy in autism: The importance of function. *Research in Autism Spectrum Disorders, 2*, 469–479.

Dahl, M., & Sundelin, C. (1986). Early feeding problems in an affluent society. *Acta Paediatrica, 75*, 370–379.

Danford, D. E., & Huber, A. M. (1982). Pica among mentally retarded adults. *American Journal of Mental Deficiency, 87*, 141–146.

Dawson, J. E., Matson, J. L., & Cherry, K. E. (1998). An analysis of maladaptive behaviors in persons with autism, PDD-NOS, and mental retardation. *Research in Developmental Disabilities, 19*, 439–448.

Deitz, D. D., & Repp, A. C. (1989). Mental retardation. In T. H. Ollendick, M. Hersen, T. H. Ollendick, & M. Hersen (Eds.), *Handbook of child psychopathology* (2nd ed., pp. 75–91). New York: Plenum Press.

DeLeon, I. G., Kahng, S., Rodriguez-Catter, V., Sveinsdóttir, I., & Sadler, C. (2003). Assessment of aberrant behavior maintained by wheelchair movement in a child with developmental disabilities. *Research in Developmental Disabilities, 24*, 381–390.

Didden, R., Duker, P. C., & Korzilius, H. (1997). Meta-analytic study on treatment effectiveness for problem behaviors with individuals who have mental retardation. *American Journal on Mental Retardation, 101*, 387–399.

Didden, R., Korzilius, H., & Curfs, L. G. (2007). Skin-picking in individuals with Prader-Willi Syndrome: Prevalence, functional Assessment, and its comorbidity with compulsive and self-injurious behaviours. *Journal of Applied Research in Intellectual Disabilities, 20*, 409–419.

Dominick, K. C., Davis, W. O., Lainhart, J., Tager-Flusberg, H., & Folstein, S. (2007). Atypical behaviors in children with autism and children with a history of language impairment. *Research in Developmental Disabilities, 28*, 145–162.

Dougher, M. J., & Hackbert, L. (1994). A behavior-analytic account of depression and a case report using acceptance-based procedures. *The Behavior Analyst, 17*, 231–333.

Durand, V., & Carr, E. G. (1987). Social influences on 'self-stimulatory' behavior: Analysis and treatment application. *Journal of Applied Behavior Analysis, 20*, 119–132.

Dykens, E. M., Cassidy, S. B., & DeVries, M. L. (2011). Prader-Willi syndrome. In S. Goldstein, C. R. Reynolds, S. Goldstein, & C. R. Reynolds (Eds.), *Handbook of neurodevelopmental and genetic disorders in children* (2nd ed., pp. 484–511). New York: Guilford.

Ebanks, M. E., & Fisher, W. W. (2003). Altering the timing of academic prompts to treat destructive behavior maintained by escape. *Journal of Applied Behavior Analysis, 36*, 355–359.

Edelson, M. (2006). Are the majority of children with autism mentally retarded? A systematic evaluation of the data. *Focus on Autism and Other Developmental Disabilities, 21*, 66–83.

English, C. L., & Anderson, C. M. (2006). Evaluation of the treatment utility of the analog functional analysis and the structured descriptive assessment. *Journal of Positive Behavior Interventions, 8*, 212–229.

Falcomata, T. S., Roane, H. S., Feeney, B. J., & Stephenson, K. M. (2010). Assessment and treatment of elopement maintained by access to stereotypy. *Journal of Applied Behavior Analysis, 43*, 513–517.

Favell, J. E., McGimsey, J. F., & Schell, R. M. (1982). Treatment of self-injury by providing alternate sensory activities. *Analysis & Intervention in Developmental Disabilities, 2*, 83–104.

Feeley, K. M., & Jones, E. A. (2006). Addressing challenging behaviour in children with Down syndrome: The use of applied behaviour analysis for assessment and intervention. *Down Syndrome: Research & Practice, 11*, 64–77.

Fisher, W. W., Lindauer, S. E., Alterson, C. J., & Thompson, R. H. (1998). Assessment and treatment of destructive behavior maintained by stereotypic object manipulation. *Journal of Applied Behavior Analysis, 31*, 513–527.

Fisher, W. W., Piazza, C. C., Bowman, L. G., Kurtz, P. F., Sherer, M. R., & Lachman, S. R. (1994). A preliminary evaluation of empirically derived consequences for the treatment of pica. *Journal of Applied Behavior Analysis, 27*, 447–457.

Flannery, K. B., & Horner, R. H. (1994). The relationship between predictability and problem behavior for students with severe disabilities. *Journal of Behavioral Education, 4*, 157–176.

Fox, R. A., Keller, K. M., Grede, P. L., & Bartosz, A. M. (2007). A mental health clinic for toddlers with developmental delays and behavior problems. *Research in Developmental Disabilities, 28*, 119–129.

Foxx, R. M., & Martin, E. D. (1975). Treatment of scavenging behavior (coprophagy and pica) by overcorrection. *Behavioral Research and Therapy, 13*, 153–162.

Franco, J. H., Lang, R. L., O'Reilly, M. F., Chan, J. M., Sigafoos, J., & Rispoli, M. (2009). Functional analysis and treatment of inappropriate vocalizations using a speech-generating device for a child with autism. *Focus on Autism and Other Developmental Disabilities, 24*, 146–155.

Freeman, K. A., Walker, M., & Kaufman, J. (2007). Psychometric properties of the Questions About Behavioral Function Scale in a child sample. *American Journal on Mental Retardation, 112*, 122–129.

Gardner, W. I., & Cole, C. L. (1990). Aggression and related conduct difficulties. In J. L. Matson (Ed.), *Handbook of behavior modification with the mentally retarded* (2nd ed., pp. 225–248). New York: Plenum Press.

Goh, H.-L., Iwata, B. A., & Kahng, S. W. (1999). Multicomponent assessment and treatment of cigarette pica. *Journal of Applied Behavior Analysis, 32*, 297–316.

Goh, H., Iwata, B. A., Shore, B. A., & DeLeon, I. G. (1995). An analysis of the reinforcing properties of hand mouthing. *Journal of Applied Behavior Analysis, 28*, 269–283.

Goldman, S., Wang, C., Salgado, M. W., Greene, P. E., Kim, M., & Rapin, I. (2009). Motor stereotypies in children with autism and other developmental disorders. *Developmental Medicine & Child Neurology, 51*, 30–38.

Graff, R. B., Lineman, G. T., Libby, M. E., & Ahearn, W. H. (1999). Functional analysis and treatment of screaming in a young girl with severe disabilities. *Behavioral Interventions, 14*, 233–239.

Hagopian, L. P., & Adelinis, J. D. (2001). Response blocking with and without redirection for the treatment of pica. *Journal of Applied Behavior Analysis, 34*, 527–530.

Hagopian, L. P., & Toole, L. M. (2009). Effects of response blocking and competing stimuli on stereotypic behavior. *Behavioral Interventions, 24*, 117–125.

Hagopian, L. P., Wilson, D. M., & Wilder, D. A. (2001). Assessment and treatment of problem behavior maintained by escape from attention and access to tangible items. *Journal of Applied Behavior Analysis, 34*, 229–232.

Hall, S., DeBernardis, M., & Reiss, A. (2006). Social escape behaviors in children with Fragile-X syndrome. *Journal of Autism and Developmental Disorders, 36*, 935–947.

Hall, S., Oliver, C., & Murphy, G. (2001). Self-injurious behaviour in young children with Lesch-Nyhan syndrome. *Developmental Medicine & Child Neurology, 43*, 745–749.

Hanley, G., Iwata, B., & McCord, B. (2003). Functional analysis of problem behavior: A review. *Journal of Applied Behavior Analysis, 36*, 147–185.

Hanley, G. P., Iwata, B. A., Thompson, R. H., & Lindberg, J. S. (2000). A component analysis of "stereotypy as reinforcement" for alternative behavior. *Journal of Applied Behavior Analysis, 33*, 285–297.

Harding, J. W., Wacker, D. P., Berg, W. K., Barretto, A., Winborn, L., & Gardner, A. (2001). Analysis of response class hierarchies with attention-maintained problem behaviors. *Journal of Applied Behavior Analysis, 34*, 61–64.

Hastings, R. P., & Noone, S. J. (2005). Self-injurious behavior and functional analysis: Ethics and evidence. *Education and Training in Developmental Disabilities, 40*, 335–342.

Hausman, N., Kahng, S., Farrell, E., & Mongeon, C. (2009). Idiosyncratic functions: Severe problem behavior maintained by access to ritualistic behaviors. *Education & Treatment of Children, 32*, 77–87.

Hill, J., & Furniss, F. (2006). Patterns of emotional and behavioural disturbance associated with autistic traits in young people with severe intellectual disabilities and challenging behaviours. *Research in Developmental Disabilities, 27*, 517–528.

Hurley, A., & Levitas, A. S. (2007). The importance of recognizing autism spectrum disorders in intellectual disability. *Mental Health Aspects of Developmental Disabilities, 10*, 157–161.

Iwata, B. A., & DeLeon, I. G. (1995). *The functional analysis screening tool (FAST)*. Unpublished manuscript, University of Florida.

Iwata, B. A., Dorsey, M. F., Slifer, K. J., & Bauman, K. E. (1994). Toward a functional analysis of self-injury. *Journal of Applied Behavior Analysis, 27*, 197–209 (Reprinted from *Analysis and Intervention in Developmental Disabilities, 2*, 3–20, 1982).

Iwata, B. A., Pace, G. M., Dorsey, M. F., & Zarcone, J. R. (1994). The functions of self-injurious behavior: An experimental-epidemiological analysis. *Journal of Applied Behavior Analysis, 27*, 215–240.

Jacobson, J. W. (1982). Problem behavior and psychiatric impairment within a developmentally disabled population: I. *Behavior frequency. Applied Research in Mental Retardation, 3*, 121–139.

Johnston, S. S., & O'Neill, R. E. (2001). Searching for effectiveness and efficiency in conducting functional assessments: A review and proposed process for teachers and other practitioners. *Focus on Autism & Other Developmental Disabilities, 16*, 205.

Jones, R. S. (1991). Stereotypy: Challenging behaviour or adaptive response. *Scandinavian Journal of Behaviour Therapy, 20*, 25–40.

Kahng, S., & Iwata, B. A. (1999). Correspondence between outcomes of brief and extended functional analyses. *Journal of Applied Behavior Analysis, 32*, 149–159.

Kahng, S., Leak, J., Vu, C., & Mishler, B. (2008). Mechanical restraints as positive reinforcers for aggression. *Behavioral Interventions, 23*, 137–142.

Kearney, C. A. (2008). School absenteeism and school refusal behavior in youth: A contemporary review. *Clinical Psychology Review, 28*, 451–471.

Kearney, C. A., Cook, L., Wechsler, A., Haight, C. M., & Stowman, S. (2008). Behavioral assessment. In M. Hersen, A. M. Gross, M. Hersen, & A. M. Gross (Eds.), *Handbook of clinical psychology* (Children and adolescents, Vol. 2, pp. 551–574). Hoboken: Wiley.

Kearney, C. A., & Silverman, W. K. (1993). Measuring the function of school refusal behavior: The School Assessment Scale. *Journal of Clinical Child Psychology, 22*, 85–96.

Kearney, C. A., & Silverman, W. K. (1999). Functionally based prescriptive and nonprescriptive treatment for children and adolescents with school refusal behavior. *Behavior Therapy, 30*, 673–695.

Kennedy, C. H. (2007). Stereotypic movement disorder. In P. Sturmey (Ed.), *Functional analysis in clinical treatment* (pp. 193–209). San Diego: Elsevier Academic Press.

Kern, L., Mauk, J. E., Marder, T. J., & Mace, F. (1995). Functional analysis and intervention for breath holding. *Journal of Applied Behavior Analysis, 28*, 339–340.

Kern, L., & Vorndran, C. M. (2000). Functional assessment and intervention for transition difficulties.

Journal of the Association for Persons with Severe Handicaps, 25, 212–216.

Kerr, P. L., & Muehlenkamp, J. J. (2010). Features of psychopathology in self-injuring female college students. *Journal of Mental Health Counseling, 32*, 290–308.

King, N. J., & Bernstein, G. A. (2001). School refusal in children and adolescents: A review of the past 10 years. *Journal of the American Academy of Child & Adolescent Psychiatry, 40*, 197–205.

Kodak, T., Grow, L., & Northup, J. (2004). Functional analysis and treatment of elopement for a child with Attention Deficit Hyperactivity Disorder. *Journal of Applied Behavior Analysis, 37*, 229–232.

Kodak, T., & Piazza, C. C. (2008). Assessment and behavioral treatment of feeding and sleeping disorders in children with autism spectrum disorders. *Child and Adolescent Psychiatric Clinics of North America, 17*, 887–905.

Kuhn, D. E., Hardesty, S. L., & Sweeney, N. M. (2009). Assessment and treatment of excessive straightening and destructive behavior in an adolescent diagnosed with autism. *Journal of Applied Behavior Analysis, 42*, 355–360.

Kurita, H. (1991). School refusal in pervasive developmental disorders. *Journal of Autism and Developmental Disorders, 21*, 1–15.

Kurtz, P. F., Chin, M. D., Huete, J. M., Tarbox, R. F., O'Connor, J. T., Paclawskyj, T. R., et al. (2003). Functional analysis and treatment of self-injurious behavior in young children: A summary of 30 cases. *Journal of Applied Behavior Analysis, 36*, 205–219.

LaBelle, C. A., & Charlop-Christy, M. H. (2002). Individualizing functional analysis to assess multiple and changing functions of severe behavior problems in children with autism. *Journal of Positive Behavior Interventions, 4*, 231–241.

Lang, R., Davis, T., O'Reilly, M., Machalicek, W., Rispoli, M., Sigafoos, J., et al. (2010). Functional analysis and treatment of elopement across two school settings. *Journal of Applied Behavior Analysis, 43*, 113–118.

Lang, R., Didden, R., Machalicek, W., Rispoli, M., Sigafoos, J., Lancioni, G., et al. (2010). Behavioral treatment of chronic skin-picking in individuals with developmental disabilities: A systematic review. *Research in Developmental Disabilities, 31*, 304–315.

Lang, R., Didden, R., Sigafoos, J., Rispoli, M., Regester, A., & Lancioni, G. E. (2009). Treatment of chronic skin-picking in an adolescent with Asperger syndrome and borderline intellectual disability. *Clinical Case Studies, 8*, 317–325.

Lang, R., Rispoli, M., Machalicek, W., White, P. J., Kang, S., Pierce, N., et al. (2009). Treatment of elopement in individuals with developmental disabilities: A systematic review. *Research in Developmental Disabilities, 30*, 670–681.

Langdon, N. A., Carr, E. G., & Owen-DeSchryver, J. S. (2008). Functional analysis of precursors for serious problem behavior and related intervention. *Behavior Modification, 32*, 804–827.

Le, D. D., & Smith, R. G. (2002). Functional analysis of self-injury with and without protective equipment.

Journal of Developmental and Physical Disabilities, 14, 277–290.

Lerman, D. C., & Iwata, B. A. (1993). Descriptive and experimental analyses of variables maintaining self-injurious behavior. *Journal of Applied Behavior Analysis, 26*, 293–319.

Lovaas, O. I., Newsom, C., & Hickman, C. (1987). Self-stimulatory behavior and perceptual reinforcement. *Journal of Applied Behavior Analysis, 20*, 45–68.

Lowe, K. K., Allen, D. D., Jones, E. E., Brophy, S. S., Moore, K. K., & James, W. W. (2007). Challenging behaviours: Prevalence and topographies. *Journal of Intellectual Disability Research, 51*, 625–636.

Luiselli, J. K. (2009). Aggression and noncompliance. In J. L. Matson & J. L. Matson (Eds.), *Applied behavior analysis for children with autism spectrum disorders* (pp. 175–187). New York: Springer.

Luiselli, J. K., & Murbach, L. (2002). Providing instruction from novel staff as an antecedent intervention for child tantrum behavior in a public school classroom. *Education & Treatment of Children, 25*, 356–365.

Lyons, E. A., Rue, H. C., Luiselli, J. K., & DiGennaro, F. D. (2007). Brief functional analysis and supplemental feeding for postmeal rumination in children with developmental disabilities. *Journal of Applied Behavior Analysis, 40*, 743–747.

Mace, F. C., & Knight, D. (1986). Functional analysis and treatment of severe pica. *Journal of Applied Behavior Analysis, 19*, 411–416.

Madden, N. A., Russo, D. C., & Cataldo, M. F. (1980). Environmental influences on mouthing in children with lead intoxication. *Journal of Pediatric Psychology, 5*, 207–216.

Marcus, B. A., Vollmer, T. R., Swanson, V., Roane, H. R., & Ringdahl, J. E. (2001). An experimental analysis of aggression. *Behavior Modification, 25*, 189–213.

Martell, C. R. (2008). Behavioral activation for depression. In W. T. O'Donohue, J. E. Fisher, W. T. O'Donohue, & J. E. Fisher (Eds.), *Cognitive behavior therapy: Applying empirically supported techniques in your practice* (2nd ed., pp. 40–45). Hoboken: Wiley.

Matson, J. (2009). Aggression and tantrums in children with autism: A review of behavioral treatments and maintaining variables. *Journal of Mental Health Research in Intellectual Disabilities, 2*, 169–187.

Matson, J. L., Dempsey, T., & Fodstad, J. C. (2009). Stereotypies and repetitive/restrictive behaviours in infants with autism and pervasive developmental disorder. *Developmental Neurorehabilitation, 12*, 122–127.

Matson, J. L., Kiely, S. L., & Bamburg, J. W. (1997). The effect of stereotypies on adaptive skills as assessed with the DASH-II and Vineland Adaptive Behavior Scales. *Research in Developmental Disabilities, 18*, 471–476.

Matson, J. L., & Rivet, T. T. (2008). Characteristics of challenging behaviours in adults with autistic disorder, PDD-NOS, and intellectual disability. *Journal of Intellectual and Developmental Disability, 33*, 323–329.

McClintock, K. K., Hall, S. S., & Oliver, C. (2003). Risk markers associated with challenging behaviours in people with intellectual disabilities: A meta-analytic study. *Journal of Intellectual Disability Research, 47*, 405–416.

McComas, J., Hoch, H., Paone, D., & El-Roy, D. (2000). Escape behavior during academic tasks: A preliminary analysis of idiosyncratic establishing conditions. *Journal of Applied Behavior Analysis, 33*, 479–493.

McComas, J. J., Thompson, A., & Johnson, L. (2003). The effects of presession attention on problem behavior maintained by different reinforcers. *Journal of Applied Behavior Analysis, 36*, 297–307.

McCord, B. E., Grosser, J. W., Iwata, B. A., & Powers, L. A. (2005). An analysis of response-blocking parameters in the prevention of pica. *Journal of Applied Behavior Analysis, 38*, 391–394.

McCord, B. E., Thomson, R. J., & Iwata, B. A. (2001). Functional analysis and treatment of self-injury associated with transitions. *Journal of Applied Behavior Analysis, 34*, 195–210.

Meyer, E. A., Hagopian, L. P., & Paclawskyj, T. R. (1999). A function-based treatment for school refusal behavior using shaping and fading. *Research in Developmental Disabilities, 20*, 401–410.

Miles, N. I., & Wilder, D. A. (2009). The effects of behavioral skills training on caregiver implementation of guided compliance. *Journal of Applied Behavior Analysis, 42*, 405–410.

Millichap, D., Oliver, C., McQuillan, S., Kalsy, S., Lloyd, V., & Hall, S. (2003). Descriptive functional analysis of behavioral excesses shown by adults with Down syndrome and dementia. *International Journal of Geriatric Psychiatry, 18*, 844–854.

Miltenberger, R. (1999). Understanding problem behaviors through functional assessment. In N. A. Wieseler & R. H. Hanson (Eds.), *Challenging behavior of persons with mental health disorders and severe developmental disabilities* (pp. 215–235). Washington, DC: American Association on Mental Retardation.

Moss, J. J., Oliver, C., Hall, S. S., Arron, K. K., Sloneem, J. J., & Petty, J. J. (2005). The association between environmental events and self-injurious behaviour in Cornelia de Lange syndrome. *Journal of Intellectual Disability Research, 49*, 269–277.

Murphy, G., Macdonald, S., Hall, S., & Oliver, C. (2000). Aggression and the termination of "rituals": A new variant of the escape function for challenging behavior? *Research in Developmental Disabilities, 21*, 43–5.

Nahgahgwon, K. N., Umbreit, J., Liaupsin, C. J., & Turton, A. M. (2010). Function-based planning for young children at-risk for emotional and behavioral disorders. *Education & Treatment of Children, 33*, 537–559.

Najdowski, A. C., Wallace, M. D., Ellsworth, C. L., MacAleese, A. N., & Cleveland, J. M. (2008). Functional analyses and treatment of precursor behavior. *Journal of Applied Behavior Analysis, 41*, 97–105.

Najdowski, A. C., Wallace, M. D., Penrod, B., Tarbox, J., Reagon, K., & Higher, T. S. (2008). Caregiver conducted experimental functional analyses of inappropriate mealtime behavior. *Journal of Applied Behavior Analysis, 41,* 459–465.

Nicholson, J., Konstantinidi, E., & Furniss, F. (2006). On some psychometric properties of the questions about behavioral function (QABF) scale. *Research in Developmental Disabilities, 27,* 337–352.

Northup, J., & Gulley, V. (2001). Some contributions of functional analysis to the assessment of behaviors associated with attention deficit hyperactivity disorder and the effects of stimulant medication. *School Psychology Review, 30,* 227–238.

Northup, J., Wacker, D., Sasso, G., & Steege, M. (1991). A brief functional analysis of aggressive and alternative behavior in an outclinic setting. *Journal of Applied Behavior Analysis, 24,* 509–522.

Nyhan, W. L. (2002). Lessons from Lesch-Nyhan syndrome. In S. R. Schroeder, M. Oster-Granite, T. Thompson, S. R. Schroeder, M. Oster-Granite, & T. Thompson (Eds.), *Self-injurious behavior: Gene-brain-behavior relationships* (pp. 251–267). Washington, DC: American Psychological Association.

Oliver, C., Arron, K., Hall, S., Sloneem, J., Forman, D., & McClintock, K. (2006). Effects of social context on social interaction and self-injurious behavior in Cornelia de Lange syndrome. *American Journal on Mental Retardation, 111,* 184–192.

Oliver, C., Murphy, G. H., Crayton, L., & Corbett, J. A. (1993). Self-injurious behavior in Rett syndrome: Interactions between features of Rett syndrome and operant conditioning. *Journal of Autism and Developmental Disorders, 23,* 91–109.

Oliver, C., & Richards, C. (2010). Self-injurious behaviour in people with intellectual disability. *Current Opinion in Psychiatry, 23,* 412–416.

Olson, L., & Houlihan, D. (2000). A review of behavioral treatments used for Lesch-Nyhan syndrome. *Behavior Modification, 24,* 202–222.

O'Neill, R. E., Horner, R. H., Sprague, J. R., Storey, K., & Newton, J. S. (1997). *Functional assessment and program development for problem behavior: A practical handbook* (2nd ed.). Florence: Brookes/Cole.

O'Reilly, M. F., Murray, N., Lancioni, G. E., Sigafoos, J., & Lacey, C. (2003). Functional analysis and intervention to reduce self-injurious and agitated behavior when removing protective equipment for brief time periods. *Behavior Modification, 27,* 538–559.

O'Reilly, M., Rispoli, M., Davis, T., Machalicek, W., Lang, R., Sigafoos, J., et al. (2010). Functional analysis of challenging behavior in children with autism spectrum disorders: A summary of 10 cases. *Research in Autism Spectrum Disorders, 4,* 1–10.

Oswald, D. P., Ellis, C. R., Singh, N. N., & Singh, Y. N. (1994). Self-injury. In J. L. Matson & J. L. Matson (Eds.), *Autism in children and adults: Etiology, assessment, and intervention* (pp. 147–164). Belmont: Thomson Brooks/Cole.

Paclawskyj, T. R., Matson, J. L., Rush, K. S., Smalls, Y., & Vollmer, T. R. (2000). Questions About Behavioral Function (QABF): A behavioral checklist for functional assessment of aberrant behavior. *Research in Developmental Disabilities, 21,* 223–229.

Paclawskyj, T. R., Matson, J. L., Rush, K. S., Smalls, Y. Y., & Vollmer, T. R. (2001). Assessment of the convergent validity of the Questions About Behavioral Function scale with analogue functional analysis and the Motivation Assessment Scale. *Journal of Intellectual Disability Research, 45,* 484–494.

Patel, M. R., Carr, J. E., Kim, C., Robles, A., & Eastridge, D. (2000). Functional analysis of aberrant behavior maintained by automatic reinforcement: Assessments of specific sensory reinforcers. *Research in Developmental Disabilities, 21,* 393–407.

Patterson, G. R., Chamberlain, P., & Reid, J. B. (1982). A comparative evaluation of a parent-training program. *Behavior Therapy, 13,* 638–650.

Patti, P. J., & Tsiouris, J. A. (2006). Psychopathology in adults with Down syndrome: Clinical findings from an outpatient clinic. *International Journal on Disability and Human Development, 5,* 357–364.

Pelios, L., Morren, J., Tesch, D., & Axelrod, S. (1999). The impact of functional analysis methodology on treatment choice for self-injurious and aggressive behavior. *Journal of Applied Behavior Analysis, 32,* 185–195.

Petursdottir, A. I., Esch, J. W., Sautter, R. A., & Stewart, K. K. (2010). Characteristics and hypothesized functions of challenging behavior in a community-based sample. *Education and Training in Autism and Developmental Disabilities, 45,* 81–93.

Peyton, R. T., Lindauer, S. E., & Richman, D. M. (2005). The effects of directive and nondirective prompts on noncompliant vocal behavior exhibited by a child with autism. *Journal of Applied Behavior Analysis, 38,* 251–255.

Piazza, C. C., Adelinis, J. D., Hanley, G. P., Goh, H., & Delia, M. D. (2000). An evaluation of the effects of matched stimuli on behaviors maintained by automatic reinforcement. *Journal of Applied Behavior Analysis, 33,* 13–27.

Piazza, C. C., Fisher, W. W., Brown, K. A., Shore, B. A., Patel, M. R., Katz, R., et al. (2003). Functional analysis of inappropriate mealtime behaviors. *Journal of Applied Behavior Analysis, 36,* 187–204.

Piazza, C. C., Fisher, W. W., Hanley, G. P., & Lindauer, S. E. (1998). Treatment of pica through multiple analyses of its reinforcing functions. *Journal of Applied Behavior Analysis, 31,* 165–189.

Piazza, C. C., Hanley, G. P., Bowman, L. G., Ruyter, J. M., Lindauer, S. E., & Saiontz, D. M. (1997). Functional analysis and treatment of elopement. *Journal of Applied Behavior Analysis, 30,* 653–672.

Piazza, C. C., Hanley, G. P., & Fisher, W. W. (1996). Functional analysis and treatment of cigarette pica. *Journal of Applied Behavior Analysis, 29,* 437–450.

Piazza, C. C., & Roane, H. S. (2009). Assessment of pediatric feeding disorders. In J. L. Matson, F. Andrasik,

M. L. Matson, J. L. Matson, F. Andrasik, & M. L. Matson (Eds.), *Assessing childhood psychopathology and developmental disabilities* (pp. 471–490). New York: Springer.

Piazza, C. C., Roane, H. S., Keeney, K. M., Boney, B. R., & Abt, K. A. (2002). Varying response effort in the treatment of pica maintained by automatic reinforcement. *Journal of Applied Behavior Analysis, 35*, 233–246.

Radstaake, M., Didden, R., Bolio, M., Lang, R., Lancioni, G. E., & Curfs, L. G. (2011). Functional assessment and behavioral treatment of skin picking in a teenage girl with Prader-Willi syndrome. *Clinical Case Studies, 10*, 67–78.

Rapp, J. T. (2006). Toward an empirical method for identifying matched stimulation for automatically reinforced behavior: A preliminary investigation. *Journal of Applied Behavior Analysis, 39*, 137–140.

Rapp, J. T., & Vollmer, T. R. (2005). Stereotypy I: A review of behavioral assessment and treatment. *Research in Developmental Disabilities, 26*, 527–547.

Rasmussen, K., & O'Neill, R. E. (2006). The effects of fixed-time reinforcement schedules on problem behavior of children with emotional and behavioral disorders in a day-treatment classroom setting. *Journal of Applied Behavior Analysis, 39*, 453–457.

Reed, D. D., Pace, G. M., & Luiselli, J. K. (2009). An investigation into the provision of choice in tangible conditions of a functional analysis. *Journal of Developmental and Physical Disabilities, 21*, 485–491.

Restori, A. F., Gresham, F. M., Chang, T., Lee, H. B., & Laija-Rodriquez, W. (2007). Functional assessment-based interventions for children at-risk for emotional and behavioral disorders. *California School Psychologist, 12*, 9–30.

Richman, D. M., & Hagopian, L. P. (1999). On the effects of 'quality' of attention in the functional analysis of destructive behavior. *Research in Developmental Disabilities, 20*, 51–62.

Ringdahl, J. E., Christensen, T. J., & Boelter, E. W. (2009). Further evaluation of idiosyncratic functions for severe problem behavior: Aggression maintained by access to walks. *Behavioral Interventions, 24*, 275–283.

Rodriguez, N. M., Thompson, R. H., & Baynham, T. Y. (2010). Assessment of the relative effects of attention and escape on noncompliance. *Journal of Applied Behavior Analysis, 43*, 143–147.

Rortvedt, A. K., & Miltenberger, R. G. (1994). Analysis of a high-probability instructional sequence and time-out in the treatment of child noncompliance. *Journal of Applied Behavior Analysis, 27*, 327–330.

Roscoe, E. M., Kindle, A. E., & Pence, S. T. (2010). Functional analysis and treatment of aggression maintained by preferred conversational topics. *Journal of Applied Behavior Analysis, 43*, 723–727.

Roscoe, E. M., Rooker, G. W., Pence, S. T., & Longworth, L. J. (2009). Assessing the utility of a demand assessment for functional analysis. *Journal of Applied Behavior Analysis, 42*, 819–825.

Sainato, D. M., Strain, P. S., Lefebvre, D., & Rapp, N. (1987). Facilitating transition times with handicapped preschool children: A comparison between peer-mediated and antecedent prompt procedures. *Journal of Applied Behavior Analysis, 20*, 285–291.

Sasso, G. M., Reimers, T. M., Cooper, L. J., & Wacker, D. P. (1992). Use of descriptive and experimental analyses to identify the functional properties of aberrant behavior in school settings. *Journal of Applied Behavior Analysis, 25*, 809–821.

Schieltz, K. M., Wacker, D. P., Harding, J. W., Berg, W. K., Lee, J. F., & Dalmau, Y. (2010). An evaluation of manding across functions prior to functional communication training. *Journal of Developmental and Physical Disabilities, 22*, 131–147.

Scott, T. M., Anderson, C., Mancil, R., & Alter, P. (2009). Function-based supports for individual students in school settings. In W. Sailor, G. Dunlop, G. Sugai, & R. Horner (Eds.), *Handbook of positive behavior support* (pp. 421–441). New York: Springer.

Scotti, J. R., Evans, I. M., Meyer, L. H., & Walker, P. (1991). A meta-analysis of intervention research with problem behavior: Treatment validity and standards of practice. *American Journal on Mental Retardation, 96*, 233–256.

Singh, N. N., Donatelli, L. S., Best, A. A., & Williams, D. E. (1993). Factor structure of the Motivation Assessment Scale. *Journal of Intellectual Disability Research, 37*, 65–74.

Skinner, B. F. (1953). *Science and human behavior*. Oxford, England: Macmillan.

Slifer, K., Iwata, B. A., & Dorsey, M. F. (1984). Reduction of eye gouging using a response interruption procedure. *Journal of Behavior Therapy and Experimental Psychiatry, 15*, 369–375.

Smith, K. M., & Matson, J. L. (2010). Behavior problems: Differences among intellectually disabled adults with co-morbid autism spectrum disorders and epilepsy. *Research in Developmental Disabilities, 31*, 1062–1069.

Stahr, B., Cushing, D., Lane, K., & Fox, J. (2006). Efficacy of a function-based intervention in decreasing off-task behavior exhibited by a student with ADHD. *Journal of Positive Behavior Interventions, 8*, 201–211.

Stage, S. A., Jackson, H. G., Moscovitz, K., Erickson, M., Thurman, S., et al. (2006). Using multimethod-multisource functional behavioral assessment for students with behavioral disabilities. *School Psychology Review, 35*, 451–471.

Stokes, J. V., & Luiselli, J. K. (2009). Applied behavior analysis assessment and intervention for health: Threatening self-injury (rectal picking) in an adult with Prader-Willi syndrome. *Clinical Case Studies, 8*, 38–47.

Strachan, R., Shaw, R., Burrow, C., Horsler, K., Allen, D., & Oliver, C. (2009). Experimental functional analysis of aggression in children with Angelman syndrome. *Research in Developmental Disabilities, 30*, 1095–1106.

Sturmey, P. (1996). *Functional analysis in clinical psychology*. Oxford, England: Wiley.

Tarbox, J., Wallace, M. D., Tarbox, R. F., Landaburu, H. J., & Williams, W. (2004). Functional analysis and treatment of low-rate problem behavior in individuals with developmental disabilities. *Behavioral Interventions, 19*, 73–90.

Tarbox, R. S. F., Wallace, M. D., & Williams, L. (2003). Assessment and treatment of elopement: A replication and extension. *Journal of Applied Behavior Analysis, 36*, 239–244.

Tarbox, J., Wilke, A. E., Najdowski, A. C., Findel-Pyles, R. S., Balasanyan, S., Caveney, A. C., et al. (2009). Comparing indirect, descriptive, and experimental functional assessments of challenging behavior in children with autism. *Journal of Developmental and Physical Disabilities, 21*, 493–514.

Tate, B. G., & Baroff, G. S. (1966). Aversive control of self-injurious behavior in a psychotic boy. *Behavior Research and Therapy, 4*, 281–287.

Taylor, L. L., & Oliver, C. C. (2008). The behavioural phenotype of Smith-Magenis syndrome: Evidence for a gene-environment interaction. *Journal of Intellectual Disability Research, 52*, 830–841.

Thompson, R. H., Fisher, W. W., Piazza, C. C., & Kuhn, D. E. (1998). The evaluation and treatment of aggression maintained by attention and automatic reinforcement. *Journal of Applied Behavior Analysis, 31*, 103–116.

Thompson, R. H., & Iwata, B. A. (2007). A comparison of outcomes from descriptive and functional analyses of problem behavior. *Journal of Applied Behavior Analysis, 40*, 333–338.

Turner, M. (1999). Annotation: Repetitive behavior in autism: A review of psychological research. *Journal of Child Psychology and Psychiatry, 40*, 839–849.

Tuten, M., Jones, H. E., Ertel, J., Jakubowski, J., & Sperlein, J. (2006, June). Reinforcement-based treatment: A novel approach to treating substance abuse during pregnancy. *Counselor Magazine*, 22–29.

Virues-Ortega, J., & Haynes, S. N. (2005). Functional analysis in behavior therapy: Behavioral foundations and clinical application. *International Journal of Clinical and Healthy Psychology, 5*, 567–587.

Volkert, V. M., & Vaz, P. C. M. (2010). Recent studies on feeding problems in children with autism. *Journal of Applied Behavior Analysis, 43*, 155–159.

Vollmer, T. R., Marcus, B. A., Ringdahl, J. E., & Roane, H. S. (1995). Progressing from brief assessments to extended experimental analyses in the evaluation of aberrant behavior. *Journal of Applied Behavior Analysis, 28*, 561–576.

Vollmer, T. R., Northup, J., Ringdahl, J. E., LeBlanc, L. A., & Chauvin, T. M. (1996). Functional analysis of severe tantrums displayed by children with language delays: An outclinic assessment. *Behavior Modification, 20*, 97–115.

Weiss, M., Fiske, K., & Ferraioli, S. (2009). Treatment of autism spectrum disorders. In J. L. Matson, F. Andrasik, & M. L. Matson (Eds.), *Treating childhood psychopathology and developmental disabilities* (pp. 287–332). New York: Springer.

Wilder, D. A., Chen, L., Atwell, J., Pritchard, J., & Weinstein, P. (2006). Brief functional analysis and treatment of tantrums associated with transitions in preschool children. *Journal of Applied Behavior Analysis, 39*, 103–107.

Wilder, D. A., Harris, C., Reagan, R., & Rasey, A. (2007). Functional analysis and treatment of noncompliance by preschool children. *Journal of Applied Behavior Analysis, 40*, 173–177.

Wilder, D. A., Normand, M., & Atwell, J. (2005). Noncontingent reinforcement as treatment for food refusal and associated self-injury. *Journal of Applied Behavior Analysis, 38*, 549–553.

Wilder, D. A., Register, M., Register, S., Bajagic, V., & Neidert, P. L. (2009). Functional analysis and treatment of rumination using fixed-time delivery of a flavor spray. *Journal of Applied Behavior Analysis, 42*, 877–882.

Williams, K. E., Field, D. G., & Sieverling, L. (2010). Food refusal in children: A review of the literature. *Research in Developmental Disabilities, 31*, 625–628.

Woodcock, K. K., Oliver, C. C., & Humphreys, G. G. (2009). Associations between repetitive questioning, resistance to change, temper outbursts and anxiety in Prader–Willi and Fragile-X syndromes. *Journal of Intellectual Disability Research, 53*, 265–278.

Methods of Defining and Observing Behaviors

6

Sarah Hurwitz and Noha F. Minshawi

Introduction

In functional analysis, the ability to track the occurrence of a target behavior is essential to being able to identify what factors maintain that behavior. This is so fundamental that to overlook the crucial step of defining and observing behaviors in designing an intervention or research study is to open the door to a large number of reliability and validity issues in our research and integrity and generalization problems in our treatments. Therefore, taking the time a priori to carefully consider the behaviors to be targeted and how best to measure these behaviors over time is the first step to sound intervention and research.

There are several reasons why creating operational definitions and recording data on behaviors is so important to social and behavioral sciences as a whole and to functional analysis in particular (Haynes & O'Brien, 2000). Defining behaviors accurately is necessary in order to make a diagnosis, and many psychological diagnoses require the presence of specific, observable behaviors.

Clear definitions of behaviors also serve to enhance communication between practitioners, caregivers, and other individuals involved in research or clinical care. Ensuring that all parties are talking about the same behavior allows for valid and reliable data to be collected by multiple people and in different settings. In addition, Haynes and O'Brien (2000) state that the most important reason to create operational definitions of behaviors is to help the clinician and the client carefully consider the behavior and clarify the way that they are thinking about this behavior. This point can be readily transferred to Applied Behavior Analysis (ABA) and other fields where multiple individuals are typically part of the assessment and treatment process, and all team members must be in agreement with the decisions being made.

The focus of this chapter is threefold: (1) to identify target behaviors for research and intervention, (2) to define these target behaviors so that they can be identified by multiple observers across settings, and (3) to illuminate methods to observe and measure the target behaviors. To be more specific, there are several factors to consider when identifying and defining a behavior for research or intervention. First, one must consider whether the behavior is clinically or socially significant enough to warrant further attention. While this is a point that is often overlooked or taken for granted, the decision of which behaviors to study is just as important as the manner in which we go about studying the behaviors.

S. Hurwitz (✉) • N.F. Minshawi
Department of Psychiatry, Indiana University School of Medicine, Indianapolis, IN, USA

Christian Sarkine Autism Treatment Center, James Whitcomb Riley Hospital for Children, Indiana University School of Medicine, Indianapolis, IN 46202, USA
e-mail: sarahbethhurwitz@gmail.com; nminshaw@iupui.edu

J.L. Matson (ed.), *Functional Assessment for Challenging Behaviors*, Autism and Child Psychopathology Series, DOI 10.1007/978-1-4614-3037-7_6, © Springer Science+Business Media, LLC 2012

The second goal of this chapter is to provide guidelines for defining these target behaviors. It is important to determine which aspects of the behavior are most important in order to ensure that the targets of the study have ecological validity and clinical significance. Once this has been determined, the behavior must be operationally defined with sufficient detail that interrater reliability can be obtained. Operational definitions for a number of commonly observed problem behaviors are included in this chapter to provide the reader with examples of different ways in which these behaviors have been defined in the recent literature.

The final goal of this chapter is to present information on different methods of data collection that are of particular relevance to functional analysis. Once it has been determined that a behavior is of significant interest to warrant data collection and the behavior has been operationally defined, the next step is to determine the appropriate data collection methodology. It is important to make a good match between the target behavior and the method that will best capture the occurrences of that behavior. Proper consideration of the strengths and weaknesses of different data collection systems is vital to ensuring that the appropriate aspects of the behavior will be captured and the data collected can be used meaningfully.

Identifying Target Behaviors

The first step in identifying target behaviors is to determine if a behavior is of significant enough concern to merit intervention. In other words, one must ask: Is this behavior important? Sometimes this important question is overlooked for a number of reasons. For example, some might think that if one person finds the behavior to be problematic, then that is sufficient reason to intervene. Others might think that if a behavior is "interesting" or "unique," then the behavior must be a worthwhile research target. While these may be appropriate rationales at times, they typically are not able to stand alone. Instead, one must consider other aspects of a behavior that may make it an appropriate target, including whether the behavior in question is socially significant, dangerous, results in restrictions being placed on the individual, and whether the behavior interferes with the acquisition of other skills (Hanley, Iwata, & McCord, 2003). In addition, it is important to keep in mind that we often want to focus our attention on the promotion of new, adaptive skills in addition to decreasing less desirable behaviors.

Social Significance

The social significance of a target behavior is one important factor to consider in evaluating a potential target behavior. Behaviors can be socially significant for a number of reasons. The behavior may be significant in that it impairs an individual's ability to interact with others in his or her community. For example, if a child engages in severe tantrum behaviors when his parents take him to church, his parents may begin to limit the amount of time the child attends church or may leave the child at home while the rest of the family attends church. Another way that a behavior can be socially significant is if the behavior results in a negative appraisal of the individual by other people. This can frequently be the case with repetitive behaviors, such as hand flapping, in individuals with Autistic Disorder. Because hand flapping is not a behavior observed in typical social interactions, the fact that an individual is flapping her hands may result in other people viewing her as "different." These negative appraisals can lead to decreased attempts by others to interact with the person with socially significant behavior issues and thereby reduce opportunities for socialization.

Dangerous Behaviors/Risk for Harm

A behavior that places an individual and those around him or her at risk for bodily harm may be reason for intervention or study. The behaviors most commonly associated with risk for harm are physical aggression and self-injurious behaviors (SIB). Physical aggression and SIB are among the most common reasons for inpatient admissions for individuals with developmental disabilities (Mandell, 2008) due to the potential for injury. As a result, these behaviors often come to the attention of researchers and clinicians so they can be addressed before they cause severe injury. Behaviors that currently cause injury or have the potential to cause injury without intervention often become high priority research and intervention targets.

Restrictive Behaviors

Many behavior problems are significant because of the degree of restriction these behaviors can place on the living, educational placements, and quality of life of individuals with developmental disabilities. Individuals with severe behavior problems are more likely to be placed in more restrictive living environments, such as group homes and residential facilities (Lakin, Hill, Hauber, Bruininks, & Heal, 1983). In addition, behavior problems can greatly limit the degree to which children with developmental disabilities and other psychiatric conditions can be integrated into classroom environments with their neuro-typically developing peers. As was previously mentioned, some behavior problems can limit the amount of social interactions and social opportunities available as well.

Interfering Behaviors

Finally, when considering whether a specific behavior problem should become the focus of an intervention or a research study, one should also consider the degree to which the behavior in question interferes with the ability to engage in or learn more appropriate behaviors. For example, parents may be concerned that their 5-year-old daughter is not yet toilet trained. But when questioned about prior toilet training attempts, the parents may report that whenever they attempt to seat the child on the toilet, she engages in tantrum behaviors that consist of crying, screaming, and dropping to the ground. These behaviors are severe enough that the parents eventually terminate the demand and allow the child to avoid sitting on the toilet. The tantrum behaviors that are initially not presented as a target for intervention clearly become more clinically relevant when one considers that these behaviors are interfering with the child's ability to learn a new, more adaptive skill. Careful consideration of the antecedents to behavior problems and the consequences evoked by the behavior will assist in determining whether the behavior is potentially interfering with acquisition or demonstration of more appropriate skills.

Adaptive Skills

While the majority of behavioral research and clinical intervention is focused on maladaptive or inappropriate behaviors, such as aggression and SIB, it is important that clinicians and researchers not forget that adaptive and appropriate behaviors should also be considered as behavioral targets. The prior discussion regarding socially significant behaviors can be applied to determining which adaptive skills that may be targeted in research or clinical intervention. While we may consider a behavior problematic if it limits opportunities for social interaction, an adaptive behavior may be targeted because of its ability to facilitate interactions with others. For example, teaching a young child to say "Hi" or "Do you want to play?" are useful adaptive skills because these two behaviors may lead to further socialization opportunities, such as a conversation or play. Furthermore, if a problem behavior leads to negative appraisals from others, then we may consider teaching adaptive behaviors that can lead to positive appraisals. Teaching appropriate hygiene skills may help to avoid negative appraisals, while teaching workplace etiquette such as how to engage in small talk in the break room may lead to coworkers viewing an individual in a more positive manner. Regardless of the skill, it is important that researchers and clinicians carefully consider the adaptive behaviors that can and should be taught to individuals with developmental disabilities.

Creating Operational Definitions of Target Behaviors

Once a target behavior has been selected based on the criteria detailed above, the prescribed process for conducting a functional assessment typically begins with the operational definition of the target behavior (Tassé, 2006). This step is crucial and without a clearly defined target behavior it is almost impossible to ensure the reliability of the data being recorded.

Kazdin (2001) recommends three criteria for creating operational definitions of target behaviors. First, the behavior should be defined *objectively*. An objective definition is one that is based on the characteristics of the behavior that can be observed. Therefore, the behavior should not be something that is unobservable, such as a thought, opinion, or motivation. In addition, one should avoid placing subjective, moral, or social judgments into the behavioral definitions. For example, stating that a behavior is "mean" or "cruel" might imply that the individual engaging in the behavior has malicious intent, which may not always be the case. This type of subjectivity in describing behaviors can also negatively influence the individuals collecting data.

Second, the definition should be *clear and unambiguous*. The rule of thumb that Kazdin (2001) provides is that an observer should be able to read the behavioral definition, repeat it, and paraphrase it with little explanation from the individual who wrote the definition. Unfortunately, many terms used to describe behavior are ambiguous. For example, a teacher might report that a child is "difficult" or "out of control." Although this is type of statement might be compelling, it is not measurable. By eliminating the subjectivity in definitions, one can ensure that all individuals involved in data collection will be taking data on the same behavior and not their subjective opinion of the behavior. Converting ambiguous terms into clear statements that can be observed and measured is a crucial component to a good operational definition.

This is an especially important point to consider when a clinician has chosen to rely on other

Table 6.1 Examples of ambiguous terms vs. quantifiable descriptions of behaviors

Ambiguous term	Quantifiable description
Disruptive behavior	Child throws his work on the floor and overturns his chair
Tantrum	Child lays on the floor, yells, and kicks her feet
Aggression	Child hits his brother with an open hand
Being mean	Child curses at her classmates

individuals, such as parents or teachers, to take behavioral data. There are many colloquial terms for problem behaviors that may have different meanings in different geographical areas and cultures. For example, one parent may say that her child has a "meltdown" when she screams and cries, while the teacher may consider these behaviors to be a "fit" or "tantrum." If both of these individuals are responsible for taking data on the screaming and crying behavior of the child but terms are not clearly and quantifiably defined, then the data will lack reliability and potentially validity. Table 6.1 provides examples of ambiguous terms for common problem behaviors and how these behaviors can be described in a quantifiable way.

Kazdin (2001) makes the final point that the operational definition of a behavior should be *complete*. All of the responses that fall within the definition should be clearly outlined, and the responses that should be included and excluded should be defined and enumerated. The completeness of a definition is important when one considers the complexity of the behaviors that are the focus of functional behavioral assessments (FBA). One way in which one can ensure that a definition is complete is to consider including all possible topographies of the behavior. The topography of a behavior is what the behavior looks like in objective terms. For example, "physical aggression" can include topographies such as hitting with an open hand, biting, kicking, head-butting, grabbing, and any number of other related behaviors. In order for an operational definition to be complete, it should include all of the topographies of the behavior that are of concern and explicitly exclude topographies that are not relevant to the target behavior. While we know that topography does not provide information as to the function of a target behavior, topography can be important in creating an operational definition that is clear, concise, and complete.

Examples of Operationally Defined Target Behaviors

In contemplating how to go about operationally defining a behavior of interest, it is sometimes helpful to consider the way that the behavior has been defined by other researchers. Table 6.2 presents examples of how several common problem behaviors have been defined in the recent literature. While many of these examples come from the field of ABA, operational definitions were also obtained from other child-focused research. By studying the definitions of problem behaviors utilized by researchers across several disciplines,

one can develop a greater appreciation for the fact that the definitions of these behaviors can vary greatly, and without proper definitions, we can never be entirely sure that we are all speaking the same language. In reviewing the definitions provided, it is significant to note that the definitions are clear, succinct, and complete and all provide sufficient detail that another individual could read the definitions and begin taking data on the behaviors without need for further clarification or explanation.

Observation Methods

Once it has been determined that a behavior is significant enough to target with an intervention and the behavior has been operationally defined, the next step is to select an appropriate observation measurement system for use throughout the intervention or research study. There are several

Table 6.2 Examples of operationally defined target behaviors

Target behavior	Operational definition	References
Tantrum	"…saying 'I don't want to' or 'no' at a volume above normal conversational level, and whining, defined as a high-pitched, unintelligible cry"	Wilder, Chen, Atwell, Pritchard, and Weinstein (2006)
Tantrum	"…excessive tantrums without aggression (tantrums that do not include aggression or violence but that included shouting, crying, and/or nondirected flailing movements)"	Belden, Thomson, and Luby (2008)
Noncompliance	"…Noncompliance was defined as refusing to carry out instructions or requests made by the mother"	Singh et al. (2006)
Noncompliance	"Verbally skilled noncompliance was defined as the child not following directions, but instead trying to talk things out reasonably and calmly with the mother"	Johnston, Murray, & Ng (2007)
Self-injury	"SIB was defined as using any part of the body to hit another part of the body, using any part of the body to hit a surface, biting self and kicking self"	Kerth, Progar, and Morales (2009)
Self-injury	"SIB was defined as any open- or closed-fist hand-to-head or fist-to-body contact; knee-to-head contact from any distance; or leg-to-leg contact"	Magnusson and Gould (2007)
Stereotypy	"Holding toy near eyes and repeatedly swinging it back and forth"	Lang et al. (2010)
Stereotypy	"*Vocal stereotypy* was defined as acontextual audible sounds or words produced with an open or closed mouth"	Lanovaz, Fletcher, and Rapp (2009)
Physical aggression	"Aggression consisted of hitting, kicking, punching, grabbing, pulling hair, and throwing objects from less than 0.3 m from another person"	Kahng, Abt, and Schonbachler (2001)
Physical aggression	"…defined as hitting, slapping, and sitting on a therapist"	Roane, Fisher, Sgro, Falcomata, and Pabico (2004)

ways to generate information about problem behaviors including parent or teacher interviews, questionnaires, standardized assessments, and direct observation. An interview or other assessment tool can provide important information about which behaviors to examine and the context(s) in which these behaviors occur. Although interviews and standardized assessments play a role in functional analysis, their utility is somewhat limited because interviews and questionnaires rely on anecdotal reports (Hanley et al., 2003), and standardized assessments cannot be repeated frequently. On the other hand, making observations directly provides clear, replicable, and reliable data about behavior. Additionally, direct observation can be conducted in the child's natural environment and provides a concrete record of what is observed there (Rogers, 2001).

Using direct observation to collect data about behavior is a key component to functional analysis. "One advantage of the direct method is that the observer is recording the antecedents, behaviors, and consequences as they occur rather than reporting them from someone's memory. This information is likely to be more objective and accurate when it is derived from direct observation" (p. 139, Barnhill, 2005). One downside to direct observation is that it can be quite time-consuming and labor intensive. The time and effort involved provides important information, but it may not be practical in all circumstances. Since direct observation is the method used most commonly in functional assessment (Hanley et al., 2003), the remainder of this chapter will focus on developing measurement systems for direct observation of behavior.

Location

One of the first issues to be addressed prior to selecting a measurement system is determining the location(s) in which behaviors will be observed. Data can be taken in the child's natural environment (i.e., in his/her classroom or home, or in the community) or in a clinic or laboratory setting. The choice of location is dependent on the conditions under which the behavior is most

likely to be seen. For example, if the target behavior is related disruptive behavior in the classroom, naturally, the observation must take place in the classroom setting. On the other hand, there are times when observations are not practical in the child's natural environment. For example, if the targeted behavior may result in harm to others, such as aggressive behavior, then the classroom, where other children may be placed in a dangerous position, may not be an appropriate setting. In these cases, a simulation of the situation in which the behavior is most commonly exhibited can be created in the clinic or laboratory instead. In the clinic or lab, the most probable antecedents and consequences of the target behavior should be employed to elicit the behavior. For whatever setting is selected, the option exists to record the data live (as it happens) or to videotape the session and code the data later.

Selecting a Measurement System

The goal of an observation session is to systematically record the occurrences of the target behavior. In functional assessment, these observations will be repeated frequently and compared over time and across social or environmental conditions to determine the function of the behavior (Herzinger & Campbell, 2007). In order for observation sessions to be comparable, the data must be recorded in the same way each time. If the data collection system, targeted behavior, or operational definition of the behavior change between observations, then the data can no longer be compared, and vast amounts of time, effort, and other resources may be lost. Therefore, before any direct observations begin, a systematic plan should be developed to ensure that the target behavior can be recorded accurately and efficiently over time, in all applicable settings, and by different observers.

The first step in choosing a measurement system is to start with a clear definition of the target behavior. The definition should include important parameters of the behavior, such as what the behavior looks like, when it begins and

Table 6.3 Characteristics of behavioral measurement systems

Measurement system	Behavioral features	Example target behavior
Event recording	High or low frequency; discrete	Aggression
Partial-interval recording	High frequency; can be difficult to count	Hand flapping
Whole-interval recording	High frequency; continuous	Being on-task in classroom
Time sampling	Low frequency; continuous	Wandering around classroom
Duration	Lasts a relatively long time; behavior has a clear beginning and end	Tantrums

ends, if it continues for a long time, and if it occurs frequently or not. Once there is an operational definition, the system that measures the behavior most effectively and usefully should be chosen. Frequency and duration of the behavior are the two most important factors to consider when choosing a recording system.

Behaviors that occur frequently may occur quickly and then be over (e.g., calling out an answer or hitting a sibling), or they may last for a longer time (e.g., wandering around the room unengaged or throwing a tantrum). Behaviors can also be very discrete, meaning they have easily recognizable beginnings and ends (like raising a hand to answer a question), or they can be more difficult to measure precisely (as in repetitive hand flapping behavior). All of these factors of the behavior should be thought about as the match between the target behavior and the measurement system is made.

Depending on the type of behavior being examined, the data will be recorded as a frequency count, a rate of occurrence, or duration of the behavior. For behaviors that are frequent, it may be important to record each incident of the behavior during a specific period of time, or it may be more important to examine the length of time that the behavior lasts. For less frequently occurring behavior, it may be impractical to have a dedicated observer wait all day to see the behavior so a sampling procedure employed by an observer who is also doing other things might be more useful. There are several coding systems commonly used for behavioral observations; four of the most commonly used systems are (1) event coding, (2) interval coding (partial and whole intervals), (3) time sampling, and (4) duration coding (Table 6.3).

Types of Measurement Systems

Event Recording

Event recording provides a frequency count of a behavior over an allotted amount of time. This means that for each observation session, one can know the exact number of times that the target behavior occurred. Event recording is best used to track discrete behaviors (behaviors that have a clear beginning and a clear end). These can be positive or negative behaviors, such as correctly using a target word, making inappropriate vocalizations during class, hitting another child, or throwing learning materials on the floor.

The first step in event recording is to determine how long an observation period will be (e.g., 10 min, an hour, the entire day, or across a week). For high frequency behaviors, a sample of time can give sufficient information, particularly if you choose the time of day that the behavior is most frequently observed or most problematic. Good times to observe might include 20 min of reading time at school, an hour session of speech therapy, or during a trip to the grocery store. For low-frequency behaviors, it may be necessary to record every instance that the behavior occurs. For example, it might be important to document each instance of aggression toward a classmate, even if the aggression happens only once every other day.

During the observation, a notation is made for each time a behavior occurs. A data sheet should include a column to record each instance of the target behavior, the start and the end time for the observation session, as well as who is observing and the date. See Table 6.4 for a sample event recording coding sheet.

Table 6.4 Sample event recording data sheet

Child's name: <u>Jamie</u>
Target behavior: <u>Yells out answer without being called on
by the teacher</u>

Date	Start time	End time	Number of vocalizations	Observer initials
1/21/2011	9:15	9:45	✓✓✓✓	EMG
1/25/2011	9:18	9:50	✓✓	EMG
1/26/2011	9:20	9:50	✓✓✓✓✓	SBH

Table 6.5 Levels of intensity for self-injurious behavior (SIB)

Level 1 intensity = SIB with no visible damage
Level 2 intensity = SIB which results in bruise
Level 3 intensity = SIB which results in breaking of skin
Level 4 intensity = SIB which results in the need for medical intervention

Rate

There are times when observation sessions are of different lengths. In this case, two approaches can be taken. First, the observation could be limited so that each session is always the same length of time. This can be done by ending observations at a specified time even if the activity is not complete or the behavior is still occurring. For example, if the frequency of tantrums during reading time is being targeted, only observe the first 10 min of reading time regardless of how long the reading lesson continues.

The other way to compare sessions of different lengths is to calculate the rate that of the behavior. Rate is the frequency of the behavior expressed as a ratio with time (Alberto & Troutman, 1995). For example, if reading time lasts for 20 min on some days and 30 min on other days, the observation would continue for the full length of reading time each day, and then, a rate of tantrums can be obtained by dividing the frequency by the number of minutes. This would create a rate of tantrums per minute and allow data to be compared across sessions.

To calculate the rate, divide the number occurrences of the behavior by the length of the session. The time element can be per minute, per hour, or some other ratio of time depending on how often the behavior occurs and how long observations are. For example, for a 30-min observation, if there are 15 episodes of the behavior, calculate the per-minute rate by dividing 15 by 30 and obtain the rate of 0.5 episodes per minute. For observation sessions that are of the same length, the rate per activity can also be determined. For example, during 10 min of reading time, if five tantrums are seen, the rate of five tantrums per reading session can be used to compare to the next 10-min observation.

Intensity

There are also scenarios where the frequency of the behavior is not as important as the severity or intensity of each instance. This can be especially valuable information for those behaviors that may occur at a low frequency but may cause varying degrees of harm or damage each time. In these situations, it may be useful to know the level of intensity of each episode of a behavior. How intense a tantrum is or how severe an aggressive event was may be just as important to track as how often the events occur. If this is a critical factor, recording the intensity for each episode of the behavior can provide illuminating information. In order to record intensity, first, develop a rubric by defining observable parameters for each level of the behavior. There can be two levels of intensity (e.g., high and low) or many levels scored on a likert-type scale (e.g., a score of 1 to 5, with 1 being none and 5 being many). Each level should be well defined so that it can be used across observers. An example of four levels of intensity for episodes of SIB is in Table 6.5. To include intensity in data recording, add a column for intensity on to the recording sheet so that for each time the behavior occurs, you note what level of intensity was observed.

Interval Recording

In interval recording, observation sessions are divided into brief time intervals of several seconds each (e.g., 10- or 15-s intervals, usually less than 30 s), and the observer records whether the target behavior occurs in each interval (Barnhill, 2005). This is different from event recording because only some incidents of the behavior will be identified, but an estimate of the behavior is still obtained. Interval recording is especially useful for behaviors that occur very frequently or behaviors that do not have obvious beginnings or ends. There are three main types

Table 6.6 Interval coding for a 5-min observation session of 20-s intervals

Mark each aspect of tantrum behavior seen during each interval
- Behavior 1: whining/crying
- Behavior 2: yelling
- Behavior 3: hitting self on head

Behavior	20	40	60	20	40	60	20	40	60	20	40	60	20	40	60
1	✓	✓	✓	✓	✓										
2		✓	✓	✓											
3			✓												

of interval recording, partial-interval recording, whole-interval recording, and momentary time sampling (see next section below).

In *partial-interval recording*, a notation is made if the behavior is seen at all during the interval. Often, this method is chosen when the target behavior occurs frequently or for behaviors that are not easily counted. For example, if a child is engaging in a repetitive behavior like hand flapping or rocking, it may difficult to count how many times the behavior is repeated. Instead, the child is observed for a short interval, and a notation is made regardless if the behavior is seen once or many times during the interval.

In order to aid data collection, the observer may set aside a few seconds after each interval to write down what happened so that they do not miss occurrences in the next interval. For example, the observer can watch the child for a standard interval of time, say 10 s, and then take the next 5 s to record what happened, return to observation for 10 s, and again record for 5 s until the observation session is complete. Alternatively, if coding via video, the video can be watched for 10 s, paused as notations are recorded, and then play can be resumed to view the next 10-s interval.

Interval recording is summarized by the percentage of total intervals in which the behavior was recorded (Furniss, 2009). For example, if the behavior was noted during 10 out of 30 intervals, there was 30% occurrence of the behavior. This provides an estimate of the total number of times the behavior was seen rather than an exact count. For many purposes, an estimate provides enough information, and an exact count is not necessary.

Whole-interval recording uses the same system as partial-interval recording; only the behavior must be present during the entire interval.

Behaviors that are continuous, like on-task behavior or being out of seat in class, are very appropriate for whole-interval recording. Whole-interval recording is especially useful when there is a behavioral goal of increased sustained behavior (Steege, Watson, & Gresham, 2009). Whole-interval recording produces a conservative estimate of the behavior because if the behavior does not persist for the entire interval, it is not recorded as present.

Table 6.6 is a sample data sheet for partial-interval recording for three aspects of tantrum behavior. In this example, the overall tantrum is divided into three related target behaviors to help identify how extreme the tantrum becomes. If a tantrum occurs during an interval, from one to three, check marks can be made depending on how many aspects of the behavior are seen. In this example, tantrum behavior was seen during 33% of the observation, and it escalated to self-injury for only one interval, about 7% of the time. A column that is left blank indicates that the target behavior was not seen during that interval.

Momentary Time Sampling

Momentary time sampling is commonly used when more frequent observation is not practical (Barnhill, 2005). Momentary time sampling is a subset of interval recording and is best used for behaviors that are not very frequently occurring. These behaviors can be discrete or last for longer periods of time. In momentary time sampling, data is taken at predetermined intervals of time. At a specific time, the observer looks up, records if the behavior is happening at that instant, and then does not make a record again until the prescribed moment of the next interval. This method provides only an estimate of the rate of the target behavior, but it can be very useful if the person recording the data is a teacher or other adult who is doing several things at once.

As an example, a teacher in her classroom is concerned that a child is constantly getting up from his desk and wandering around the room during math lessons. In this case, an interval of five minutes might be used. At the very beginning (or end) of the interval, the teacher looks at the child, records if the child is sitting in his/her seat at that moment, and then continues with her teaching. When another five minutes pass, the teacher again looks at the child and repeats the observation and recording. During a 30-min lesson, the teacher would have six data points recorded about the child's in-seat behavior. However, if the child left his or her seat between observations and then sat back down, this information would be missed. On the other hand, there is enough data to have a good sense of how disruptive the out-of-seat behavior was during the lesson, and the data could be collected without the expense of a dedicated observer. The benefits of time sampling can often outweigh the potential loss of information in settings or with observers who are not able to devote all of their time to collecting data or when data must be collected on multiple individuals at the same time.

Duration Coding

The duration of a behavior refers to how long the behavior lasts. This is important for behaviors that take a long time to resolve, like screaming and crying during an elongated tantrum, or behaviors that are not lasting long enough, like staying on-task during homework time. Some of the same behaviors that can be measured using event recording can also be measured using duration recording. Therefore, a choice of priority must be made: is it more important to know how many times a child engages in the behavior or how long they are spending engaging in the behavior. For example, a child may rock and flap his hands in front of his eyes on four distinct occasions in an hour observation session, but each episode may last for 3 or 4 min. In this case, the duration of time spent during the hour (i.e., 15 min) may be more valuable to know than the number of episodes (i.e., four times), so a dura-

Table 6.7 Duration recording data sheet

Child's name: <u>Jamie</u>
Target behavior: <u>Amount of time child gets out of seat until she is seated again</u>
Date: <u>1/11/2011</u>
Observation start time: <u>11:00 am</u> Observation end time: <u>12:30 pm</u> = Total (mins): <u>90</u>

Episode	Start time	End time	Duration
1	11:03	11:08	5 min
2	11:42	11:50	7 min
3	12:20	12:24	4 min
		Total Duration:	16 min

tion recording would be the measurement system of choice.

Duration can be measured in seconds, minutes, or even hours. A stopwatch or a clock with a second hand is a good tool for measuring duration. As soon as the behavior begins, the stopwatch is clicked on, or the start time is recorded. Time then passes, and when the behavior ends, the stopwatch is clicked off or the end time is recorded. This is repeated for every time the behavior is seen during the observation session. If using the stopwatch, the total cumulative amount of time spent in the behavior will be apparent at the end of the session. If using a clock or watch to record the duration of each episode of the behavior, the total time spent can be added up to give you the duration for the session. A sample recording sheet for duration can be seen in Table 6.7.

In Table 6.7, each episode of the behavior is recorded on a separate line. Using this type of recording sheet also provides a count of frequency because for each duration that is recorded, one occurrence of the behavior is also noted (Glasberg, 2006). Using a stopwatch to time duration does not supply the frequency count, but it is more parsimonious.

Rate

The length of time that a child engages in a behavior can be measured in two ways for duration coding: the average duration and the total duration (Alberto & Troutman, 1995). The average duration is the average time that the child engages in a behavior across the course of a day (or other period of time). For example, if the child cries three times in a day for 15, 5, and 10 min each, then the average crying duration for that day would be 10 min. The total duration gives the total amount of time a child engages in a behavior over the course of an observation session. For example, if the child wanders around the room unengaged for 2-, 3-, and 5-min episodes during an hour of observation, the total duration would be 10 min of aimless wandering per hour.

Latency

Latency is another time-based system that measures the interim between behaviors. Latency is the length of time between an environmental event and the start of a behavior. For example, how long it takes a child to get started on a task after being told to start or how much time elapses between when the child is asked to sit down and the child actually sits in the seat. Latency is useful to know when the goal is to reduce the amount of time between a request and the behavior.

A–B–C Analysis

Another way to collect direct observation data is by using the Antecedent–Behavior–Consequence, or A–B–C, analysis. In this system, when the behavior is observed, the events occurring immediately prior to and following the behavior are recorded. This information can then be used to form hypotheses about the events that are provoking and maintaining the target behavior (Gresham, Watson & Skinner, 2001). If the goal of functional analysis is to identify a causal relationship between environmental factors and the target behavior (Asmus, Franzese, Conroy & Dozier, 2003), having a record of this series of events sheds light on the situation in which the behavior occurs.

Recording so much information can be quite time-consuming, so the A–B–C analysis can be used in conjunction with the other measurement systems discussed earlier in this chapter to provide context to support the data taken on duration or rate of occurrence of the target behavior. That is, the A–B–C data can be taken for enough time to clarify causes of the behavior, and the other methods can be used to track the behavior over time. Table 6.8 is a sample A–B–C recording form for a child who talks to himself, loudly and off-topic, during a therapeutic social-skills group.

When planning intervention, the A–B–C data can then be quite useful. The context provided by this observation suggests the antecedent or consequent events that appear to trigger the behavior. These environmental factors can be manipulated and data on the occurrence of the target behavior taken. This systematic manipulation of antecedents or consequences can be continued until a reduction in the challenging behavior and/or an increase in an appropriate replacement behavior is seen (Stichter, 2001). Additional information on intervention will be provided in another chapter of this book.

Table 6.8 Sample A–B–C recording form

Date: <u>January 12, 2011</u>
Behavior: <u>Child talks aloud to himself about movies or TV shows during group activities during social-skills group</u>

Time	Antecedent	Behavior	Consequence
4:05	Therapist says, "It's time to put toys away and gather for circle time"	Child starts talking to himself in agitated voice about Transformers	Therapist asks him to stop talking or go to the break area until he can be quiet; child goes to break area
4:15	Therapist asks children to take turns reading	Child mumbles to himself and looks upset	Therapist says he does not have to read aloud
4:40	Children are eating snack together, they are prompted to engage in conversation with peers	Child talks for 5 min about Pokemon without asking questions or pausing to allow others to comment	Therapist finally asks him who he is talking to and child is quiet for the rest of snack

Conclusion

Direct observation of behavior is a valuable, although time-consuming, step in providing important insights about the function of challenging behavior. A well-defined behavior can be reliably measured and tracked over time. By determining the measurement system that provides the most accurate information about a target behavior, data can be systematically collected and used for several purposes in functional analysis. Behavioral data can be used to identify the cause(s) that maintain a behavior, to develop an intervention that will address the behavior, and to track the occurrence of that behavior over time to determine if the intervention is successful. When carefully considered, this methodological step of observing behavior can provide insights and utility across many settings for many individuals involved.

References

Alberto, P. A., & Troutman, A. C. (1995). *Applied behavior analysis for teachers*. Englewood Cliffs: Prentice Hall.

Asmus, J. M., Franzese, J. C., Conroy, M. A., & Dozier, C. L. (2003). Clarifying functional analysis outcomes for disruptive behaviors by controlling consequence delivery for stereotypy. *School Psychology Review, 32*, 624–630.

Barnhill, G. P. (2005). Functional behavioral assessment in schools. *Intervention in School and Clinic, 40*, 131–143.

Belden, A. C., Thomson, N. R., & Luby, J. L. (2008). Temper tantrums in healthy versus depressed and disruptive preschoolers: Defining tantrum behaviors associated with clinical problems. *The Journal of Pediatrics, 152*, 117–122.

Furniss, F. (2009). Assessment Methods. In J. L. Matson (Ed.), *Applied behavior analysis for children with autism spectrum disorders*. New York: Springer.

Glasberg, B. A. (2006). *Functional behavior assessments for people with autism: Making sense of seemingly senseless behavior*. Bethesda: Woodbine House.

Gresham, F. M., Watson, T. S., & Skinner, C. H. (2001). Functional behavioral assessment: Principles, procedures, and future directions. *School Psychology Review, 30*, 156–172.

Hanley, G. P., Iwata, B. A., & McCord, B. E. (2003). Functional analysis of problem behavior: A review. *Journal of Applied Behavior Analysis, 36*, 147–185.

Haynes, S. N., & O'Brien, W. H. (2000). *Principles and practice of behavioral assessment*. New York: Springer.

Herzinger, C. V., & Campbell, J. M. (2007). Comparing functional assessment methodologies: A quantitative synthesis. *Journal of Autism and Developmental Disorders, 37*, 1430–1445.

Johnston, C., Murray, C., & Ng, L. (2007). Types of noncompliance in boys with Attention-Deficit/Hyperactivity Disorder with and without oppositional behavior. *Child and Family Behavior Therapy, 29*, 1–20.

Kahng, S., Abt, K. A., & Schonbachler, H. E. (2001). Assessment and treatment of low-rate high-intensity problem behavior. *Journal of Applied Behavior Analysis, 34*, 225–228.

Kazdin, A. E. (2001). *Behavior modification in applied settings* (6th ed.). Belmont: Wadsworth Publishing.

Kerth, D. M., Progar, P. R., & Morales, S. (2009). The effects of non-contingent self-restraint on self-injury. *Journal of Applied Research in Intellectual Disabilities, 22*, 187–193.

Lakin, K., Hill, B., Hauber, F., Bruininks, R., & Heal, L. (1983). New admissions and readmissions to a national sample of public residential facilities. *American Journal on Mental Deficiency, 88*, 13–20.

Lang, R., O'Reilly, M., Sigafoos, J., Machalicek, W., Rispoli, M., Lancioni, G., et al. (2010). The effects of an abolishing operation intervention component on play skills, challenging behavior, and stereotypy. *Behavior Modification, 34*, 267–289.

Lanovaz, M. J., Fletcher, S. E., & Rapp, J. T. (2009). Identifying stimuli that alter immediate and subsequent levels of vocal stereotypy: A further analysis of functionally matched stimulation. *Behavior Modification, 33*, 682–704.

Magnusson, A. F., & Gould, D. D. (2007). Reduction of automatically-maintained self-injury using contingent equipment removal. *Behavioral Interventions, 22*, 57–68.

Mandell, D. S. (2008). Psychiatric hospitalization among children with autism spectrum disorders. *Journal of Autism and Developmental Disorders, 38*, 1059–1065.

Roane, H. S., Fisher, W. W., Sgro, G. M., Falcomata, T. S., & Pabico, R. R. (2004). An alternative method of thinning reinforcer delivery during differential reinforcement. *Journal of Applied Behavior Analysis, 37*, 213–218.

Rogers, E. (2001). Functional behavioral assessment and children with autism: Working as a team. *Focus on Autism and Other Developmental Disabilities, 16*, 228–231.

Singh, N. N., Lancioni, G. E., Winton, A. S. W., Fisher, B. C., Wahler, R. G., Mcaleavey, K., et al. (2006). Mindful parenting decreases aggression, noncompliance, and self-injury in children with autism. *Journal of Emotional and Behavioral Disorders, 14*, 169–177.

Steege, M. W., Watson, T. S., & Gresham, F. M. (2009). *Conducting school-based functional behavioral assessments*. New York: Guilford.

Stichter, J. P. (2001). Functional analysis: The use of analogues in applied settings. *Focus on Autism and other Developmental Disabilities, 16*, 232–239.

Tassé, M. J. (2006). Functional behavioural assessment in people with intellectual disabilities. *Current Opinion in Psychiatry, 19*, 475–480.

Wilder, D. A., Chen, L., Atwell, J., Pritchard, J., & Weinstein, P. (2006). Brief functional analysis and treatment of tantrums associated with transition in preschool children. *Journal of Applied Behavior Analysis, 39*, 103–107.

Interview and Observation Methods in Functional Assessment

7

Alison M. Kozlowski and Johnny L. Matson

Introduction

Challenging behaviors are evinced by individuals who have a variety of disabilities including those with intellectual disability (ID; McClintock, Hall, & Oliver, 2003; Poppes, van der Putten, & Vlaskamp, 2010) and/or autism spectrum disorders (ASD; Matson, Wilkins, & Macken, 2009; Mudford et al., 2008; Murphy, Healy, & Leader, 2009), as well as those individuals who have mild disabilities or do not possess any documented disabilities (Gettinger & Stoiber, 2006; Kinch, Lewis-Palmer, Hagan-Burke, & Sugai, 2001). When formulating treatment plans for these individuals, clinicians often state that conducting a functional behavioral assessment is an integral part of the process and assists in treatment planning. In fact, federal law in the USA currently mandates that treatment of all challenging behaviors is based on the results of a functional behavioral assessment as stated in the Individuals with Disabilities Education Act Amendments of, 1997 and 2004 (Individuals with Disabilities Education

Act Amendments of, 1997, 20 U.S.C. Section 1400 et seq, 1997; Individuals with Disabilities Education Act Amendments of, 2004, 11 Stat. 37 U.S.C. Section 1401, 2004). However, the methods of conducting a functional behavioral assessment need not be identical across cases. Techniques are often individualized depending on the frequency and severity of the challenging behavior, availability of resources, and information that has already been acquired regarding the challenging behavior and its function(s).

Functional behavioral assessment, in general, refers to methods of ascertaining the maintaining variables of challenging behaviors through both experimental and nonexperimental means, and it comprises three main categories: indirect or anecdotal assessments, descriptive or naturalistic observational assessments, and experimental functional analysis (EFA) (Iwata, Vollmer, Zarcone, & Rodgers, 1993; Neidert, Dozier, Iwata, & Hafen, 2010). Although only the former two is discussed in this chapter, it is first critical to understand the difference between functional behavioral assessment in general and EFA. While these terms may seem synonymous and are often confused as such, they are not and should not be used interchangeably. Functional behavioral assessment includes a group of possible strategies used to determine the function(s) of challenging behavior, whereas EFA, which is one type of functional behavioral assessment, refers solely to the experimental manipulation of environmental variables to achieve this same information.

A.M. Kozlowski (✉)
Louisiana State University, Baton Rouge,
LA 70803, USA
e-mail: alikoz@gmail.com

J.L. Matson
Department of Psychology, Louisiana State University,
Baton Rouge, LA 70803, USA
e-mail: johnmatson@aol.com

J.L. Matson (ed.), *Functional Assessment for Challenging Behaviors*,
Autism and Child Psychopathology Series, DOI 10.1007/978-1-4614-3037-7_7,
© Springer Science+Business Media, LLC 2012

The remaining functional behavioral assessment techniques do not incorporate experimental manipulation of variables.

EFA is commonly viewed as the hallmark of functional behavioral assessment (Hanley, Iwata, McCord, 2003; Iwata, Dorsey, Slifer, Bauman, & Richman, 1982/1994; Neidert et al., 2010). This is largely in part due to the fact that EFA is the only established way in which a causal relationship can be determined between different functions and behaviors, while other functional behavioral assessment strategies only indicate which functions and behaviors correlate with one another. An earlier chapter of this book provides an in depth review of EFA and its components, so it will not be discussed thoroughly here. However, it is important to note here that, despite its elite status, EFA is not always practical or safe to employ. In these circumstances, other functional behavioral assessment methods, such as those that will be reviewed here, are necessary.

Instances in which EFA would not be deemed appropriate include when the behavior is not occurring frequently enough to adequately assess it in such a setting (Matson & Minshawi, 2007). If the challenging behavior is occurring only rarely, the chances of it occurring within a contrived setting are also low. The safety of the individual and others also needs to be given consideration when conducting a functional behavioral assessment. Severe behaviors that may cause injury to the self or others are not ideally assessed through EFA. This is because an EFA requires that the challenging behavior occurs without interruption. Therefore, safety parameters frequently employed in the naturalistic setting would actually interfere with identifying the function of the behavior. Another concern with EFA is that factors related to the challenging behavior may be unable to be integrated into the assessment process, such as the behavior occurring with specific caregivers (English & Anderson, 2004). Furthermore, EFA typically requires large amounts of resources including trained staff, significant periods of time, reinforcers, and work space that is not always readily available to clinicians or facilities (Matson & Minshawi, 2007). Therefore, alternative functional behavioral assessment methods tend to be necessary and/or preferred in many cases.

The focus of this chapter is on interview and observations methods that may be completed as a part of the functional behavioral assessment process. First, overall interview methods is addressed with descriptions of some of the most commonly used and most researched interviews currently available being provided. Next, a similar overview is given for direct observation methods and their examples. Then, since many studies exploring the psychometrics of both interviews and direct observation methods are in comparison to one another as well as other functional behavioral assessment methods, psychometric data, advantages, and disadvantages of these tools are offered and compared in subsequent sections.

Interview Methods

Interviews are among the most common functional behavioral assessment strategies employed (Ellingson, Miltenberger, & Long, 1999; Rojahn, Whittaker, Hoch, & González, 2007). Use of interviews allows clinicians to collect a variety of information regarding the challenging behavior(s) and bypasses many of the concerns with EFA. Such methodology does not require the target behavior to be exhibited during the assessment process, which permits assessment of less frequently occurring behaviors and those behaviors that pose serious danger or risk to the self or others. Furthermore, an interview of this kind could be viewed as a broadband functional assessment measure. In contrast to EFA and many scaling methods such as the *Questions About Behavioral Function* (QABF; Matson & Vollmer, 1995) and *Motivation Assessment Scale* (MAS; Durand & Crimmins, 1992), all of which are thoroughly reviewed in other chapters of this book, the results provide clinicians with comprehensive information surrounding the target behavior that may otherwise not be considered. Responses are typically open-ended and are, therefore, not limited or restricted by confounding variables or specific categories of functions. However, as will be discussed later on with respect to the interviews reviewed herein, there are also drawbacks with functional behavioral assessment interviews, as with any other assessment strategy.

Teacher/Caregiver Interviews

Functional Analysis Interview Form

The Functional Analysis Interview Form (FAIF) is one of the most popular and frequently used interview measures for assessing the function(s) of challenging behaviors. The interview is administered to someone familiar with the individual being assessed (e.g., parent and caregiver) and takes approximately 45–90 min to complete (O'Neill et al., 1997). The FAIF is a paper-and-pencil interview and primarily elicits information through open-ended questions related to the behaviors in question. It comprises 11 sections which probe for information regarding the following: (1) descriptions of the behaviors, (2) potential bioenvironmental events that may affect the behaviors, (3) events and situations that predict the presence of the behaviors, (4) the functions or consequences maintaining the behaviors, (5) the efficiency of the behaviors, (6) functional alternative behaviors the individual already displays, (7) the individual's communicative abilities, (8) things to do and avoid when working with the person to increase their success, (9) reinforcing items, activities, or events for the individual, (10) behavior and treatment history, and (11) a diagram to summarize the information collected regarding predictors and/or consequences of challenging behaviors. Interviewers pose the questions to respondents and record the respondent's answers in the appropriate space. Follow-up questions may be asked as needed throughout the interview.

Functional Assessment Checklist: Teachers and Staff

Although its name may imply otherwise, the Functional Assessment Checklist: Teachers and Staff (FACTS) (March et al., 2000) is a semi-structured interview to be used for functional behavioral assessments with student populations.

The interview was created by modifying the FAIF (O'Neill et al., 1997) and is administered in a similar fashion. However, rather than requiring 45–90 min to complete, the FACTS only requires 10–25 min, with administration time dependent on how knowledgeable the informant is with respect to the student being assessed and the number and complexity of challenging behaviors in question (McIntosh et al., 2008). The interview comprises two parts: Part A begins by collecting narrative information regarding strengths of the individual, identifying problem behaviors, and identifying routines during which the behaviors most commonly occur (e.g., when, where, and with whom). The last section is completed by asking the respondent to provide the interviewer with the student's daily schedule including activities, individuals present during different activities, the specific problem behaviors elicited at different times, and the likelihood of these behaviors occurring during these times, which is rated on a scale from 1 (low) to 6 (high). Up to three routines are then selected for further assessment in Part B based on similar behaviors being likely to occur during certain conditions.

During Part B, each routine identified during Part A is examined separately. Therefore, up to three Part B assessments may be conducted for the individual. After identifying which routine will be examined during each specific Part B assessment, more details regarding the problem behavior are gather through open-ended questions (e.g., operationally defining the behavior, frequency, duration, and intensity). Next, predictors/antecedents and then consequences are explored with many options being made available as well as giving the respondent the opportunity to include self-identified predictors and/or consequences. A summary of the behavior is then compiled, which integrates the antecedents, behavior, and consequences. This information is later used for development of a treatment plan. The respondent rates their confidence in the compiled summary statement on a scale of 1 (not very confident) to 6 (very confident). Lastly, strategies previously and/or currently used for preventing and treating the problem behavior are named.

Functional Assessment and Intervention Program

The Functional Assessment and Intervention Program (FAIP) is a computer-based functional behavioral interview program originally developed for use in school settings (University of Utah, Utah State University, & Utah State Department of Education, 1999 as cited in Hartwig, Tuesday Heathfield, & Jenson, 2004). The program guides the interviewee through five sections pertaining to a specific individual and his/her targeted challenging behavior. In the first three sections, the interviewee is asked to provide information regarding identifying and setting information, antecedents, and consequences. Prior to continuing, the interviewee is then prompted to confirm or disconfirm all antecedents and consequences the program has identified based on the information provided. In the fourth section, the program integrates the identified antecedents and consequences to formulate hypothesized functions. Up to four possible functions may be elicited from the program: gain attention, obtain access to tangibles, escape/avoid demands, and sensory stimulation. At this time, the interviewee either confirms or disconfirms each hypothesized function. In the last section, the interviewee is given function-based and research-supported interventions that are specific to the individual based on identifying information provided earlier. The interviewee is then able to choose from these options.

Student Interviews

Although the majority of functional behavioral assessment interviews rely on parents, caregivers, or teachers as informants, a more recent development in the field has incorporated gathering information from students/individuals engaging in challenging behaviors. Being able to derive information from this source allows clinicians better insight into challenging behaviors including the potential for a wider breadth of data. To date, several variations of a student-guided functional assessment interview exist which are commonly adapted from one another.

Student-Assisted Functional Assessment Interview

The *Student-Assisted Functional Assessment Interview* (Kern, Dunlap, Clarke, & Childs, 1994) was the first interview of its kind. The interview is divided into four sections and takes approximately 20–30 min to administer. The first section contains 12 questions regarding the student's schoolwork and classroom to which the student can respond "always," "sometimes," or "never." In the second section, open-ended questions are posed to the student to assess why and when the targeted challenging behavior occurs, what changes could be made within the school setting to alleviate the student's difficulties and to identify rewards/activities that the student enjoys. Next, the student is asked to rate all of their classes in terms of how much they enjoy the subject using a Likert scale with ratings 1–5 where 1 indicates "not at all" and 5 corresponds to "very much." In the final section, what the student likes and dislikes about each subject is explored through a series of open-ended questions.

Student-Guided Functional Assessment Interview

The *Student-Guided Functional Assessment Interview* (Reed, Thomas, Sprague, & Horner, 1997) was developed for use in school settings when children are engaging in challenging behaviors within the classroom, mainly talking out of turn, teasing/bullying, not following directions, and not completing work. The interview is broken down into multiple sections and typically administered to both the student and teacher. First, the individual is asked to define the target behaviors. Next, problematic settings and/or classes are noted by instructing the individual to complete a daily schedule. The schedule contains each class or other activity the student participates in throughout the day as well as the instructor for that class or activity. The individual is then asked to rate the likelihood and intensity of the student engaging in the target behavior during that class or activity on a scale of 1 (least difficult) to 6 (most difficult). A blank diagram is then presented to be completed by the individual with respect to events surrounding the target behavior (e.g., class demands, teacher demands, receiving attention, and noise/distractions). Events are documented in the order in which they occur before or after the target behavior. Lastly, a support plan is developed in a similar diagram where setting events and predictors are manipulated, replacement behaviors are contrived, and consequences are given for engagement in the challenging behavior versus the desired behavior.

Direct Observation Methods

Although interviews provide clinicians with a wealth of information, best practice suggests that multiple methods of functional behavioral assessment be integrated to determine the function(s) of challenging behaviors. Observation methods are yet another option frequently incorporated into comprehensive functional behavioral assessments. While observations certainly involve direct examination of the individual, it is important to understand that observation methods are not synonymous with EFA. However, in contrast to EFA, direct observations occur within the natural environment of the individual thus allowing clinicians the ability to assess situations in which challenging behaviors actually occur. Furthermore, unlike alternative methods of functional behavioral assessment, direct observations do not rely on retrospective report or memory, thereby eliminating confounds associated with such reports.

Contingency Event Recording (A–B–C Data/Recording)

Contingency event recording, more commonly referred to as Antecedent–Behavior–Consequence (A–B–C) data/recording, is by far the most prevalent form of nonexperimental observation methods used in functional behavioral assessment. This method was actually one of the first functional behavioral assessment techniques introduced in applied settings and was developed by Bijou, Peterson, and Ault (1968). Contingency event recording involves direct observation of the individual being assessed in their natural environ-

ment. While conducting this observation, real-time data is recorded, thereby eliminating the biased effects of retrospective report. Contingency event recording was originally developed to be completed in an unstructured format where data is collected by documenting the date, time, antecedent event(s), target behavior (i.e., the challenging behavior), and consequent event(s) in separate columns. Antecedents refer to the events occurring prior to the display of the target behavior, while consequent events are those occurring after the individual has already begun engaging in the target behavior. The data is descriptive in nature detailing the sequence of events in the observer's own words; therefore, it is commonly dubbed the *descriptive* or *narrative* recording format (Cooper, Heron, & Heward, 2007; Miltenberger, 2001). Additional columns may be included depending on the goal of the assessment with data in other categories related to the challenging behavior, such as other individuals present at the time of the challenging behavior or the location in which the behavior occurred, being recorded (Rojahn, Schroeder, & Hoch, 2008). For an example of a blank A–B–C recording sheet of this kind, refer to Appendix A.

Subsequently, contingency event recording was expanded to include A–B–C checklists, also known as structured A–B–C data collection. The premise of the data collection is synonymous with the original A–B–C recording sheets except that now narrative report for the antecedent event(s), target behavior, and consequent event(s) is replaced with options for the observer to simply check-off based on occurrence. An example of an A–B–C checklist is presented in Appendix B. One such checklist was developed by O'Neill and colleagues (1997), named the *Functional Assessment Observation Form* (FAOF). This specific observation form contains eight sections. First, the individual being observed and dates of observation are noted, with the possibility of observations spanning over more than just 1 day. Next, predetermined time intervals are decided upon and labeled on the form. These time intervals are dependent on the individual being observed and may coincide with specific activities throughout the day, similar to scatter plot data collection which will be discussed shortly. This form actually differs from traditional contingency event recordings by including this component. The next sections (i.e., behaviors, predictors, perceived functions, and actual consequences) are presented in a checklist format. All targeted challenging behaviors are listed followed by predictors, also known as antecedents. The perceived functions section, which also differs from typical contingency event recordings, prompts the observer to endorse which listed function he/she believes to have brought about the behavior. Finally, in the actual consequences section, the observer checks the column aptly describing what occurred following the individual engaging in the targeted challenging behavior. The authors encourage clinicians to first conduct an interview to choose which behaviors, predictors, perceived functions, and actual consequences should be displayed as options on the data collection form. With more recent advances in technology, additional contingency event recording strategies using a structured format have become available. For example, similar to A–B–C checklists documenting information on paper, personal data assistants have been used to electronically collect observational data (Tarbox et al., 2009). When using these devices, antecedents, behaviors, and consequences are documented similar to a paper-and-pencil checklist format.

Both contingency event recording formats have advantages and disadvantages that clinicians should be aware of prior to choosing which specific data collection method to utilize. Ideally, individuals with a strong background in functional behavioral assessment will be called upon for the collection of behavioral data. Unfortunately, this is seldom possible in practice, and parents and teachers are commonly required to collect the appropriate data. Therefore, one of the more immediate considerations should be the competency of the observer who will be collecting the data. When using the unstructured, narrative format, observers are able to describe in their own words what events occurred prior to and following the target challenging behavior. This eliminates the confound of the observer not understanding specific terms commonly located

on A–B–C checklists, and it also provides the observer with the ability to describe all of the events regardless of their perceived effect on the target behavior. However, structured checklists may cue the observer to notice specific antecedents or consequences that they may have otherwise overlooked or considered irrelevant to the situation. Another clearly positive property of checklists is that they are easy and quick to complete. If an observer collecting A–B–C data is also working with the individual who is exhibiting the challenging behavior, which is quite common since parents, teachers, and therapists are often those collecting the data, it may not be feasible to expect the observer to provide a narrative on the events. This would be especially true if there is a greater frequency of the challenging behavior.

Despite the advantages and disadvantages of each A–B–C data collection method, very little research has yet to examine the differences between structured and unstructured A–B–C data. Based on the results of one study assessing the accuracy and preference of both formats among 16 special education teachers and paraprofessionals, the structured format yielded slightly greater accuracy and was more preferred among teachers (Lerman, Hovanetz, Strobel, & Tetreault, 2009). Overall, the accuracy of data collected across both methods was only modest due to the teachers' lack of knowledge regarding functional behavioral assessment. Therefore, further training in functional behavioral assessment is necessary for teachers, especially those working with children who display behavioral difficulties.

Contingency event recording data is commonly interpreted in one of two ways. The simplest method is based on a correlational visual inspection of the frequencies of the antecedents and consequences related to specific challenging behaviors (Tarbox et al., 2009). If the antecedents and consequences serve the same function for the same behavior, it is sufficient to say that the occurrence of the behavior served that single function. Then, the most frequently occurring of those functions for that specific behavior may be hypothesized to maintain the behavior. If antecedents and consequences do not coincide during a single occurrence of a behavior, the interpretation becomes more complicated. In these cases, the behavior may be maintained by multiple functions or irrelevant correlating antecedents and consequences may be coinciding with the behavior. As such, interpretations should be made with caution. On the other hand, contingency event recording data may also be analyzed by calculating conditional probabilities (Lerman & Iwata, 1993; Mace & Lalli, 1991). First, the proportion of times the target behavior followed each antecedent out of all of the times the target behavior occurred is calculated. In addition, the percentage of times each consequence followed the target behavior is also calculated. As will be discussed in the next section, conditional probabilities may also be calculated for continuous event recording with additional calculations possible.

Continuous Event Recording

Based on Bijou and colleagues' (1968) original work on contingency event recording, continuous event recording was subsequently developed (Mace, Lalli, & Lalli, 1991). Data collection begins by an individual first compiling a list of possible antecedents, challenging behaviors, and consequences during observation periods. All categories may be broad or narrow depending on the specific individual being assessed. Then predetermined time intervals for data collection are established and divided into equal time segments for data collection. Mace and colleagues suggest that 15–60-min observation periods be used with 10-s time intervals. Therefore, if the designated observation period is 15 min, the entire period can be divided into 90 10-s time intervals. During the direct observation periods, observers use a partial-interval recording procedure. If any of the antecedents or behaviors occur during a 10-s period, the appropriate box is marked. This is the distinguishing difference between contingency and continuous event recording – all antecedents are recorded regardless of if they are following by engagement in the target behavior. Consequences are documented somewhat differently; only consequences occurring up to 30 s following challenging behaviors are documented.

Once again, the 30-s window is a suggestion which may be modified. As was discussed with respect to interpretation of contingency event recording data, conditional probabilities may also be calculated for continuous event recordings. Also, due to the nature of continuous event recording data collection allowing for additional variables to be collected, other calculations may also be possible. For example, intervals during which a specific antecedent preceded the target behavior divided by the number of intervals containing that specific antecedent can also be calculated since all antecedents are documented regardless of whether they are antecedents to the target behavior. Therefore, this data allows the clinician to determine how often the target behavior actually followed the antecedent—perhaps the antecedent occurred frequently without a subsequent occurrence of the target behavior. Information of this kind can be quite valuable.

Scatter Plot Analysis

While slightly less direct than data collected through contingency or continuous event recordings, scatter plot analysis is yet another observational method of collecting data related to the function(s) of challenging behavior. To collect this type of data, predetermined time intervals are decided upon before beginning data collection (Touchette, MacDonald, & Langer, 1985). Although these time intervals can be as simple as hour or half-hour blocks of time throughout the day, it is strongly suggested that the time periods represent different activities occurring during the day or even other changes in the environment, such as staff shift changes. Recording data according to differing environmental aspects will allow for easier interpretation of the data. Scatter plot data is simpler to collect in comparison to contingency or continuous event recording data because its collection only requires that an individual denote whether the target behavior occurred during the specified time interval rather than supply a descriptive narrative account or determine the antecedents or consequences of the behavior. Data collection can be implemented in two ways: either frequency data can be collected with a tally mark being placed in the time period during which the target behavior occurred or data can be plotted on a grid during the observation period. If the tally mark method is chosen, the data is later compiled into a graph with the time period along the *X*-axis and the frequency of the challenging behavior along the *Y*-axis similar to the visual presentation of the grid data collection method. This method may also be more feasible in settings where training in data collection is limited since frequency data is often collected to monitor progress regardless of its inclusion in a scatter plot.

Utilizing the grid option eliminates the need for two steps in the scatter plot process; however, it requires greater time investment during actual data collection. On the grid, successive days are presented along the *X*-axis, while the time periods are displayed on the *Y*-axis. Then for each time period over the course of each day, the appropriate block is shaded accordingly. Typically, an empty cell indicates that the target behavior was absent, while a filled cell marks presence of the behavior. However, depending on the frequency of the target behavior, variations of this method can be used (Kahng et al., 1998; Touchette et al., 1985). For example, a blank cell may represent an absence of the behavior, while a shaded cell denotes low frequencies of the behavior and a filled cell indicates high frequencies of the behavior. The difference between low and high frequencies of the behavior would be based on predetermined criteria. Although more than three different codes can be used, some have found this to compromise the interpretability of the data (Touchette et al.).

Interpretation of scatter plot data involves inspection of the visual display to determine time periods, which correlate with specific events, during which the target behavior is more likely to occur. Although some researchers find scatter plots to be advantageous in that they are easily interpreted visually, simple visual interpretation of scatter plot data does not always arrive at a conclusion regarding temporal periods during which the target behavior is most likely to occur (Kahng et al., 1998). However, this is not to say that these

conclusions cannot be derived from scatter plot data. When Kahng et al. were unable to decipher a temporal pattern from several visual displays of scatter plot data, the authors constructed a control chart (Pfadt & Wheeler, 1995) for each scatter plot to statistically interpret the data. Control charts are commonly used as one of many statistical procedures to improve industrial organization production. However, Pfadt and Wheeler suggest that these statistical procedures may also be applied to the behavioral sciences to analyze behavior patterns. The statistical analysis aims to identify patterns of variability that are considered "out of statistical control." That is, they are statistically sufficiently deviant from the mean so as to be significantly different. Applying this statistical analysis to the same 15 sets of data which had been impervious to scatter plot analyses resulted in a temporal pattern being identified for 12 of the 15 data sets. Although Kahng et al. state that needing to apply this statistical analysis to scatter plot data compromises one of the main advantages of scatter plot analysis (i.e., being able to visually interpret the data with ease), its addition still allows clinicians to identify temporal patterns of behavior, which is the goal of scatter plot analysis.

Psychometric Properties of Interview and Direct Observation Methods

Since the current chapter focuses on two functional behavioral assessment methods (i.e., interviews and direct observations), and these two methods are often compared to one another in studies, data regarding the reliability and validity of the aforementioned methods will be discussed in a similar fashion. First, some examples of studies only addressing one form of functional behavioral assessment will be presented. Subsequently, examples of studies examining multiple functional behavioral assessment strategies will be reviewed. Please note that the review of psychometric properties presented is not an all inclusive compilation of studies regarding the specific assessment method, but rather a demonstration of recent research.

Interviews

FACTS

An excellent review completed by McIntosh et al. (2008) provides a wealth of information on the psychometric properties of the FACTS. The review aggregated the results of nine separate studies assessing the properties of the FACTS in a total of 41 children attending public preschools, elementary schools, and middle schools. The test–retest reliability was found to be strong with respect to antecedents, functions, and total behavioral hypotheses, while the test–retest reliability for setting events was moderate. Inter-rater reliability was also moderate across respondents. In terms of validity, convergent validity has been most commonly explored by comparing the FACTS to either direct observations or an EFA. Complete agreement between the FACTS and direct observations reached 90%, while the FACTS and EFA agreed on functions for 53% of the cases. However, it should be noted that there were some instances in which there was partial agreement between assessment methods. For example, for 5% of validation cases between the FACTS and direct observations, the direct observations pointed toward multiple functions, one of which was consistent with the function identified by the FACTS. Similarly, for 24% of the validation cases between the FACTS and EFA, the EFA indicated multiple functions, one of which was also indicated by the FACTS. Validity based on treatment utility was also explored for 15 students. All treatment plans developed based on the identified function from the FACTS resulted in a decrease in targeted challenging behaviors. The majority of students experienced at least a 50% reduction in problem behaviors.

FAIP

A sample of 59 school psychologists, social workers, and teachers participated in the standardization of the FAIP using a sample of children in the third through sixth grades who engaged in challenging behaviors within the classroom setting (Hartwig et al., 2004). For inter-rater reliability, 19 pairs of participants were asked to complete the FAIP on 19 separate students. Inter-rater reliability for the entire FAIP averaged 63.9% agreement, while inter-rater reliability for the derived functions averaged 70.96% agreement across participants. Test–retest reliability was calculated by having one set of 19 participants complete the FAIP for a second time, approximately 30 days following its first administration. Test–retest reliability averaged 72.66% for the entire FAIP and 81.4% agreement for the derived functions. Concurrent validity was assessed by having multiple respondents complete the FAIP, MAS, and FAIF. There was 69.44% agreement between the FAIP and MAS, and 76.34% agreement between the FAIP and FAIF. The clinical utility of all three assessments was also measured, with results indicating that professionals most preferred the FAIP overall when compared with the MAS and FAIF.

Student-Guided Functional Assessment Interview

Reed and colleagues (1997) assessed the inter-rater reliability of the *Student-Guided Functional Assessment Interview* by administering the interview to ten students in the fifth through eighth grades, and their corresponding teachers, who had a history of exhibiting challenging behaviors within the school setting. All interviews were administered first to teachers and then to the corresponding students within 3 days of the original interview. When conducting interviews with the students, prompting questions were frequently incorporated as students often needed guidance throughout the assessment. These were used as follow-up questions to the main questions asked during the interview and were standard for all interviews with students.

Taken collectively, there was 60% teacher–student agreement on the entire functional behavioral assessment portion of the interview. When breaking down the results according to the different aspects of the functional behavioral assessment section, agreement was variable. Teachers and students demonstrated agreement on 81.5% of challenging behaviors, with students identifying more behaviors than did teachers. The behaviors that were reported only by the students and not the teachers appear to be those that were not necessarily observable to teachers within the classroom setting (e.g., possession of inappropriate items), thus at least minimally explaining the discrepancy. While there was 77% agreement for predictors and consequences of challenging behaviors, there was only 23% agreement on setting events. Overall, there was 38% agreement on the support plan portion of the interview, with agreement varying between 25% and 48% across prevention strategies, teaching strategies, consequences, and setting changes. However, consistency between the functional assessment and support plan portions for teacher and student interviews was 78% and 70%, respectively, suggesting that there was moderate to good ability on behalf of the informants to develop treatment plans consistent with their hypothesized functions. Taken collectively, there was a 22% agreement across the entire interview between teachers and students.

Direct Observations

Continuous Event Recording

Lerman and Iwata (1993) investigated the ability of continuous event recordings to identify the function of self-injurious behaviors in six adults with profound intellectual disability. For five of the individuals, continuous event recordings were completed for a total of 24 h. For one individual, assessment was conducted for a total of 48 h to determine whether a lengthier assessment period would clarify the results. In addition, EFAs were completed for all participants independent of the continuous event recording results. While EFAs were found to identify the maintaining variables of self-injurious behavior in all of the participants, continuous event recordings appeared to be successful only in differentiating social versus nonsocial functions. Whether attention, escape, or another social contingency maintained the behavior could not be discerned through the descriptive assessment. Additionally, a lengthier assessment period did not prove effective in further clarifying the results of a descriptive assessment. However, it should be noted that EFA was held as the gold standard in this assessment and its results were not validated. Therefore, it is

possible that the results derived through the EFAs were similarly invalid.

Scatter Plot Analysis

Touchette and colleagues (1985) reported excellent inter-rater reliability between observers in collection of data that was used in scatter plot analyses for three individuals with ASD. For two of the three children assessed, functions maintaining the challenging behavior were identified through scatter plot analysis, thereby causing function-based interventions to be implemented. A subsequent reduction in challenging behaviors was observed for all clients.

Symons, McDonald, and Wehby (1998) used scatter plot analysis in two behavior management classrooms in Canada for two boys who engaged in challenging behaviors frequently throughout the day (i.e., more than 10 times per day). Each of the two classroom teachers was instructed to collect frequency data for each 30-min interval throughout the school day. During the study, the first author (Symons) collected interobserver agreement data with each teacher for a minimum of 20% of school days to ensure inter-rater reliability; the average agreement was 93.0%. The first author then made a scatter plot visual display of each student's behavior data using symbols to denote low, medium, and high frequencies of the behavior based on preestablished criteria for each individual student. These scatter plots were updated on a weekly basis. To assess the validity of scatter plot data, team meetings were held approximately once each week with the first author, teacher, and teacher's aide present to analyze the data and identify time periods of concern, if any. Once one or more time periods of concern were noted, hypotheses regarding the elevation in the presence of the target behavior during these time periods were proposed, and an appropriate intervention was then implemented for one of the time periods based on this hypothesis. For both students, implementation of an intervention based on scatter plot analysis resulted in a moderate decrease in challenging behaviors, thereby supporting the effectiveness of scatter plot analysis in functional behavioral assessment within the classroom setting.

Maas, Didden, Bouts, Smits, and Curfs (2009) used scatter plot analysis to determine the temporal characteristics of excessive daytime sleepiness and disruptive behaviors in seven adults with Prader-Willi Syndrome. Frequency data were collected by parents and/or caregivers across a 4-week period between normal waking hours. Time periods were broken down into 2-h intervals, and within the 2-h time period the presence of behaviors was rated across two separate situations—activities versus no activities. Each behavior received one of three scores; 0 indicated not sleepy/no disruptive behavior, 1 indicated somewhat sleepy/somewhat disruptive behavior, and 2 indicated very sleepy or asleep/severe disruptive behavior. All codes were operational defined for the observers. Interobserver agreement for data collection was deemed good. Separate scatter plots for excessive daytime sleepiness and disruptive behaviors were then constructed for each participant during activities and during the absence of activities. The time intervals were segmented vertically with activity and non-activity periods separated, and successive days were segmented horizontally. Scatter plot analysis indicated that individuals with Prader-Willi Syndrome exhibited excessive daytime sleepiness more commonly during the late afternoon and evening hours, especially when no activities were planned. Excessive daytime sleepiness was also more common on Saturdays, also increasing when there was no activity involvement. A less distinct pattern emerged for disruptive behaviors; engagement in disruptive behavior was relatively consistent across days and activity involvement. However, there was a slight elevation during weekends when no activities were provided. The results of this study have many implications for the use of scatter plot analysis. First, as the authors themselves point out, more concrete results may have been obtained through the use of shorter time intervals (e.g., Touchette et al., 1985). Secondly, since the authors based much of their analysis on the hypothesis that the targeted behaviors would increase during periods of inactivity, the information obtained through the analysis was somewhat limited. Specific activities were not considered nor were other possible influential factors, such as staff preference.

Comparisons of Multiple Assessment Methods

Arndorfer, Miltenberger, Woster, Rortvedt, and Gaffaney (1994) used a multi-assessment method to assess the maintaining variables of challenging behaviors in five children ages 2–13 years who had varying levels of intellectual impairment, developmental delays, and/or other psychological disorders. The first phase of the study was termed the "descriptive assessment" and included assessment methods such as administration of the MAS and FAIF, as well as contingency event recording data collected through direct observations independently by the parents and researchers. For one child, all four assessments arrived at the same function. For the remaining four children, the FAIF and A–B–C data indicated identical functions while the MAS was inconsistent. The descriptive assessment data was then compiled for each child, so that hypotheses regarding the function(s) of the challenging behaviors could be made, with the hypothesized function being chosen as the one supported by the most assessments. As such, the FAIF's and A–B–C data's identified function was always the one chosen for manipulation. EFAs were then completed to assess the validity of the hypothesized functions derived through the descriptive assessments. All children's descriptive assessment results were validated through 90–120 min EFAs. Functional Communication Training (FCT), a treatment protocol frequently implemented to teach individuals to appropriately communicate to achieve the same function their challenging behavior had been maintained by, was then implemented for two of the children according to the validated function. Teaching these children to verbally request the attention or tangible they desired significantly decreased the rate of their challenging behaviors. Thus, implementation of FCT further validated the results of both these children's descriptive assessments and EFAs. Therefore, both the results of the FAIF and contingency event recordings were validated through the findings in this study.

Cunningham and O'Neill (2000) conducted a similar study with three boys aged 3–5 years who were diagnosed with an ASD. Each child engaged in challenging behaviors to include biting self, physical aggression, and tantrums. Four functional behavioral assessment techniques were compared: EFA, an interview (FAIF), contingency event recording (FAOF), and a scaling method (MAS). While multiple functions were identified for each child, all four assessment methods arrived at the same primary function for two of the children. For the third child, the EFA and FAIF arrived at the same primary function, while contingency event recording and the MAS arrived at another identical primary function. In this example, the secondary function identified by the EFA and FAIF was also the same and served as the primary function identified by contingency event recording and the MAS, and vice versa. Therefore, although the sample size within the study was quite small, a limitation that will be discussed later, these findings suggest that the aforementioned functional behavioral assessment methods were able to reliably identify the same function albeit at different rankings.

Alter, Conroy, Mancil, and Haydon (2008) implemented four different functional behavioral assessment techniques with four children who were at risk for emotional and behavioral disorders. The FAIF, MAS, and A–B–C recordings were all compared to EFA, which was designated as the most valid method of assessment. When compared, the FAIF, MAS, and A–B–C recording methods all demonstrated low agreement with one another. Furthermore, the FAIF and MAS also demonstrated low consistency with EFA. Therefore, within this sample, the FAIF was not deemed a valid assessment of maintaining variables of challenging behaviors. On the other hand, A–B–C recordings were designated as the only assessment method which corroborated the findings of an EFA for all four children. Therefore, although contingency event recording does not involve experimental manipulation of variables present within the individual's immediate environment as does EFA, this study indicated that the results of these two assessments are quite similar.

Murdock, O'Neill, and Cunningham (2005) assessed the reliability and validity of teacher interviews, student interviews, and contingency event recordings. Eight boys ages 12–15 participated in the study, all of which were receiving services for a behavior disorder. The teacher and student interviews were developed specifically for the study, while the FAOF was used to collect contingency event recording data. The interviews were administered separately to groups of teachers and individual students, and they solicited information regarding the behaviors, their antecedents, and their consequences. Summary statements were then derived based on the information collected, and teachers and students were then individually asked to rank these statements as to which scenarios were the most problematic, thus the most likely to be maintaining the challenging behavior. With respect to data collected through the FAOF, rankings were made similarly by calculating the percent occurrence of each function across all observations. Interobserver agreement was also calculated for the direct observations, with an average agreement of 80%. Results indicated a significant discrepancy between the challenging behaviors identified by teachers and students with only a 30% rate of agreement. Much like the study conducted by Reed and colleagues (1997), teachers were less likely to identify behaviors that were not easily observable within the classroom setting. Overall, there was a 64% agreement across all three functional behavioral assessment methods (i.e., teacher interview, student interview, and contingency event recording) with respect to accuracy of identified function as well as rank order of that function with respect to other noted functions. The remaining 36% of cases displayed agreement between teacher interviews and contingency event recording data but not with student interviews.

Newcomer and Lewis (2004) investigated the validity of descriptive assessment methods (i.e., teacher interviews, student interviews, scatter plots, and A–B–C recordings) in three children ages 9–11 years old attending public elementary schools who were displaying behavioral difficulties putting them at risk for failure that school year. Assessment occurred in three phases—the first phase explored functions utilizing the aforementioned descriptive assessment methods, the second phase generated hypotheses based on the descriptive assessment methods, and an EFA was conducted during the third phase to confirm the hypotheses generated. Across all three children, the A–B–C recordings, scatter plots, student interviews, and EFA demonstrated convergent validity. The teacher interview, which was conducted using an adapted FAIF, corroborated the findings for two of the three children, while the third child's FAIF indicated the child's primary function as his secondary one. Therefore, taken together, it appears that all of the descriptive assessment methods were valid in identifying the maintaining variable of these three children's challenging behaviors. Based on these maintaining variables, function-based treatments and nonfunction-based treatments were implemented. For all children, function-based treatments resulted in a significant decrease in challenging behaviors when compared with baseline. Nonfunction-based treatments were met with increases and significant variability in challenging behaviors for two of the students, and a slight decrease in one student. However, for the student who experienced decreases in challenging behaviors both during function- and nonfunction-based treatments, the gains were greater with the former.

Mueller and Kafka (2006) completed a comprehensive functional behavioral assessment for a 4-year-old girl who engaged in object mouthing within the classroom setting. Techniques employed included parent and teacher interviews, contingency event recording, and EFA. The interviews conducted were not according to a specified protocol, but did elicit information regarding antecedents and consequences of object mouthing. Taken together, the parent and teacher interviews were relatively inconclusive in identifying specific antecedents likely to precede object mouthing. However, an attention function was hypothesized based on information acquired regarding consequences since the consequence to mouthing was always a verbal reprimand. Based on contingency event recordings, mouthing was only potentially maintained by attention in the form of verbal reprimands, but most likely maintained by a nonsocial function as it occurred across various situations without discrimination. Finally, an EFA was conducted with attention and alone conditions to distinguish whether object mouthing was maintained by attention or nonsocial variables. No discernable pattern of object mouthing was seen across conditions, thereby confirming the results of contingency event recordings in that the behavior was maintained by nonsocial variables.

Ervin, DuPaul, Kern, and Friman (1998) utilized a teacher interview, student interview (*Student Assisted Functional Assessment Interview*), and direct observations to formulate hypotheses regarding the function of two teenage boys' off-task behavior within the classroom. Both boys met diagnostic criteria for attention-deficit/hyperactivity disorder and oppositional defiant disorder at the time of the study. Based on the cumulative results of the descriptive assessments, which all pointed toward identical functions, function-based intervention plans were implemented for both of the boys. A significant decrease was seen in the off-task behavior of both boys during intervention phases with an increase in the behaviors occurring during reversal procedures. Therefore, the cumulative results of the comprehensive functional behavioral assessment appeared valid in identifying the variables maintaining both of the boys' off-task behavior, allowing for appropriate interventions to be put in place.

Overview of Interviews in Functional Behavioral Assessment

Given that interviews are among the most popular method of functional behavioral assessment, attention needs to be given to their potential use in identifying maintaining variables of challenging behaviors and aiding in implementation of appropriate interventions. To date, minimal research has been conducted on the psychometric properties of various interviews, and the results of studies that have been completed are relatively inconsistent with one another. While some have found parent, caregiver, and/or teacher interviews to be quite beneficial in identifying the function of challenging behaviors (e.g., Cunningham & O'Neill, 2000; McIntosh et al., 2008; Newcomer & Lewis, 2004), others tend to find that these assessment methods are invalid (e.g., Alter et al., 2008).

Many variables may play a role in the differences found between studies. O'Neill and colleagues (1997) assert that the FAIF should be administered by a professional with training in functional assessment. Although this is a relatively undisputable claim with respect to all functional assessment methods, it appears appropriate to say that this may hold even more truth for functional assessment interviews, as opposed to rating scales, due to the unstructured nature of the assessment process as well as the clinical judgment needed to interpret the results. While the FAIF and other interview methods are exceedingly thorough, they produces a much more complex set of data when compared with rating scales due to the open-ended format of the interview as well as the lack of a scoring algorithm (Sturmey, 1994). Therefore, it is possible that the findings of studies differed based on the training of those administering the interviews. In fact, despite its popular use, research has also identified interviews to be the assessment method with which clinicians have had the least amount of training (Ellingson et al., 1999). Furthermore, when asked to rate how easy different functional behavioral assessment strategies were to use, interviews were rated as being more difficult to use than scaling methods and direct observations. Interviews were also rated less effective in determining the function(s) of behavior and less useful when compared with EFA and direct observation, but to be more effective and more useful in comparison to rating scales. In addition to these concerns about interviews overall, another major limitation of interviews is that they rely on retrospective report.

The utility of interviews in functional behavioral assessment does not solely rely on the specific interview administered nor its psychometrics but also the respondent participating in the interview process. Borgmeier and Horner (2006) investigated the predictive validity of confidence ratings made by the respondents. A total of 63 teachers and staff participated in completing the FACTS for nine students. Five to eight teachers or staff completed the interview for each of the nine students, all of whom varied in their exposure to the student during the school day, exposure to the student during periods when the targeted

challenging behavior most commonly occurred, and self-assessed experience with functional behavioral assessment. At the conclusion of the interview, the teachers and staff were asked to rate how confident they were that their interview had identified the correct function on a 6-point Likert scale ranging from 1 (not confident) to 6 (very confident). Then, an EFA was conducted to identify the function of the behavior.

Although the vast majority of informants reported possessing little to no experience with conducting a functional behavioral assessment or developing a treatment plan, it was found that 91.4% of respondents rated their confidence as a 4 or higher. However, the only significant finding was that those individuals who were highly confident and identified the correct function had significantly more exposure to the student both throughout the school day and during times in which the student engaged in the targeted behavior. Therefore, when choosing a respondent for a functional behavioral assessment interview, it seems appropriate that those being interviewed should be individuals who have considerable exposure to the student. However, exposure is not sufficient. The respondent must also indicate that they are confident in their ratings. Unfortunately, confidence ratings cannot be obtained until the interview is complete. Though this is without question a limitation of this finding, this information is still valuable in determining if the already administered interview is likely valid. Clearly, more research needs to be conducted to investigate this relationship. In the meantime, it is suggested that informants be those who are familiar with the individual both during and outside of behavioral challenges. Furthermore, if confidence ratings are later found to be weak, those conducting the interview are advised to interpret the results with caution or to weigh the results of other interviews more heavily.

Experience with functional behavioral assessment is another factor that may affect the validity of interview results. Although Borgmeier and Horner (2006) did not find a correlation between the validity of interview results and experience with functional behavioral assessment, a significant flaw with this finding is that the experience of functional behavioral assessment was self-assessed on a Likert scale. Therefore, it may be that participants rated their experience and knowledge with functional behavioral assessment based on different factors. Other research has found that training informants on aspects of functional behavioral assessment actually does lead to an increased ability to accurately identify the functions of challenging behaviors (McNeill, Watson, Henington, & Meeks, 2002). Therefore, conducting interviews with informants who have at least some background in functional behavioral assessment would prove to be beneficial.

The strong suggestion to choose informants who have knowledge of functional behavioral assessment clearly speaks against the idea of including students or individuals engaging in the challenging behaviors in the interview process. However, this is not necessarily the case. Collecting information from those engaging in challenging behaviors may be quite beneficial, with students having the ability to identify intervention strategies that may assist them personally. Furthermore, as was commonly seen when conducting student interviews, students are likely to identify more behavior problems than teachers due to exposure limitations on the part of teachers (Murdock et al., 2005; Reed et al., 1997). Yet, there was some discrepancy between studies with respect to teacher and student interviews corroborating each other's findings (Ervin et al., 1998; Murdock et al.; Newcomer & Lewis, 2004; Reed et al.). Additionally, despite the possible advantages of including the student or individual engaging in the challenging behavior in the functional behavioral assessment interview process, this assessment method may not be appropriate for all populations. At present, research has only documented its use among individuals, primarily students, who have either a mild disability or no diagnostic label. Therefore, future research needs to explore whether individuals with intellectual and/or developmental disabilities would benefit from participation in this form of functional behavioral assessment. It is likely that deficits associated with intellectual and/or developmental disabilities may hinder the individual's ability to provide accurate information, thus causing this

type of functional behavioral assessment to be deemed inappropriate. Therefore, it is highly suggested that although the effectiveness of student interviews should continue to be explored, they should not be used in isolation, even with individuals without intellectual impairments.

With respect to standard parent, teacher, and caregiver interviews, the FAI and FACTS both have moderate to strong research support with respect to their reliability and validity. At the same time, this is not to say that some research has not suggested otherwise or that a sufficient amount of research has been conducted as of yet. For example, all studies exploring these interviews have only included a small number of participants. Therefore, reliability and validity findings need to be interpreted with caution. However, although these interviews may be less systematic and have less research to support their psychometric reliability and validity, they are not without their advantages. As was previously stated, interviews do not require the individual in question to be present nor that the targeted behavior, which may pose danger to the individual and/ or others, be exhibited. Interviews also require significantly less time to complete than EFAs. The majority of functional behavioral assessments likely include at least a minor interview regardless of its effectiveness in identifying functions. This is because interviews prompt informants to supply basic information that EFA, direct observations, and scaling methods do not. Most interviews, such as the FAIF and FACTS, require the respondent to operationally define the targeted behavior, a critical piece of information that other functional behavioral assessment methods do not incorporate. It is not that these alternative methods are overlooking the importance of this information, but rather that it is assumed that this information has already been gathered through an interview. Therefore, at least a brief interview should be mandatory when beginning a functional behavioral assessment as it may be seen as a starting point to any functional behavioral assessment, especially when the function(s) of behavior are elusive to the assessor.

Although very little research has been conducted on the FAIP to date, the results of the preliminary study are exciting and provide initial evidence that the FAIP may be a useful interview assessment for use when conducting functional behavioral assessments. It differs from the majority of other interviews by interpreting the narrative reports from respondents, thus formulating hypotheses regarding the function(s) of behaviors. Since the lack of a scoring algorithm is one of the more prominent disadvantages to functional behavioral assessment interviews, the FAIP's built in scoring program is a major advantage. Not only does it sidestep the difficulty in interpretation of the results, but also it does not require significant expertise in the area of functional behavioral assessment. Furthermore, since the FAIP is administered by a computer as opposed to a professional, its use significantly reduces the need for personnel resources that may not be available. The cost of administering the FAIP is also another likely advantage of the interview due to less resources being needed and because a one-time fee would be in place as opposed to purchasing of multiple assessment measures. However, this is not to say that the FAIP is not without its disadvantages. Clearly, a great deal of more research is needed. Also, in contrast to other interviews which appear to be more broad based in nature, as they will probe about many different factors within the individual's environment that may be affecting his/her behavior, the FAIP narrows its results down to four general hypotheses. It should also be noted that although the FAIP makes a significant contribution to treatment by providing function- and research-based interventions, a professional is needed to implement and monitor the effectiveness of these treatments.

Overview of Direct Observation Methods in Functional Behavioral Assessment

Direct observation data, including contingency event recordings, continuous event recordings, and scatter plots, can greatly assist in the functional behavioral assessment process despite their status as correlational assessment methods. In comparison to EFA, these methods require considerably less resources. Relatively little training is required to collect and interpret the data, and supplies needed are of little or no cost. Furthermore, since direct observation data is collected during the individual's regular activities, it does not often require extra personnel or time to complete. Although direct observations are critiqued for only being able to identify correlations between behaviors and antecedents/consequences, a major limitation of EFAs, the fact that the behaviors are not occurring in the natural environment, is overcome by this method of assessment.

Despite the similarity in the overall method of collecting direct observation data, there are significant differences between the three methods discussed within this chapter that warrant consideration. Direct observations vary in their simplicity, range of data, and validity. While scatter plot data is the simplest to collect, its results are more ambiguous than either contingency or continuous event recordings since the presence of targeted behaviors is merely correlated with different time periods, which is in turn correlated with different activities occurring throughout the day. Though some have found the results of such analyses to be beneficial and helpful in formulating treatment plans, results are somewhat speculative in nature. On the other hand, contingency and continuous event recordings provide significantly more information to the clinician and can also actually integrate some aspects of a scatter plot analysis since the time of day can similarly be documented. However, contingency and continuous event recordings also require more training in the area of functional behavioral assessment to ensure that accurate data is being collected. Furthermore, these methods require more time and attention be given to data collection while conducting observations since significantly more documentation is required. Although continuous event recordings would appear to be superior over contingency event recordings, the former may be just as unreasonable to conduct as EFAs since it requires constant documentation throughout a predetermined observation period. In fact, it is rather unlikely that staff working with an individual to be observed would be capable of completing a continuous event recording while working with the individual.

Based on the advantages and disadvantages of the three direct observation methods discussed here in comparison to one another, it is not surprising that contingency event recordings are often chosen in lieu of either of the other two methods. This, of course, means that there has also been less research conducted on either of the other two methods. The research that has been conducted on scatter plot analyses and continuous event recordings to date is at best inconsistent. However, the most common of the direct observation methods, contingency event recording, is also the direct observation method with the most evidence to support its use in functional behavioral assessment (e.g., Alter et al., 2008; Newcomer & Lewis, 2004). Although contingency event recording cannot be considered synonymous with EFA by any means, the results have repeatedly been found to corroborate those found through an EFA. Therefore, contingency event recordings should routinely be completed when conducting a functional behavioral assessment, especially if resources do not permit that an EFA or more comprehensive assessment be conducted.

Conclusion

EFA, which is often deemed the gold standard of functional behavioral assessment methods, is not always practical, safe, or even possible. Therefore, alternative functional behavioral assessment techniques are often deemed necessary. Within this chapter, various interview and direct observation methods commonly used to aid in functional behavioral assessment have been reviewed. All of these assessments have their own strengths and weaknesses, which have been addressed accordingly. Based on the information presented herein, it should be apparent that although many alternative functional behavioral assessment techniques exist, none are without their flaws. While each of these overall methods and their specific strategies have different advantages and disadvantages to consider prior to beginning any functional behavioral assessment, the key to a comprehensive functional behavioral assessment does not rely on only one method but rather a collaboration of different methodologies to assist in the treatment planning process. Furthermore, functional behavioral assessments should be individualized so that one set protocol is unlikely to be appropriate for all cases.

Didden (2007) suggests a seven-step plan for conducting a thorough functional behavioral assessment: (1) identify and operationally defined the targeted challenging behaviors, (2) utilize direct observation methods such as contingency event recordings and scatter plots, (3) administer interviews and scales to those familiar with the individual, (4) complete an EFA, (5) integrate results from functional behavioral assessment to formulate hypotheses regarding the function(s) of targeted challenging behaviors, (6) develop a treatment plan based on the derived function maintaining the targeted challenging behavior(s), and (7) monitor effectiveness of treatment interventions. Although this seven-step plan appears to be without question the ideal assessment, in most cases it is not practical. Therefore, in cases in which a comprehensive functional behavioral assessment involving an EFA or solely an EFA cannot be conducted, it is proposed that alternative, brief functional behavioral assessment strategies be used initially with a progression to more time-consuming and labor-intensive methods as deemed necessary (Vollmer et al., 1995). With this progression as the basis to functional behavioral assessment, a brief interview and some form of direct observation, preferably contingency event recordings, should undoubtedly be included with more intense methods being incorporated when needed. In this manner, the most parsimonious way of identifying functions maintaining challenging behaviors can be accomplished.

Appendix A

Date/ time	Antecedents (what happened right before?)	Target behavior	Consequence (what happened right after?)

Appendix B

Date/time								
Staff initials								
Behavior								
Physical aggression								
Out of seat								
Location								
Classroom								
Hallway								
Bathroom								
Cafeteria								
Playground								
Antecedents								
Direction given								
Preferred item removed								
Transition								
Denied request								
No staff attention								
Other (write on back)								
Consequences								
Verbal reprimand								
Redirection to current task								
Ignored								
Given tangible								
Allowed to escape activity								
Other (write on back)								

References[1]

Alter, P. J., Conroy, M. A., Mancil, G. R., & Haydon, T. (2008). A comparison of functional behavior assessment methodologies with young children: Descriptive methods and functional analysis. *Journal of Behavioral Education, 17*, 200–219.

Arndorfer, R. E., Miltenberger, R. G., Woster, S. H., Rortvedt, A. K., & Gaffaney, T. (1994). Home-based descriptive and experimental analysis of problem behaviors in children. *Topics in Early Childhood Special Education, 14*, 64–87.

*Bergstrom, M. K. (2003). *Efficacy of school-based teams conducting functional behavioral assessment in the general education environment.* Unpublished doctoral dissertation, University of Oregon.

Bijou, S. W., Peterson, R. F., & Ault, M. H. (1968). A method to integrate descriptive and experimental field studies at the level of data and empirical concepts. *Journal of Applied Behavior Analysis, 1*, 175–191.

*Borgmeier, C. & Horner, R. H. (2006). An evaluation of the predictive validity of confidence ratings in identifying accurate functional behavioral assessment hypothesis statements. *Journal of Positive Behavior Interventions, 8*, 100–105.

*Carter, D. L. & Horner, R. H. (2007). Adding functional behavioral assessment to First Step to Success: A case study. *Journal of Positive Behavior Interventions, 9*, 229–238.

Cooper, J. O., Heron, T. E., & Heward, W. L. (2007). *Applied behavior analysis* (2nd ed.). Upper Saddle River: Pearson.

Cunningham, E., & O'Neill, R. E. (2000). Comparison of results of functional assessment and analysis methods with young children with autism. *Education and Training in Mental Retardation and Developmental Disabilities, 35*, 406–414.

Didden, R. (2007). Functional analysis methodology in developmental disabilities. In P. Sturmey (Ed.), *Functional analysis in clinical treatment* (pp. 65–86). Burlington: Academic.

Durand, V. M., & Crimmins, D. B. (1992). *The Motivation Assessment Scale administrative guide.* Topeka: Monaco & Associates.

Ellingson, S. A., Miltenberger, R. G., & Long, E. S. (1999). A survey of the use of functional assessment procedures in agencies serving individuals with developmental disabilities. *Behavioral Interventions, 14*, 187–198.

[1] References marked with an asterisk indicate studies included in the McIntosh et al. (2008) review paper discussed within.

English, C. L., & Anderson, C. M. (2004). Effects of familiar versus unfamiliar therapists on responding in the analog functional analysis. *Research in Developmental Disabilities, 25,* 39–55.

Ervin, R. A., DuPaul, G. J., Kern, L., & Friman, P. C. (1998). Classroom-based functional and adjunctive assessments: Proactive approaches to intervention selection for adolescents with attention deficit hyperactivity disorder. *Journal of Applied Behavior Analysis, 31,* 65–78.

*Filter, K. J., & Horner, R. H. (2009). Function-based academic interventions for problem behavior. *Education and Treatment of Children, 11,* 222–234.

Gettinger, M., & Stoiber, K. C. (2006). Functional assessment, collaboration, and evidence-based treatment: Analysis of a team approach for addressing challenging behaviors in young children. *Journal of School Psychology, 44,* 231–252.

Hanley, G. P., Iwata, B. A., & McCord, B. E. (2003). Functional analysis of problem behavior: A review. *Journal of Applied Behavior Analysis, 36,* 147–185.

Hartwig, L., Tuesday Heathfield, L., & Jenson, W. R. (2004). Standardization of the Functional Assessment and Intervention Program (FAIP) with children who have externalizing behaviors. *School Psychology Quarterly, 19,* 272–287.

Individuals with Disabilities Education Act Amendments of 1997, 20 U.S.C. Section 1400 et seq. (1997).

Individuals with Disabilities Education Act Amendments of 2004, 11 Stat. 37 U.S.C. Section 1401. (2004).

Iwata, B. A., Dorsey, M. F., Slifer, K. J., Bauman, K. E., & Richman, G. S. (1994). Toward a functional analysis of self-injury. *Journal of Applied Behavior Analysis, 27,* 197–209 (Reprinted from *Analysis and Intervention in Developmental Disabilities, 2,* 3–20, 1982).

Iwata, B. A., Vollmer, T. R., Zarcone, J. R., & Rodgers, T. A. (1993). Treatment classification and selection based on behavioral function. In R. Van Houten & S. Axelrod (Eds.), *Behavior analysis and treatment* (pp. 102–125). New York: Plenum.

Kahng, S., Iwata, B. A., Fischer, S. M., Page, T. J., Treadwell, K. R. H., Williams, D. E., et al. (1998). Temporal distributions of problem behavior based on scatter plot analysis. *Journal of Applied Behavior Analysis, 31,* 593–604.

Kern, L., Dunlap, G., Clarke, S., & Childs, K. E. (1994). Student-assisted functional assessment interview. *Diagnostique, 19,* 29–39.

Kinch, C., Lewis-Palmer, T., Hagan-Burke, S., & Sugai, G. (2001). A comparison of teacher and student functional behavior assessment interview information from low-risk and high-risk classrooms. *Education and Treatment of Children, 24,* 480–494.

Lerman, D. C., Hovanetz, A., Strobel, M., & Tetreault, A. (2009). Accuracy of teacher-collected descriptive analysis data: A comparison of narrative and structured recording formats. *Journal of Behavioral Education, 18,* 157–172.

Lerman, D. C., & Iwata, B. A. (1993). Descriptive and experimental analyses of variables maintaining self-injurious behavior. *Journal of Applied Behavior Analysis, 26,* 293–319.

Maas, A. P. H. M., Didden, R., Bouts, L., Smits, M. G., & Curfs, L. M. G. (2009). Scatter plot analysis of excessive daytime sleepiness and severe disruptive behavior in adults with Prader-Willi syndrome: A pilot study. *Research in Developmental Disabilities, 30,* 529–537.

Mace, F. C., & Lalli, J. S. (1991). Linking descriptive and experimental analyses in the treatment of bizarre speech. *Journal of Applied Behavior Analysis, 24,* 553–562.

Mace, F. C., Lalli, J. S., & Lalli, E. P. (1991). Functional analysis and treatment of aberrant behavior. *Research in Developmental Disabilities, 12,* 155–180.

*March, R. E. & Horner, R. H. (2002). Feasibility and contributions of functional behavioral assessment in schools. *Journal of Emotional and Behavioral Disorders, 10,* 158–170.

March, R. E., Horner, R. H., Lewis-Palmer, T., Brown, D., Crone, D., Todd, A. W., et al. (2000). *Functional Assessment Checklist: Teachers and Staff (FACTS).* Eugene: Educational and Community Supports.

Matson, J. L., & Minshawi, N. F. (2007). Functional assessment of challenging behavior: Toward a strategy for applied settings. *Research in Developmental Disabilities, 28,* 353–361.

Matson, J. L., & Vollmer, T. (1995). *Questions About Behavioral Function (QABF).* Baton Rouge: Disability Consultants, LLC.

Matson, J. L., Wilkins, J., & Macken, J. (2009). The relationship of challenging behaviors to severity and symptoms of autism spectrum disorders. *Journal of Mental Health Research in Intellectual Disabilities, 2,* 29–44.

McClintock, K., Hall, S., & Oliver, C. (2003). Risk markers associated with challenging behaviours in people with intellectual disabilities: A meta-analytic study. *Journal of Intellectual Disability Research, 47,* 405–416.

McIntosh, K., Borgmeier, C., Anderson, C. M., Horner, R. H., Rodriguez, B. J., & Tobin, T. J. (2008). Technical adequacy of the Functional Assessment Checklist: Teachers and Staff (FACTS) FBA interview measure. *Journal of Positive Behavior Interventions, 10,* 33–45.

*McKenna, M. K. (2006). *The role of function-based academic and behavior supports to improve reading achievement.* Unpublished doctoral dissertation. University of Oregon.

McNeill, S. L., Watson, T. S., Henington, C., & Meeks, C. (2002). The effects of training parents in functional behavior assessment on problem identification, problem analysis, and intervention design. *Behavior Modification, 26,* 499–515.

Miltenberger, R. G. (2001). *Behavior Modification: principles and procedures* (2nd ed.). Belmont: Wadsworth/Thomson Learning.

Mudford, O. C., Arnold-Saritepe, A. M., Phillips, K. J., Locke, J. M., Ho, I. C. S., & Taylor, S. A. (2008).

Challenging behaviors. In J. L. Matson (Ed.), *Clinical assessment and intervention for autism spectrum disorders* (pp. 267–297). London: Elsevier.

Mueller, M. M., & Kafka, C. (2006). Assessment and treatment of object mouthing in a public school classroom. *Behavioral Interventions, 21*, 137–154.

Murdock, S. G., O'Neill, R. E., & Cunningham, E. (2005). A comparison of results and acceptability of functional behavioral assessment procedures with a group of middle school students with emotional/behavioral disorders (E/BD). *Journal of Behavioral Education, 14*, 5–18.

Murphy, O., Healy, O., & Leader, G. (2009). Risk factors for challenging behaviors among 157 children with autism spectrum disorder in Ireland. *Research in Autism Spectrum Disorders, 3*, 474–482.

Neidert, P. L., Dozier, C. L., Iwata, B. A., & Hafen, M. (2010). Behavior analysis in intellectual and developmental disabilities. *Psycholgoical Services, 7*, 103–113.

Newcomer, L. L., & Lewis, T. J. (2004). Functional behavioral assessment: An investigation of assessment reliability and effectiveness of function-based interventions. *Journal of Emotional and Behavioral Disorders, 12*, 168–181.

O'Neill, R. E., Horner, R. H., Albin, R. W., Sprague, J. R., Storey, K., & Newton, J. S. (1997). *Functional assessment and program development for problem behavior: A practical handbook*. Pacific Grove: Brooks/Cole.

Pfadt, A., & Wheeler, D. J. (1995). Using statistical process control to make data-based clinical decisions. *Journal of Applied Behavior Analysis, 28*, 349–370.

Poppes, P., van der Putten, A. J. J., & Vlaskamp, C. (2010). Frequency and severity of challenging behaviour in people with profound intellectual and multiple disabilities. *Research in Developmental Disabilities, 31*, 1269–1275.

*Preciado, J. A. (2006). *Using a function-based approach to decrease problem behavior and increase reading academic engagement for Latino English language learners*. Unpublished doctoral dissertation. University of Oregon.

Reed, H., Thomas, E., Sprague, J. R., & Horner, R. H. (1997). The Student Guided Functional Assessment Interview: An analysis student and teacher agreement. *Journal of Behavioral Education, 7*, 33–49.

Rojahn, J., Schroeder, S. R., & Hoch, T. A. (2008). *Self-injurious behavior in intellectual disabilities*. Amsterdam: Elsevier.

Rojahn, J., Whittaker, K., Hoch, T., & González, M. L. (2007). Assessment of self-injurious and aggressive behavior. In L. Glidden & J. L. Matson (Eds.), *International review of research in mental retardation* (Handbook of assessment in persons with intellectual disability, Vol. 34, pp. 281–319). Amsterdam: Elsevier.

*Salentine, S. P. (2003, May). The impact of "contextual fit" on the selection of behavior support plan procedures. In R. H. Horner (Chair), *Moving from functional assessment to the design of behavior support*. Symposium conducted at the conference of the International Association for Behavior Analysis, San Francisco.

*Schindler, H. R. & Horner, R. H. (2005). Generalized reduction of problem behavior of young children with autism: Building transsituational interventions. *American Journal of Mental Retardation, 110*, 36–47.

Sturmey, P. (1994). Assessing the functions of aberrant behaviors: A review of psychotropic instruments. *Journal of Autism and Developmental Disorders, 24*, 293–304.

Symons, F. J., McDonald, L. M., & Wehby, J. H. (1998). Functional assessment and teacher collected data. *Education and Treatment of Children, 21*, 135–159.

Tarbox, J., Wilke, A. E., Najdowski, A. C., Findel-Pyles, R. S., Balasanyan, S., Caveney, A. C., et al. (2009). Comparing indirect, descriptive, and experimental functional assessments of challenging behavior in children with autism. *Journal of Developmental and Physical Disabilities, 21*, 493–514.

Touchette, P. E., MacDonald, R. F., & Langer, S. N. (1985). A scatter plot for identifying stimulus control of problem behavior. *Journal of Applied Behavior Analysis, 18*, 343–351.

University of Utah, Utah State University, & Utah State Department of Education. (1999). *Functional Assessment and Intervention Program*. Longmont: Sopris West.

Vollmer, T. R., Marcus, B. A., Ringdahl, J. E., & Roane, H. S. (1995). Progressing from brief assessments to extended experimental analyses in the evaluation of aberrant behavior. *Journal of Applied Behavior Analysis, 28*, 561–576.

Experimental Functional Analysis

8

Timothy R. Vollmer, Henry S. Roane,
and Amanda B. Rone

Introduction

Terminology

Experimental functional analysis, as it relates to the assessment of severe behavior disorders, refers to behavioral assessment procedures that involve manipulation of variables hypothesized to maintain problematic behavior (e.g., Iwata, Dorsey, Slifer, Bauman, & Richman, 1982/1994). For example, the assessment could involve intentionally providing attention as a consequence to problematic behavior in one test condition to test whether such attention increases (i.e., reinforces) the problem behavior. By testing for sensitivity to attention (and other consequences) as reinforcement, an experimental functional analysis has utility distinct from other forms of behavioral assessment insofar as the variables hypothesized to maintain behavior are directly manipulated rather than inferred.

There are some redundancies in the terminology. "Experimental" is used to indicate that independent variables are introduced and withdrawn to evaluate the effects on behavior (a commonly cited analogy is the allergy test, during which the patient is intentionally exposed to hypothesized allergens). "Functional" is used to indicate that the goal is to identify changes in behavior as a function of the variables introduced; however, "functional" has also come to refer to the operant function (roughly akin to "purpose of" or "reason for" behavior). To identify the operant function of behavior means to identify the variables, such as reinforcers, responsible for its occurrence. "Analysis" is used in the sense of Baer, Wolf, and Risley (1968) to indicate that the procedure shows a reasonable demonstration of events responsible for the occurrence or nonoccurrence of behavior. Thus, it is difficult to see how an analysis (in this restricted sense of the term) could be nonexperimental or nonfunctional. Further, some people are confused by the use of the term "experimental" because of the term's association with research studies. Although an experimental functional analysis may, in fact, be a part of a research study, it is also a standard clinical procedure for the assessment of severe behavior disorders and is not experimental in the sense of "undergoing preliminary testing." This confusion may be problematic because, for example, insurance companies may be disinclined to pay for an assessment if it is considered experimental rather than routine, and a university institutional review board

T.R. Vollmer (✉) • A.B. Rone
Psychology Department, University of Florida,
Gainesville, FL 32611, USA
e-mail: vollmera@ufl.edu;
arone@heartlandforchildren.org

H.S. Roane
State University of New York Upstate
Medical University, Syracuse, NY, USA
e-mail: roaneh@upstate.edu

J.L. Matson (ed.), *Functional Assessment for Challenging Behaviors*,
Autism and Child Psychopathology Series, DOI 10.1007/978-1-4614-3037-7_8,
© Springer Science+Business Media, LLC 2012

may require further elaboration of procedures if the methods are viewed as anything other than commonly accepted practice (as may be implied by the term experimental). Thus, although it probably would suffice to say that the procedure to which we refer represents an "analysis" of behavior, we will use the term "functional analysis" hereafter both to maintain convention and to avoid unnecessary redundancy and a possible misinterpretation of the term "experimental."

Historical Overview

The functional analysis approach stems originally from behavioral assessments and treatments of self-injurious behavior (SIB). Carr (1977) reviewed studies suggesting that SIB was sometimes maintained by positive reinforcement in the form of attention or other tangible items (e.g., Lovaas & Simmons, 1969), negative reinforcement in the form of escape from instructional activity (e.g., Carr, Newsom, & Binkoff, 1976), or (what is now called) automatic reinforcement in the form of sensory stimulation (e.g., Baumeister & Forehand, 1973). Automatic reinforcement merely refers to behavior that is reinforced independent of social mediation (i.e., produces its own source of reinforcement).

The literature review by Carr (1977), coupled with clinical exigencies, seems to have set the occasion for Iwata et al. (1982/1994) to test the social positive, social negative, and automatic reinforcement hypotheses with individual participants who were hospitalized for severe SIB. Nine participants were exposed to each of four conditions: social disapproval (to test for positive reinforcement in the form of attention), academic demand (to test for negative reinforcement in the form of escape), alone (to test for automatic reinforcement), and toy play (to serve as a control for the test conditions). The format and logic behind these conditions will be discussed in additional detail later. The four conditions were presented in a multielement format, in which a separation in data paths by condition indicates a reinforcement effect in that condition, and session duration was 15 min. Results showed that one participant

engaged in differentially higher levels of SIB in the social disapproval (attention) condition, two engaged in differentially higher levels of SIB in the academic demand (escape) condition, and three engaged in differentially higher levels of SIB in the alone (automatic reinforcement) condition. In total, six of the nine participants engaged in differentially higher levels of SIB in one of the test conditions relative to the other test conditions. In addition, some participants engaged in differentially high levels of SIB in all conditions, an outcome that now usually leads to a conclusion that the behavior is maintained by automatic reinforcement.

Shortly after the original publication of Iwata et al. (1982/1994), Carr and Durand published a series of studies using logic similar to that of Iwata et al. but with a different experimental approach (e.g., Carr & Durand, 1985; Durand & Carr, 1987). Whereas Iwata et al. manipulated both antecedents to and consequences for the occurrence of problem behavior, Carr and Durand manipulated antecedents only. If the target behavior was hypothesized to be reinforced by attention (i.e., if problem behavior occurred during a period of attention deprivation), the participants were taught appropriate ways to gain attention through functional communication training (FCT). If the target behavior was hypothesized to be reinforced by escape (i.e., if problem behavior occurred following an instructional demand), the participants were taught appropriate ways to gain assistance in completing instructional activities, also via FCT. The experimenters did not manipulate any consequences following the occurrence of problem behavior, resulting in a less convincing demonstration of the operant function of the problem behavior. For this reason, the procedures used by Carr and Durand (i.e., antecedent-only manipulations) are not commonly employed in current assessments; however, these studies are of historical significance because they were among the first to adopt the logic of linking assessment to treatment.

The true utility and versatility of the functional analysis approach became increasingly clear over the past two decades, when literally hundreds of treatment studies and methodological refinements (e.g., Kahng, Iwata, DeLeon, & Worsdell, 1997) were published. Treatment studies routinely used functional analysis as a pretreatment screening method, demonstrating its utility for both research and clinical assessment. Methodological refinements have included evaluating brief assessments (e.g., Bloom, Iwata, Fritz, Roscoe, & Carreau, 2011; Northup et al., 1991), modified experimental designs (e.g., Iwata, Duncan, Zarcone, Lerman, & Shore, 1994), and inclusion of idiosyncratic test conditions (e.g., Vollmer et al., 1998), among others.

Common Test and Control Conditions

Functional analyses are usually conducted as a series of sessions, comprising experimental conditions. In some cases, the conditions are presented in a planned order, but in other cases they are presented randomly or in alternating order (Hanley, Iwata, & McCord, 2003). The logic of a planned sequence is that one session can serve as an establishing operation for the subsequent session in the series. For example, in an alone session, the participant receives no attention, so attention should have high value in a subsequent attention session. Most commonly, the functional analyses are conducted using a multielement format wherein conditions are alternated and sessions usually last anywhere from 5 to 15 min. The most common conditions of a functional analysis are attention, demand, alone, tangible, and play. Each will be discussed briefly below.

Attention

The attention condition is designed to test for socially mediated positive reinforcement in the form of attention (Iwata et al., 1982/1994). This condition attempts to address the question, "Does the participant engage in the behavior because it produces attention from others?" During this condition, a therapist is in the room with the participant but directs his or her attention away from the participant. The absence of attention is the establishing operation for attention as reinforcement.

For example, the therapist might say, "I need to do some work," and then begin shuffling through papers or a book while "ignoring" the participant. The participant receives no attention from the therapist unless a target response occurs. If a target response occurs, the therapist delivers attention, usually in the form of a reprimand, comfort statements, physical blocking, or some combination thereof, immediately following the target response. Therefore, in this context, the participant is deprived of attention until he/she engages in a targeted problem behavior. Usually, the specific form of attention delivered is designed to mimic the type of attention the participant was observed to receive during natural interactions (e.g., Piazza et al., 1999), and although the attention usually takes the form of a brief statement or interaction, the duration of attention is sometimes designed to match the duration of reinforcement in other conditions (e.g., Fisher, Piazza, & Chiang, 1996).

Demand

The demand condition is designed to test for socially mediated negative reinforcement in the form of escape (Iwata et al., 1982/1994). This condition attempts to address the question, "Does the participant engage in the behavior because it produces escape from or avoidance of non-preferred tasks?" During this condition, a therapist presents some type of instructional demand to the participant. The form of the demand can be academic, self-care, or any instruction that has been observed to be potentially non-preferred to the participant; however, potentially non-preferred demands should be restricted to those commonly or necessarily presented to the participant in their natural environment (e.g., teeth brushing, completing a math worksheet). This restriction is important to ensure that demands are constrained to those that are socially valid instructional activities, and not just demands that the individual may find to be extremely aversive. The instructional demands are the establishing operation for escape as reinforcement. The therapist presents instructions either continuously or on a set schedule (such as once every 30 s) and usually follows a three-step sequence involving a verbal instruction, a model or gestural prompt, and physical guidance to complete the instruction. The instructional sequence is always completed unless a target response occurs, at which time the therapist terminates the instructional sequence until the next scheduled demand or after a programmed break interval, such as 20 or 30 s.

Alone

The alone condition is designed to test whether behavior persists in the absence of social reinforcement (i.e., is automatically reinforced). This condition attempts to address the question, "Does the participant engage in the behavior if there are no social consequences for the behavior?" The participant is placed in a room alone with no toys or preferred activities and is ideally observed through a one-way window (Iwata et al., 1982/1994). The general absence of stimulation is considered to be an establishing operation for automatic reinforcement. In some school and home settings, a one-way window arrangement is not available, so experimenters have modified the condition to be a "no consequence" condition. During a no consequence condition, an observer is present in the room with the participant, but the target behavior produces no social consequences. When behavior persists in an alone condition, there is strong evidence to conclude that the target behavior is operant behavior maintained by automatic reinforcement (for a more detailed discussion, see Vollmer, 1994).

Tangible

A tangible condition was not included in the original Iwata et al. (1982/1994) study. The tangible condition is designed to test for socially mediated positive reinforcement in the form of contingent access to preferred items or activities. This condition attempts to address the question, "Does the participant engage in the behavior because it produces access to a preferred item or activity?"

Typically, the participant is allowed access to preferred items or activities, which are then removed when the session begins. Contingent on occurrences of the target behavior, the items or activities are returned to the participant for a scheduled period of time, such as 20 or 30 s. The tangible condition is usually used only when there is evidence to suggest that a target behavior commonly produces such a consequence, otherwise there is potential for false-positive outcomes (Shirley, Iwata, & Kahng, 1999).

Control

The control condition, described as "toy play" in the Iwata et al. (1982/1994) study, is designed to eliminate establishing operations and reinforcement contingencies used in the test conditions. To control for the effects of positive reinforcement, the participant is provided with continuous attention, attention delivered on a dense schedule (e.g., one statement delivered every 30 s), or attention provided on a brief differential reinforcement schedule (e.g., attention provided if the participant has not engaged in a target behavior for 5 s). In addition, the participant is provided with ample stimulation in the form of preferred tangible items. To control for the effects of escape, the participant is not presented with any demands. Characteristically, low rates of the target behavior are obtained in the control condition.

Sample Outcomes

Figure 8.1 is adapted from Vollmer, Iwata, Smith, Zarcone, and Mazaleski (1993).In this study, each data point represents a single session lasting 15 min. Note that the behavior rates are elevated in the attention condition relative to all other conditions, providing an example of SIB reinforced by attention (positive reinforcement).

Figure 8.2 is adapted from Vollmer, Marcus, and Ringdahl (1995a). In this study, each data point represents a single session lasting either 10 (upper panel) or 5 min (lower panel). In the upper

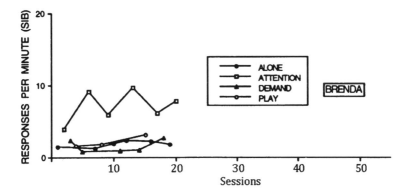

Fig. 8.1 An example of a functional analysis showing attention as reinforcement for SIB. Brenda was an adult woman living in a residential facility. Adapted from Vollmer, Iwata, Smith, et al. (1993)

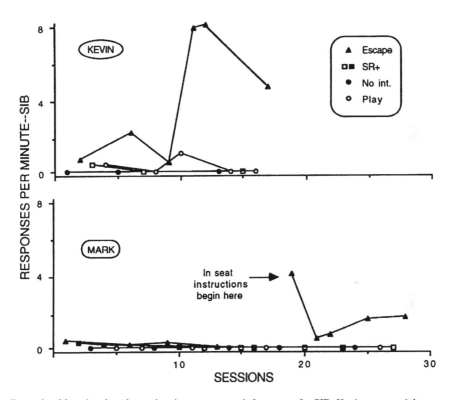

Fig. 8.2 Example of functional analyses showing escape as reinforcement for SIB. Kevin was an adolescent and Mark was a preschooler. Adapted from Vollmer, Marcus, and Ringdahl (1995a)

panel, the participant was allowed brief breaks from walking contingent on SIB. Note that the behavior rates are elevated in the escape (demand) condition relative to all other conditions, providing one example of SIB reinforced by escape. In the lower panel, the participant was allowed brief breaks from table work contingent on SIB. At the point in the assessment where table work started (denoted by an arrow), SIB occurred at differentially higher rates during the escape condition, providing a second example of SIB reinforced by escape (negative reinforcement).

Figure 8.3 is adapted from Ringdahl, Vollmer, Marcus, and Roane (1997). In this study, each data point represents the level of responding during a single 10-min session, and both assessments are for the same child. In the upper panel, one topography of SIB (hand banging) occurred in all conditions and persisted when consecutive no interaction conditions were conducted, and in the lower panel, a second topography of SIB (hand and body hitting) occurred only during the no interaction conditions. Both of these outcomes provide examples of SIB reinforced by automatic reinforcement.

Figure 8.4 is adapted from Athens and Vollmer (2010). In this study, each data point represents

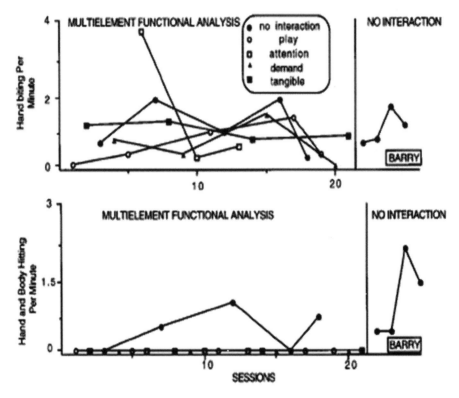

Fig. 8.3 Examples of functional analyses showing SIB maintained by automatic reinforcement. Barry was a preschooler. In the *upper panel*, hand banging occurred in all conditions and persisted in the no interaction condition. In the *lower panel*, hand and body hitting occurred exclusively in the no interaction condition. Both outcomes are indicative of an automatic reinforcement effect. Adapted from Ringdahl et al. (1997)

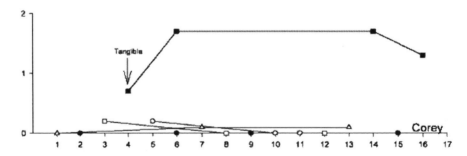

Fig. 8.4 An example of a functional analysis showing an outcome where tangible items (toys) reinforced Corey's disruptive behavior. Adapted from Athens and Vollmer (2010)

the level of responding in a single 10-min session. Note that the behavior rates are differentially higher in the tangible condition when compared with the other conditions, providing an example of disruptive behavior reinforced by the delivery of tangible items.

The Utility of Functional Analysis

Functional Analysis as Clinical Assessment

Dozens of the leading behavioral treatment institutes and programs do currently, or have historically, used functional analysis as an initial assessment for the purposes of treatment development. To list just a few examples, functional analysis is or was a requisite assessment in the following behavior analytic programs: Kennedy Krieger Institute/Johns Hopkins School of Medicine, Marcus Autism Center/Children's Healthcare of Atlanta, Monroe-Meyer Institute/University of Nebraska Medical Center, University of Iowa Children's Hospital, Florida Center for Self-Injury, Children's Seashore House/University of Pennsylvania School of Medicine, Family Behavior Analysis Clinic/Upstate Medical University among many others. The typical model is that once an individual is admitted to the program, they participate in a functional analysis prior to the development of a treatment program (Iwata, Pace et al., 1994).

Functional analysis is so commonly used by expert practitioners because it directly prescribes treatment. A clinical premise of functional analysis is that behavior disorders are not best evaluated solely on the basis of response topography. For example, two different clients might engage in exactly the same form of behavior, but the behavior might be maintained by negative reinforcement for one person and maintained by positive reinforcement for the other. Therefore, even though these individuals may engage in topographically identical behavior, the treatments for each individual may differ significantly because of the functional, rather than topographical, treatment prescription. The treatment classification

should not be viewed as a treatment for a particular form of behavior (e.g., hand biting); rather, it should be viewed as a treatment for behavior maintained by a particular source of reinforcement (e.g., social positive reinforcement). A second clinical premise is that behavior disorders are best classified according to behavioral functions. For example, one individual might engage in property destruction maintained by negative reinforcement and another person might engage in SIB maintained by negative reinforcement. The treatment for those two individuals could be more similar than a treatment for two individuals who engage in exactly the same form of SIB (Vollmer & Smith, 1996), because an emphasis is placed on the function rather than the form of the behavior.

The clinical goal of a functional analysis is to match the treatment to the assessment outcome. For example, if behavior is found to be maintained by positive reinforcement in the form of attention, attention can either be withheld (extinction), provided contingent on some alternative behavior (differential reinforcement), provided noncontingently, or some combination, to reduce motivation to engage in problem behavior and to break the contingency between problem behavior and attention (e.g., Vollmer, Iwata, Zarcone, Smith, & Mazaleski, 1993). Similarly, if behavior is maintained by negative reinforcement in the form of escape, escape can either be withheld during extinction (e.g., Iwata et al., 1990), provided contingent on some alternative behavior during differential reinforcement (e.g., Marcus & Vollmer, 1995), provided noncontingently (e.g., Vollmer, Marcus, & Ringdahl, 1995a), or some combination.

When behavior is maintained by automatic reinforcement, the treatment prognosis is not as good as when behavior is maintained by social reinforcement because the therapist often cannot directly control the automatic reinforcer. Nonetheless, when behavior is maintained by automatic reinforcement, treatment could involve identifying substitutable reinforcers to provide either contingently or noncontingently (e.g., Vollmer, Marcus, & LeBlanc, 1994). Further, the automatic reinforcement produced by the behavior can be blocked, either by equipment or by physical means, as a form of extinction (e.g., Lerman & Iwata, 1996).

If a functional analysis is not conducted, there is a degree of guesswork involved in treatment development. For example, if the reinforcer(s) maintaining problematic behavior are not identified, a therapist might prescribe an irrelevant treatment or, even worse, a "treatment" that actually exacerbates the behavior. An example of an irrelevant treatment would be ignoring behavior that is maintained by automatic reinforcement. Even if the prescribed treatment is implemented with complete integrity, the behavior will not extinguish because the reinforcer that is maintaining the behavior has not been withheld. Yet, professional therapists might be inclined to ignore the behavior based on their experience with extinction being effective with socially reinforced behavior. An example of a treatment that might exacerbate problematic behavior could be timeout for behavior that is maintained by escape from instructional demands. In this situation, it is likely that the behavior would get worse because timeout might actually serve as negative reinforcement (Iwata, Pace, Cowdery, & Miltenberger, 1994). Yet, professional therapists might be inclined to implement timeout based on their experience with timeout being an effective punishment procedure.

Functional Analysis as a Research Method

Hundreds of published studies have demonstrated the utility of functional analysis as a research method. Vollmer and Smith (1996) discussed three distinct contributions of the approach as a research method, and these contributions are summarized below.

Understanding Diverse Response Topographies

Since the publication of Iwata et al. (1982/1994), dozens of studies have systematically replicated the approach to identify the operant function of seemingly inexplicable problematic behavior, including classroom disruption (Northup et al.,

1995), breath holding (Kern, Mauk, Marder, & Mace, 1995), pica (Mace & Knight, 1986), schizophrenic vocalizations (Wilder, Masuda, O'Conner, & Baham, 2001), and coprophagia (Ing, Roane, & Veenstra, 2011) just to name of few. Thus, the use of functional analysis in research may provide new information on previously misunderstood or little understood behavior disorders.

However, the systematic replication of functional analysis methods to identify the function of other diverse forms of behavior should proceed with caution. Recall that the functional analysis of SIB was based on decades of prior research pointing to attention, escape, and automatic reinforcement as specific sources of reinforcement for the disorder (Carr, 1977). However, these specific sources of reinforcement may need to be refined in some cases (such as when peer rather than adult attention might function as reinforcement; e.g., Northup et al., 1995) or when phylogenic variables possibly play a role. For example, it is now widely known that aggression serves operant functions (e.g., Marcus, Vollmer, Swanson, Roane, & Ringdahl, 2001); however, there is evidence that animals (presumably including humans) will behave aggressively in response to extreme aversive stimulation (e.g., Ulrich & Azrin, 1962) and there is clear evidence of a role of imitation and modeling in aggression (e.g., Bandura & Waiters 1963). Thus, the expansion of the functional analysis approach to topographies other than SIB should progress as cautiously and systematically as possible, taking into account a range of potential influences.

Translational Research

Prior to the development of functional analysis assessment methodology, there was a degree of guesswork involved in identifying putative reinforcers maintaining problematic behavior. With the advent of functional analysis procedures, reinforcers can be identified explicitly. By so doing, principles of reinforcement that have been widely studied in basic research can be usefully applied to the human situation. Although it is beyond the scope of this chapter to detail the range of translational research made possible by functional analysis, we will highlight one area to demonstrate the role of functional analysis in translational research: the matching law.

The matching law is a widely accepted principle of reinforcement that posits proportional behavior rates on two or more alternatives will match proportional reinforcement rates on those alternatives. For example, if you had two buttons to press and one of the buttons produced money twice as often as the other (on average), after a period of time you will tend to press that button almost twice as often as the other button. We have found that the same was true of children allocating problematic and appropriate behavior (Borrero & Vollmer 2002; Borrero et al., 2010).

In one study (Borrero & Vollmer, 2002), we first observed children interacting with their parents and teachers in natural settings such as the home or classroom. Observers scored whether certain events, such as attention, access to tangibles, or escape from instructions, tended to follow either problematic behavior or appropriate behavior. Next, we conducted a functional analysis to identify specific sources of reinforcement for the problematic behavior. Finally, we revisited our observational data and scored the frequency with which reinforcers identified during the functional analysis following appropriate versus problematic behavior during the naturalistic observations. We found that if the problematic behavior produced greater frequencies of reinforcement, the participants tended to engage in proportionally more problematic behavior. This finding has clinical value insofar as the goal of parent or teacher training then becomes one of reversing the reinforcement contingencies to favor appropriate behavior. In a subsequent study (Borrero et al., 2010), we found that problematic and appropriate behavior rates essentially reversed as contingencies of reinforcement were reversed. In both of these matching law studies, it would have been impossible to know for certain that particular events functioned as reinforcers if we had not conducted a functional analysis.

Participant Screening

Many behavioral treatment studies are preceded by a pretreatment functional analysis to screen for individuals whose behavioral functions are appropriate for the research question at hand. Part one of behavioral studies commonly involves showing via functional analysis that behavior is reinforced by a particular consequence. Part two of the study (if a treatment study) then goes on to evaluate the efficacy of one or more treatments for behavior *given* a particular operant function. A prototype for this approach was published by Iwata, Pace, Kalsher, Cowdery, and Cataldo (1990). First, Iwata et al. showed that the SIB of seven individuals was reinforced by escape from instructional activity. Next, the experimenters implemented escape extinction (i.e., eliminated escape as a consequence by guiding the participants through the instructed task even when SIB occurred) and showed that the SIB was reduced in six of seven cases. It was important to first show that the behavior in question was in fact maintained by escape, otherwise the subsequent extinction procedure would not have been a logical next step. For example, if the behavior had been reinforced by attention or physical contact, escape extinction in the form of guided compliance might have actually strengthened the behavior.

Preassessment Considerations

Informed Consent

The Iwata et al. (1982/1994) paper provided detailed information on informed consent and medical protection for the participants who participated. In recent years, such detail is often omitted from functional analysis studies; however, we recommend that informed consent should always be obtained before beginning any functional analysis involving dangerous behavior. One reason for this suggestion is that to nonprofessionals (and in some cases other professionals), a functional analysis may be counterintuitive unless it is carefully explained. For example, it may not be immediately clear why it is important to intentionally reinforce dangerous behavior before commencing with treatment. An additional reason for obtaining informed consent is that the parents or guardians should be aware of the potential risks and should have knowledge of the assessment procedures. For example, the alone condition of a functional analysis involves having an individual alone in a room to test for problem behavior maintained by automatic reinforcement, and the rationale for the condition may not be readily apparent to an untrained individual.

Medical Monitoring and Protection

In order for a functional analysis to identify the variables maintaining problem behavior, it is necessary for problem behavior to occur during one or more of the assessment conditions. With SIB, in particular, such situations may place the participant at a risk for harm, and it is important to obtain a medical opinion and to collaborate with medical personnel to determine the extent to which the SIB is allowable. For some individuals, a single blow to the head or eyes may be deemed unacceptable, in which case they would likely be excluded from a functional analysis unless protective equipment is used; however, for other individuals, what might appear to be severe and dangerous may actually be judged by medical personnel to be relatively harmless in the short term. For example, face slapping may be loud and cause redness, but observing this behavior for relatively short periods of time, such as the 5–15 min typical of a functional analysis session, is often deemed by medical personnel as not overly dangerous, especially when weighed against the possibility of successful treatment for the behavior. When conducting a functional analysis of SIB, it is important to weigh the "pros" of the assessment (i.e., identifying a treatment that will ultimately reduce the occurrence of the behavior) to the "cons" (i.e., permitting the repeated occurrence of SIB). To date, there have been few attempts to standardize protective procedures for functional analyses (see Weeden, Mahoney, & Poling, 2010 for a discussion).

When protective equipment or response blocking is required, it is important to recognize the potential confounding influence of those variables. For example, protective equipment can potentially extinguish or punish SIB (e.g., Dorsey,

Iwata, Reid, & Davis, 1982; Mazaleski, Iwata, Rodgers, Vollmer, & Zarcone, 1994). In addition, physical contact in the form of blocking can potentially produce an extinction effect (Lerman & Iwata, 1996), a punishment effect (Smith, Russo, & Le, 1999), or even a reinforcement effect (Vollmer, Iwata, Smith, & Rodgers, 1992). Access to self-restraining materials can also influence the outcome of a functional analysis (Smith, Iwata, Vollmer, & Pace, 1992; Smith, Lerman, & Iwata, 1996). In short, although protection in the form of equipment or blocking may be medically necessary, the potential confounds should be recognized.

During functional analyses of aggression, it is common for therapists to wear protective equipment, including shin guards, long sleeves, arm pads, etc. (Marcus et al., 2001). We are aware of no studies to date that have shown protective equipment to alter the outcome of functional analyses of aggression. Thus, it is considered standard best practice to ensure protection of the therapist conducting the assessment, and we recommend the use of protective equipment when necessary.

Session Duration

In the Iwata et al. (1982/1994) study, sessions were 15 min in duration; however, Wallace and Iwata (1999) demonstrated that assessment outcomes for 10-min sessions were nearly identical to session outcomes for 15-min sessions (the 10-min "sessions" were actually the first 10 min of the 15-min sessions). Interestingly, even 5-min sessions were shown to yield very few discrepancies when compared with the results of the 15-min sessions. Thus, most current applications of functional analyses involve relatively brief, usually 10-min, sessions. The duration of the session should be determined prior to beginning the analysis and should remain constant unless a participant reaches some predetermined termination criterion.

Response Topography

Many individuals with severe behavior disorders display multiple topographies of problematic behavior, and it is best to preselect the specific form or forms of behavior that will produce the test consequences during the functional analysis. Researchers have shown that reinforcing one topography of behavior can greatly alter the probability of another topography occurring (e.g., Lalli, Mace, Wohn, & Livezy, 1995; Richman, Wacker, Asmus, Casey, & Andelman, 1999); thus, reinforcing too many topographies of behavior might in fact "disguise" the function of the most problematic form of behavior. If an individual engages in several topographies of serious problem behavior, multiple (i.e., separate) functional analyses can be conducted to help ensure the accurate identification of the variables maintaining each specific problem behavior. For example, if an individual engages in SIB and aggression, a separate functional analysis should be conducted for each behavior rather than combining the topographies.

Experimental Design

Most commonly, a multielement design is used in the context of a functional analysis to demonstrate experimental control. Some researchers have used the logic of a multielement design but in a much briefer format, either by using brief reversals (e.g., Northup et al., 1991) or by using within-session data analyses (e.g., Vollmer, Iwata, Zarcone, et al., 1993). When the multielement approach yields undifferentiated outcomes, some researchers have used either a sequential test-control format in which a single test condition is juxtaposed against the control condition (e.g., Iwata, Duncan, et al., 1994) or a reversal design to isolate the test conditions and minimize multiple-condition interference (e.g., Vollmer, Iwata, Duncan, & Lerman, 1993).

Previously we have described a model for progressing from brief assessments to extended experimental analyses to clarify outcomes in the most efficient manner possible without sacrificing clear outcomes (Vollmer, Marcus, Ringdahl, & Roane, 1995b). In that model, the assessment begins with a brief evaluation in which the conditions are rapidly alternated in a multielement format, but the (within session) minute-by-minute

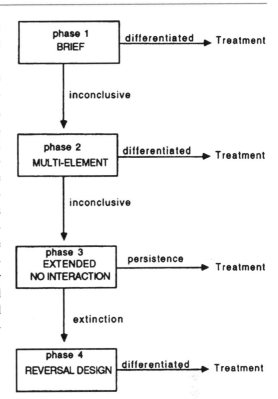

Fig. 8.5 A model for progressing from brief to extended functional analyses. Figure adapted from Vollmer, Marcus, Ringdahl, et al. (1995)

response rates are plotted to more rapidly detect response patterns. If the within-session response rates are differentiated by condition, the participant then moves on to treatment. If they are not differentiated by condition, the assessment becomes a standard multielement assessment as described by Iwata et al. (1982/1994). If the multielement assessment is differentiated, the participant then moves on to treatment; however, if the assessment is undifferentiated, the participant is then exposed to several consecutive alone or no consequence sessions to determine whether the behavior will persist in the absence of social reinforcement. If the behavior does maintain in the alone or no interaction condition, the assessment is concluded and behavior is determined to be maintained by automatic reinforcement; however, if the behavior extinguishes in the alone or no interaction condition, the social reinforcement test conditions (attention, demand, and tangible) are presented in isolation in a reversal design format. The progression is summarized in Fig. 8.5, which is adapted from the Vollmer, Marcus, Ringdahl, et al. (1995) paper.

Limitations and Future Directions

Inconclusive Outcomes

Iwata, Pace et al. (1994) reported that inconclusive outcomes were obtained in 4.6% of their functional analyses of SIB. Although not a high percentage, it can be expected that almost 1 in 20 assessments will not yield useful outcomes. For these cases, it is possible that extraneous or uncontrolled sources of reinforcement influence the behavior. It may also be possible that the variables maintaining the behavior are highly specific. For example, it is possible that behavior maintained by social positive reinforcement in the form of attention is only reinforced by the attention of a particular person (and not the therapist), making it unlikely that the problem behavior will maintain during the assessment. Epidemiological data have not been reported on the function for behavior disorders other than SIB, such as aggression; however, it stands to reason that assessments of other topographies of problem behavior are also sometimes inconclusive. Future research should be aimed at clarifying inconclusive outcomes, possibly taking into account other factors such as elicitation. For example, basic research has shown that humans will bite down reflexively in response to pain (Hutchinson, 1977), so some self-biting might occur in response to undetected aversive stimulation. Also, basic research has shown that organisms will behave aggressively in response to reinforcer loss or aversive stimulation (Ulrich & Azrin, 1962); thus, it is possible that some human aggression is elicited in that fashion.

Apart from elicitation, it is unknown whether a history of reinforcement, even when the reinforcement is no longer in place, might influence the current occurrence of some forms of aberrant behavior, in a manner similar to when an organism's behavior does not quickly extinguish despite no longer producing reinforcement. Because most functional analyses involve exposure to each test condition fewer than a dozen or so times, residual target behavior could occur in some or all conditions even though the maintaining reinforcer is not being presented. It is also possible that unidentified sources of automatic reinforcement contribute to the maintenance of behavior (Vollmer, 1994).

Difficult Treatment Implementation

At times the outcome of a functional analysis prescribes a behavioral treatment that is difficult, if not impossible, to implement successfully. For example, if a functional analysis shows that severe aggression displayed by an adult, very strong man is reinforced by escape from instructional activity, it will likely be difficult to implement an extinction component while maintaining the safety of both the individual and the therapist. Another example might involve severe SIB that is reinforced by physical contact in the form of blocking. If the SIB is sufficiently dangerous, it is difficult to develop a treatment involving extinction (i.e., the removal of blocking) because the person might get severely hurt if blocking procedures were to be removed.

Although such situations do arise, we contend that there is nothing about the functional analysis per se that creates the problem of difficult treatment implementation. Irrespective of the method used to prescribe or develop treatment, the situation would be difficult given the types of examples provided above. In fact, it is possible that by shedding light on the variables maintaining problem behavior, a functional analysis provides information for treatment development that could circumvent some of the problems associated with an extinction component. For example, Lalli et al. (1999) showed that the use of positive reinforcement for compliance successfully competed with escape for severe aggression and SIB, such that escape extinction was unnecessary. Similarly, Athens and Vollmer (2010) manipulated several reinforcement parameters such that, even when problematic behavior was still being reinforced, the "pay off" for engaging in appropriate behavior was greater along the dimensions of reinforcer immediacy, duration, and quality. Accordingly, response allocation shifted toward appropriate behavior despite the absence of an extinction component.

Time and Resource Constraints

Some have argued that a functional analysis is time consuming and cumbersome, requiring too much expertise and personnel (e.g., Sturmey, 1995). In one sense, this criticism is most unfortunate because individuals with or without disabilities spend incredible resources on other life-threatening illnesses such as cancer or heart disease. It is unlikely that anyone would ever question the resource requirements to treat such illness, and we would argue that when SIB or aggression is life threatening, resource limitations should also not govern decision making. When the target behavior is not life threatening, but greatly reduces the quality of life for the individual or the individual's family, perhaps the issue is a bit more complicated, and the following bear consideration.

Is a functional analysis time consuming? If an assessment requires (for example) six exposures to each condition, and there are four conditions, a total of 24 sessions would be required to complete the assessment. Suppose there is equal time in set up, breaks between sessions, and so on, the total (and we would consider this to be liberal time consumption) is 480 min or 8 h of assessment time. If an effective treatment can be identified in 8 h, this time allocation should be contrasted with the time allocation spent on inadvertently reinforcing the behavior, repairing/replacing destroyed items, the cost of purchasing new items, treating injuries, and so on. Further, some research has shown that clear functional analyses can take as little as 90 total minutes (e.g., Northup et al., 1991; Vollmer, Marcus, Ringdahl & Roane, 1995b).

Is a functional analysis cumbersome and does it require extensive expertise? Iwata et al. (2000) showed that undergraduate psychology students, given approximately 2 h of training, implemented functional analysis procedures with greater than

95% accuracy. Although it is true that in some cases sophisticated decision making is required when analyzing data in a functional analysis, the same is true for virtually any type of psychology assessment or medical assessment.

Does a functional analysis require high numbers of staff? Usually a functional analysis requires one therapist and one observer (with a second observer for about 20% of the sessions). Some variations of functional analysis have used a parent or teachers as the therapist or observer (e.g., Cooper, Wacker, Sasso, Reimers, & Donn, 1990). Also, because only a few general classes of reinforcement maintain a high percentage of behavior disorders, it is possible that future research could involve functional analyses during ongoing activities. For example, a parent or teacher could be taught the rule: Do not change what you are doing if the problem behavior occurs. Given that reinforcement requires stimulus change, at a minimum, social sources of reinforcement could be ruled in or out with essentially no additional personnel costs simply by having a parent or teacher follow the rule.

Are there alternatives available? If some briefer form of assessment was shown to be as reliable and as convincing as a functional analysis, most would agree that a functional analysis would not always be required. Indirect forms of assessment are reviewed elsewhere in this volume, but in short, although moving in a favorable direction, no indirect assessment methods to date have been conclusively shown to identify the operant function of behavior with consistency and reliability.

Covert Behavior

Some serious behavior problems displayed by individuals with intellectual disabilities occur either especially or exclusively when they are alone (or when they believe that they are alone; Chapman, Fisher, Piazza, & Kurtz, 1993). The covert nature of the behavior can make an assessment difficult to complete in some settings; however, a functional analysis can be accomplished when a true alone condition can be implemented (i.e., using a one-way window). An example can be seen in Cowdery, Iwata, and Pace (1990), in which the researchers showed that the severe SIB (skin picking and scratching) displayed by a young boy occurred exclusively when he was alone. They observed the behavior through a one-way window and, during treatment, provided feedback based on his wounds (although they had actually conducted direct behavioral observations). A differential reinforcement schedule was successfully implemented to treat the behavior.

Low Frequency Behavior

A related problem occurs when the target behavior occurs at such a low frequency that it is rarely observed. However, it is possible that the behavior occurs rarely because people in the environment make sure that the establishing operation is avoided. For example, staff might learn to avoid asking a resident to brush her teeth because oral hygiene sessions produce high rates of problematic behavior (e.g., Shore, Iwata, Vollmer, Lerman, & Zarcone, 1995). If so, merely conducting a functional analysis may increase the probability of observing the behavior in context because the establishing operation is intentionally presented.

Kahng, Abt, and Schonbachler (2001) reported another interesting approach. Because aggression was not observed during typical 10-min functional analysis sessions, they increased the observation period and functional analysis test contingencies to a 7-h period wherein one test condition was conducted per day. By so doing, the experimenters were able to identify the operant function of aggression insofar as it clearly occurred most frequently during the protracted attention condition. Thus, although low-rate behavior is somewhat problematic for a functional analysis approach, the procedures can be adapted to accommodate the difficulty.

High-Intensity Behavior

At times, the target behavior is so intense and dangerous that not even a single response can be allowed to occur. In these cases, the behavior

analyst might need to restrict the assessment to an interview format or records review to develop hypotheses about the function of the behavior. Another approach that has emerged in recent research involves the functional analysis of "precursor" behavior, or behavior that reliably predicts the onset of more dangerous behavior (Borrero & Borrero, 2008; Herscovitch, Roscoe, Libby, Bourret, & Ahearn, 2009; Najdowski, Wallace, Ellsworth, MacAleese, & Cleveland, 2008; Smith & Churchill, 2002). The notion behind assessing precursor behavior is that if an earlier response form is reinforced, a later response in a hierarchy need not occur

Conclusions

The functional analysis approach was based on decades of research showing that severe behavior disorders are sensitive to operant contingencies of reinforcement. The assessment method developed by Iwata et al. (1982/1994) has come to be known as an "experimental functional analysis." We have argued that the term "functional" analysis is a sufficient descriptor and is in keeping with current usage. The functional analysis approach is ideally suited to identify cause and effect relations between environmental events and behavior. As a result, this type of assessment directly prescribes treatments and serves as a useful research method. Although several potential limitations of the approach have been cited, recent research has addressed many of them. We conclude that the functional analysis approach does as should remain as a standard for behavioral assessment.

References

Athens, E., & Vollmer, T. R. (2010). An evaluation of differential reinforcement of alternative behavior without extinction. *Journal of Applied Behavior Analysis, 43*, 569–589.

Baer, D. M., Wolf, M. M., & Risley, T. R. (1968). Some current dimensions of applied behavior analysis. *Journal of Applied Behavior Analysis, 1*, 91–97.

Bandura, A., & Waiters, R. H. (1963). *Social learning and personality development*. New York: Holt, Rinehart & Winston.

Baumeister, A., & Forehand, R. (1973). Stereotyped acts. In N. R. Ellis (Ed.), *International review of research in mental retardation* (Vol. 6, pp. 55–96). New York: Academic.

Bloom, S. E., Iwata, B. A., Fritz, J. N., Roscoe, E. M., & Carreau, A. B. (2011). Classroom application of a trial-based functional analysis. *Journal of Applied Behavior Analysis, 44*, 19–31.

Borrero, C. S. W., & Borrero, J. C. (2008). Descriptive and experimental analyses of potential precursors to problem behavior. *Journal of Applied Behavior Analysis, 41*, 83–96.

Borrero, J. C., & Vollmer, T. R. (2002). An application of the matching law to severe problem behavior. *Journal of Applied Behavior Analysis, 35*, 13–27.

Borrero, C. S. W., Vollmer, T. R., Borrero, J. C., Bourret, J. C., Sloman, K. N., Samaha, A. L., et al. (2010). Concurrent reinforcement schedules for problem behavior and appropriate behavior: Experimental applications of the matching law. *Journal of the Experimental Analysis of Behavior, 93*, 455–469.

Carr, E. G. (1977). The motivation of self-injurious behavior: A review of some hypotheses. *Psychological Bulletin, 84*, 800–816.

Carr, E. G., & Durand, V. M. (1985). Reducing behavior problems through functional communication training. *Journal of Applied Behavior Analysis, 18*, 111–126.

Carr, E. G., Newsom, C. D., & Binkoff, J. A. (1976). Stimulus control of self-destructive behavior in a psychotic child. *Journal of Abnormal Child Psychology, 4*, 139–153.

Chapman, S., Fisher, W., Piazza, C. C., & Kurtz, P. F. (1993). Functional assessment and treatment of life-threatening drug ingestion in a dually diagnosed youth. *Journal of Applied Behavior Analysis, 26*, 255–256.

Cooper, L., Wacker, D., Sasso, G., Reimers, T., & Donn, L. (1990). Using parents as therapists to evaluate appropriate behavior of their children: Application to a tertiary diagnostic clinic. *Journal of Applied Behavior Analysis, 23*, 285–296.

Cowdery, G. E., Iwata, B. A., & Pace, G. M. (1990). Effects and side effects of DRO as treatment for self-injurious behavior. *Journal of Applied Behavior Analysis, 23*, 497–506.

Dorsey, M. F., Iwata, B. A., Reid, D. H., & Davis, P. A. (1982). Protective equipment: Continuous and contingent application in the treatment of self-injurious behavior. *Journal of Applied Behavior Analysis, 15*, 217–230.

Durand, V. M., & Carr, E. G. (1987). Social influences on "self-stimulatory" behavior: Analysis and treatment application. *Journal of Applied Behavior Analysis, 20*, 119–132.

Fisher, W. W., Piazza, C. C., & Chiang, C. L. (1996). Effects of equal and unequal reinforcer duration during functional analysis. *Journal of Applied Behavior Analysis, 29*, 117–120.

Hanley, G. P., Iwata, B. A., & McCord, B. E. (2003). Functional analysis of problem behavior: A review. *Journal of Applied Behavior Analysis, 36*, 147–185.

Herscovitch, B., Roscoe, E. M., Libby, M. E., Bourret, J. C., & Ahearn, W. H. (2009). A procedure for identifying precursors to problem behavior. *Journal of Applied Behavior Analysis, 42*, 697–702.

Hutchinson, R. R. (1977). By-products of aversive control. In W. K. Honig & L. L. Staddon (Eds.), *Handbook of operant behavior* (pp. 415–431). Englewood Cliffs: Prentice-Hall.

Ing, A. D., Roane, H. S., & Veenstra, R. A. (2011). Functional analysis and treatment of coprophagia. *Journal of Applied Behavior Analysis, 44*, 151–155.

Iwata, B. A., Dorsey, M. F., Slifer, K. J., Bauman, K. E., & Richman, G. S. (1994). *Journal of Applied Behavior Analysis, 27*, 197–209 (Reprinted from *Analysis and Intervention in Developmental Disabilities, 2*, 3–20, 1982).

Iwata, B. A., Duncan, B. A., Zarcone, J. R., Lerman, D. C., & Shore, B. A. (1994). A sequential, test-control methodology for conducting functional analyses of self-injurious behavior. *Behavior Modification, 18*, 289–306.

Iwata, B. A., Pace, G. M., Cowdery, G. E., & Miltenberger, R. G. (1994). What makes extinction work: An analysis of procedural form and function. *Journal of Applied Behavior Analysis, 27*, 131–144.

Iwata, B. A., Pace, G. M., Dorsey, M. F., Zarcone, J. R., Vollmer, T. R., Smith, R. G., et al. (1994). The functions of self-injurious behavior: An experimental-epidemiological analysis. *Journal of Applied Behavior Analysis, 27*, 215–240.

Iwata, B. A., Pace, G. M., Kalsher, M. J., Cowdery, G. E., & Cataldo, M. F. (1990). Experimental analysis and extinction of self-injurious escape behavior. *Journal of Applied Behavior Analysis, 23*, 11–27.

Iwata, B. A., Wallace, M. D., Kahng, S., Lindberg, J. S., Roscoe, E. M., Conners, J., et al. (2000). Skill acquisition in the implementation of functional analysis methodology. *Journal of Applied Behavior Analysis, 33*, 181–194.

Kahng, S., Abt, K., & Schonbachler, H. (2001). Assessment and treatment of low-rate high-intensity problem behavior. *Journal of Applied Behavior Analysis, 34*, 225–228.

Kahng, S., Iwata, B. A., DeLeon, I. G., & Worsdell, A. S. (1997). Evaluation of the "control over reinforcement" component in functional communication training. *Journal of Applied Behavior Analysis, 30*, 267–277.

Kern, L., Mauk, J. E., Marder, T. J., & Mace, E. C. (1995). Functional analysis and intervention for breath-holding. *Journal of Applied Behavior Analysis, 28*, 339–340.

Lalli, J. S., Mace, F. C., Wohn, T., & Livezy, K. (1995). Identification and modification of a response-class hierarchy. *Journal of Applied Behavior Analysis, 28*, 551–559.

Lalli, J. S., Vollmer, T. R., Progar, P. R., Wright, C., Borrero, J., Daniel, D., et al. (1999). Competition between positive and negative reinforcement in the treatment of escape behavior. *Journal of Applied Behavior Analysis, 32*, 285–295.

Lerman, D. C., & Iwata, B. A. (1996). A methodology for distinguishing between extinction and punishment effects associated with response blocking. *Journal of Applied Behavior Analysis, 29*, 231–234.

Lovaas, O. I., & Simmons, J. Q. (1969). Manipulation of self-destruction in three retarded children. *Journal of Applied Behavior Analysis, 2*, 143–157.

Mace, F. C., & Knight, D. (1986). Functional analysis and treatment of severe pica. *Journal of Applied Behavior Analysis, 19*, 411–416.

Marcus, B. A., & Vollmer, T. R. (1995). Effects of differential negative reinforcement on disruption and compliance. *Journal of Applied Behavior Analysis, 28*, 229–230.

Marcus, B. A., Vollmer, T. R., Swanson, V., Roane, H. R., & Ringdahl, J. E. (2001). An experimental analysis of aggression. *Behavior Modification, 25*, 189–213.

Mazaleski, J. L., Iwata, B. A., Rodgers, T. A., Vollmer, T. R., & Zarcone, J. R. (1994). Protective equipment as treatment for stereotypic hand mouthing: Sensory extinction or punishment effects? *Journal of Applied Behavior Analysis, 27*, 345–355.

Najdowski, A. C., Wallace, M. D., Ellsworth, C. L., MacAleese, A. N., & Cleveland, J. M. (2008). Functional analyses and treatment of precursor behavior. *Journal of Applied Behavior Analysis, 41*, 97–105.

Northup, J., Broussard, C., Jones, K., George, T., Vollmer, T. R., & Herring, M. (1995). The differential effects of teacher and peer attention on the disruptive classroom behavior of three children with a diagnosis of attention deficit hyperactivity disorder. *Journal of Applied Behavior Analysis, 28*, 227–228.

Northup, J., Wacker, D., Sasso, G., Steege, M., Cigrand, K., Cook, J., et al. (1991). A brief functional analysis of aggressive and alternative behavior in an outclinic setting. *Journal of Applied Behavior Analysis, 24*, 509–522.

Piazza, C. C., Bowman, L. G., Contrucci, S. A., Delia, M. D., Adelinis, J. D., & Goh, H. (1999). An evaluation of the properties of attention as reinforcement for destructive and appropriate behavior. *Journal of Applied Behavior Analysis, 32*, 437–449.

Richman, D. M., Wacker, D. P., Asmus, J. M., Casey, S. D., & Andelman, M. (1999). Further analysis of problem behavior in response class hierarchies. *Journal of Applied Behavior Analysis, 32*, 269–283.

Ringdahl, J. E., Vollmer, T. R., Marcus, B. A., & Roane, H. S. (1997). An analog evaluation of environmental enrichment as treatment for aberrant behavior. *Journal of Applied Behavior Analysis, 30*, 203–216.

Shirley, M. J., Iwata, B. A., & Kahng, S. (1999). False-positive maintenance of self-injurious behavior by access to tangible reinforcers. *Journal of Applied Behavior Analysis, 32*, 201–204.

Shore, B. A., Iwata, B. A., Vollmer, T. R., Lerman, D. C., & Zarcone, J. R. (1995). Pyramidal staff training in the extension of treatment for severe behavior disorders. *Journal of Applied Behavior Analysis, 28*, 323–332.

Smith, R. G., & Churchill, R. M. (2002). Identification of environmental determinants of behavior disorders through functional analysis of precursor behaviors. *Journal of Applied Behavior Analysis, 35*, 125–136.

Smith, R. G., Iwata, B. A., Vollmer, T. R., & Pace, G. M. (1992). On the relationship between self-injurious behavior and self-restraint. *Journal of Applied Behavior Analysis, 25*, 433–445.

Smith, R. G., Lerman, D. C., & Iwata, B. A. (1996). Self-restraint as positive reinforcement for self-injurious behavior. *Journal of Applied Behavior Analysis, 29*, 99–102.

Smith, R. G., Russo, L., & Le, D. D. (1999). Distinguishing between extinction and punishment effects of response blocking: A replication. *Journal of Applied Behavior Analysis, 32*, 367–370.

Sturmey, P. (1995). Analog baselines: A critical review of the methodology. *Research in Developmental Disabilities, 16*, 269–284.

Ulrich, R. E., & Azrin, N. H. (1962). Reflexive fighting in response to aversive stimulation. *Journal of the Experimental Analysis of Behavior, 5*, 511–520.

Vollmer, T. R. (1994). The concept of automatic reinforcement: Implications for behavioral research in developmental disabilities. *Research in Developmental Disabilities, 15*, 187–207.

Vollmer, T. R., Iwata, B. A., Duncan, B. A., & Lerman, D. C. (1993). Extensions of multi element functional analyses using reversal-type designs. *Journal of Developmental and Physical Disabilities, 5*, 311–325.

Vollmer, T. R., Iwata, B. A., Smith, R. G., & Rodgers, T. A. (1992). Reduction of multiple aberrant behaviors and concurrent development of self-care skills with differential reinforcement. *Research in Developmental Disabilities, 13*, 287–299.

Vollmer, T. R., Iwata, B. A., Smith, R. G., Zarcone, J. R., & Mazaleski, J. L. (1993). The role of attention in the treatment of attention-maintained self-injurious behavior: Noncontingent reinforcement (NCR) and differential reinforcement of other behavior (DRO). *Journal of Applied Behavior Analysis, 26*, 9–21.

Vollmer, T. R., Iwata, B. A., Zarcone, J. R., Smith, R. S., & Mazaleski, J. L. (1993). Within-session patterns of self-injury as indicators of behavioral function. *Research in Developmental Disabilities, 14*, 479–492.

Vollmer, T. R., Marcus, B. A., & LeBlanc, L. (1994). Treatment of self-injury and handmouthing following inconclusive functional analyses. *Journal of Applied Behavior Analysis, 27*, 331–344.

Vollmer, T. R., Marcus, B. A., & Ringdahl, J. E. (1995a). Noncontingent escape as treatment for self-injury maintained by negative reinforcement. *Journal of Applied Behavior Analysis, 28*, 15–26.

Vollmer, T. R., Marcus, B. A., Ringdahl, J. E., & Roane, H. S. (1995b). Progressing from brief assessments to extended experimental analyses in the evaluation of aberrant behavior. *Journal of Applied Behavior Analysis, 28*, 561–576.

Vollmer, T. R., Progar, P. R., Lalli, J. S., VanCamp, C. M., Sierp, B. J., Wright, C. S., et al. (1998). Fixed-time schedules attenuate extinction-induced phenomena in the treatment of severe aberrant behavior. *Journal of Applied Behavior Analysis, 31*, 529–542.

Vollmer, T. R., & Smith, R. G. (1996). Some current themes in functional analysis research. *Research in Developmental Disabilities, 17*, 229–249.

Weeden, M., Mahoney, A., & Poling, A. (2010). Self-injurious behavior and functional analysis: Where are the descriptions of participant protections? *Research in Developmental Disabilities, 31*, 299–303.

Wallace, M. D., & Iwata, B. A. (1999). Effects of session duration on functional analysis outcomes. *Journal of Applied Behavior Analysis, 32*, 175–183.

Wilder, D. A., Masuda, A., O'Conner, C., & Baham, M. (2001). Brief functional analysis and treatment of aberrant vocalizations in an adult with schizophrenia. *Journal of Applied Behavior Analysis, 34*, 65–68.

In Vivo Assessment: Issues of Real-Time Data

Max Horovitz and Johnny L. Matson

One of the fundamental elements of functional assessment for challenging behaviors is the collection of data. Data are used to help determine the nature of the problem, create a case formulation, carry out the functional assessment, and monitor the progress of interventions (Hartmann, Barrios, & Wood, 2004). All decisions made during the course of a functional assessment are based off of data. Most data collected during this process are collected in vivo. That is to say, most data are collected through real-time observations of individuals in their natural environment.

There are a number of advantages to in vivo data collection, primarily that observations are carried out in the same setting in which the behavior naturally occurs (Gardner, 2000). Take, for example, an individual who engages in self-injurious behavior when he is hungry. In vivo assessment allows for data to be collected in this individual's home, where he or she typically engages in the behavior. Were the individual brought into a clinic for observation, the properties of the behavior, such as frequency, intensity, and duration, may differ due to the novel environment.

Therefore, in vivo data collection has its primary advantage in its ability to be collected in the natural environment in which the behavior typically occurs. It does not require experimental manipulation of the environment, which can create an artificial setting and reduce the external validity of the data (Martens, DiGennaro, Reed, Szczech, & Rosenthal, 2008).

In vivo data collection also allows for greater specificity of data, as definitions of challenging behavior can be modified to fit each individual's unique pattern of behavior (Matson & Nebel-Schwalm, 2007). This makes in vivo data collection procedures very flexible, as they can be adapted to target a variety of behaviors in a variety of settings (Hartmann et al., 2004; Martens et al., 2008). Due to this specificity and flexibility, real-time data are more sensitive to treatment effects than data collected via scaling methods (Matson & Nebel-Schwalm, 2007).

Another advantage is that observers are able to directly see interactions between an individual and his or her environment (Gardner, 2000; Iwata, Vollmer, & Zarcone, 1990). Indirect assessments from outside informants, such as parent reports, may be susceptible to personal biases, such as expectations, attributions, and mood (Eddy, Dishion, & Stoolmiller, 1998; Fergusson, Lynskey, & Horwood, 1993). In contrast, real-time data collection allows for direct observations, thereby bypassing the need for an informant. In vivo data collection, in principle, allows for objective evaluation of the effects of treatment

M. Horovitz (✉)
Louisiana State University, Baton Rouge, LA 70803, USA
e-mail: maxh13@gmail.com

J.L. Matson
Department of Psychology, Louisiana State University,
Baton Rouge, LA 70803, USA
e-mail: johnmatson@aol.com

J.L. Matson (ed.), *Functional Assessment for Challenging Behaviors*,
Autism and Child Psychopathology Series, DOI 10.1007/978-1-4614-3037-7_9,
© Springer Science+Business Media, LLC 2012

(Iwata et al., 1990; Lipinski & Nelson, 1974). However, as we will see later in this chapter, that is not always the case.

While in vivo data collection has a number of advantages and clear utility, there are a number of problems that must be considered. This chapter discusses a variety of problems associated with the collection and use of real-time data that must be addressed. These problems are broken into five general categories: Defining the behavior, collecting the data, reliability, validity, and the interpretation and use of the data. Problems common to each of these areas are discussed in depth.

Defining the Behavior

The first step in data collection is to determine and define on what behavior data will be collected. In order for this to be done, an accurate, operational definition must be established for the behavior. For the purposes of in vivo data collection, the behavior must be defined in clearly observable terms (Bijou, Peterson, & Ault, 1968). Hawkins and Dobes (1977) suggest three characteristics of a well-formed operational definition: (1) the definition should include objective terms and refer only to observable characteristics of the behavior; (2) the definition should be unambiguous and clear to experienced observers; and (3) the definition should be complete, defining what should be included and what should be excluded, thereby reducing inference on the part of the observer. Additionally, they suggest that the definition be explicitly stated to data collectors, as implicit definitions are more prone to error. These guidelines help prevent multiple observers from using varying definitions and allow for replication of data collection.

Barrios (1993) provides a four-step process for creating such an operational definition. The first step is to research how the behavior has previously been operationalized, as it may be possible to adopt a similar definition. The second step is to construct a definition appropriate for the current behavior in the current setting. Next, the definition should be reviewed by people with knowledge on the subject matter, as well as by those who will be using it for observation. Finally, if the definition is found to be appropriate and clear, it should then be field tested by two observers who only have the definition. If high agreement is found, the definition is ready to be used; if not, additional revisions may be required.

Finally, it is necessary that the criteria used to operationally define the behavior easily distinguish the target behavior from similar behaviors. For example, if the target behavior is hitting, the criteria must clearly distinguish this from other similar behaviors, such as pushing (Bijou et al., 1968). A lack of clarity in definitions will often lead to a decrease in reliability, as will be discussed later (Bijou et al., 1968).

Collecting the Data

After defining the target behavior, the next step is to determine how data will be collected. There are many ways of classifying data collection techniques. Two primary categories of in vivo data collection procedures will be discussed in this chapter: event recording and time sampling. There are a number of methods of collecting data within each of these categories, each of which will be discussed along with associated problems.

Event Recording

Event recording involves counting the number of times a specific behavior occurs during an interval (Sulzer-Azaroff & Mayer, 1977). This is most appropriate for collecting data on discrete behaviors that have clear beginning and end points (Sulzer-Azaroff & Mayer, 1977). The most basic type of event recording is to simply write down what behavior is occurring during certain periods of times (Lipinski & Nelson, 1974). This method involves writing a descriptive account of everything relevant that is occurring during an observation. Although this method can provide a very thorough description of what has occurred, there are a number of problems with its use. Firstly, it can be very difficult to complete such recordings, as the observer is required to accurately note everything that is occurring. This requires the observer to direct the majority of their attention toward actually recording the behavior, rather than toward the individual's behavior (Lipinski & Nelson, 1974). This can result in the observer failing to fully observe the behavior, leading to inaccuracies in the recording. Additionally, as the recording is a narrative account of the behavior, it is difficult to compare findings with other researchers and clinicians (Bijou et al., 1968). As described above, a properly operationalized target behavior is necessary for communication between researchers and clinicians. A narrative summary does not allow for such communication. Moreover, as there is no clear structure, different observers might record different information. For example, one observer might record the location of the observation, whereas another may omit this information. Finally, it can be difficult, if not impossible, to objectively determine the duration, latency, or intensity of a behavior from a narrative account (Bijou et al., 1968). Without the use of standardized language and recording procedures, there is too much room for subjective interpretation.

To combat many of these weaknesses, one can add behavioral codes to the above method. Behavioral codes identify target behaviors that can either be specific or general (Bijou et al., 1968). A specific code lists specific, operationally defined behaviors to be observed. In contrast, a general code lists a class of behaviors, allowing for the recording of multiple behaviors (e.g., verbal responses). Specific symbols can be used to represent the operationally defined target behavior, making the recording process much simpler (Lipinski & Nelson, 1974). Additionally, the frequency of target behaviors can be recorded with a checklist, hand counters, or electronic counters (Sulzer-Azaroff & Mayer, 1977). This methodology improves upon the previous one, primarily by standardizing the definitions and procedures. This reduces the subjectivity involved, thereby allowing for the communication and comparison of results. As the behaviors are discretely and operationally defined, constructs such as duration, latency, and intensity can be objectively recorded. For example, if the target behavior is

tantrum behavior, defined as crying and pounding fists, the observer could easily record how long the behavior lasts and how much time lapses between occurrences. Additionally, in comparison to the previous method, much less attention needs to be directed toward the actual recording, allowing the data collector to more accurately and thoroughly observe the behavior.

Despite these improvements, there are still a number of problems associated with this methodology. Firstly, it requires prior selection of behaviors to be recorded (Goldfried, 1982; Lipinski & Nelson, 1974). Any other behaviors that occur during the observation are not recorded. For example, if tantrums are selected as the target behavior, the occurrences of other challenging behaviors during the observation are not recorded. Potentially valuable information can be lost because of this. Challenging behaviors that occur at low frequencies can also be problematic for this type of event recording (Singh et al., 2006; Tarbox et al., 2009). If observations are carried out at specific times for data collection, the behavior must occur during the observation for any information to be recorded. Take, for example, an individual who engages in self-injury when hungry. If he or she is not hungry during the observation period, it is unlikely the behavior will occur, and therefore no information can be gathered on the behavior. This has been noted to be especially problematic in mental illness, as challenging behaviors typically occur at low frequencies but high intensities in this population (Singh et al., 2006). A final problem, especially with respect to functional assessment, is that event recording says nothing about the function of the behavior (Bijou et al., 1968). No information is provided about the antecedents and consequences that may be influencing the behavior.

This final limitation can be addressed through the use of Antecedent–Behavior–Consequence (ABC) cards or sequence analysis (Bijou et al., 1968; Sulzer-Azaroff & Mayer, 1977). In addition to recording the occurrence of a behavior, the events that occur immediately before and after the behavior are recorded. Similar to the recording of the behavior itself, the antecedents and consequences can either be recorded in a narrative fashion, or target antecedents and consequences can be selected beforehand and included on a checklist. This provides considerably more information than the previous methods, as it begins to provide information about possible functions of the behavior. However, one should keep in mind that this method only describes interactions between behaviors and environmental events; this does not, in and of itself, establish a functional relationship (Bijou et al., 1968). An additional problem with this method is that it may difficult to quantify the data obtained through this method (Lerman & Iwata, 1993). It is difficult to determine if the antecedent events are similarly correlated with nonoccurrences of the target behavior. For example, suppose being asked to complete a task is identified as an antecedent. While this may frequently occur before the target behavior, it may just as frequently, or more frequently, occur without being followed by the target behavior. As data are only collected on occurrences, it is not possible to make this comparison. Finally, while some strategies for examining sequential data have been proposed (Martens et al., 2008), there is no consensus within the field on how such data should be analyzed (Tarbox et al., 2009). Additional problems with the use of ABC data will be discussed below in the section discussing use and interpretation of data.

Time Sampling

A second category of in vivo data collection is termed time sampling (Bijou et al., 1968; Sulzer-Azaroff & Mayer, 1977). Time sampling involves recording the occurrence or nonoccurrence of a behavior in a specified time interval. Time sampling, in contrast to event recording, can be appropriate for both discrete and nondiscrete behaviors (Sulzer-Azaroff & Mayer, 1977). For example, take an individual who engages in self-injury by hitting his or her head. If this individual hits his or her head twice, pauses for 20 s, and then hits his or her head again two more times should this be counted as one or two occurrences? While this is a problem for event recording, it is not at all problematic for time sampling. Additionally,

unlike event recording, time sampling allows for quantification of data (Lerman & Iwata, 1993). For example, a 30-min data collection session on self-injury could be broken into 30, 1-min intervals. If self-injury occurs during 15 intervals, this can be quantified, allowing one to say that the behavior occurred during 50% of the intervals. This number can then be compared to subsequent observations to determine if there is an increase or decrease in the behavior. Given these advantages, time sampling has frequently been used in a variety of settings with a variety of challenging behaviors (Lerman & Iwata, 1993)

Similar to event recording, there are a number of methods of collecting time-sampling data. The three primary methods of time sampling are whole-interval time sampling, partial-interval time sampling, and momentary time sampling (Sulzer-Azaroff & Mayer, 1977). Whole-interval time sampling requires the behavior to occur throughout the interval. In the above example, the individual must engage in self-injury for the entire minute for it to be scored. Conversely, in partial-interval time sampling, only one instance of the behavior must occur during the interval. In the above example, if the individual engages in self-injury, even for just 1 s during the interval, it is scored. Finally, momentary time sampling requires the behavior to occur at the end of the interval.

While time sampling clearly has some advantages, as with event recording, there are a number of problems that must be considered. Firstly, time sampling is not practical for infrequent behaviors (Sulzer-Azaroff & Mayer, 1977). For example, take an individual who engages in self-injury approximately once a week. While this behavior can be very serious, time-sampling procedures will provide little to no information on the behavior. Again, as this is often case in those with mental illness, the effectiveness of this approach is limited (Singh et al., 2006). Additionally, it is much more difficult to identify antecedents and consequences with time-sampling procedures. Specific incidences of the behavior are not recorded, thus it is not feasible to record antecedent and consequences to the behavior. This limits the utility of this method for establishing functional relationships.

Another problem is that time-sampling procedures do not record all behaviors that occur during an observation (Johnston & Pennypacker, 1993). For example, in momentary time sampling, no recording occurs until the end of the interval. However, this results in a large period of nonobservation time. The data collected will, therefore, typically be under- or over-representative of the true behavior. There is no way to assess the extent to which the data is inaccurately representing the data (Johnston & Pennypacker, 1993). Johnston and Pennypacker (1993), therefore, suggest limiting the amount of nonobservation time that occurs during a session. They also recommend limiting the interpretation of data collected through time sampling, periodically assessing for accuracy of data, and matching procedures with the distribution of responding.

A considerable amount of research has examined the various methods of time sampling, highlighting problems inherent with each. One set of researchers compared frequency recording (i.e., event recording), interval recording (i.e., partial-interval time sampling), and time sampling (i.e., momentary time sampling) for use with different rates of behavior (Repp, Roberts, Slack, Repp, & Berkler, 1976). Results showed that momentary time sampling did not produce representative data, particularly when the behavior did not occur at a constant rate and was frequently occurring. Partial-interval recording was more accurate for behaviors that occurred at low and medium rates; however, it underestimated behaviors that occurred at high rates.

Powell, Martindale, and Kulp (1975) compared all three methods of time sampling with frequency recording for measuring in-seat behavior. For frequency recording, the behavior was continuously measured over the course of the session. Whole-interval time sampling was found to consistently underestimate the frequency of the behavior, partial-interval time sampling was found to consistently overestimate the frequency of the behavior, and momentary time sampling both over-and underestimated the frequency of the behavior. However, it was noted that as the intervals were made shorter (i.e., more observations were made), the time sampling methods

became more accurate. A follow-up study (Powell, Martindale, Kulp, Martindale, & Bauman, 1977) similarly found that partial-interval time sampling overestimated the frequency of behavior, while whole-interval time sampling underestimated the frequency of behavior. As error occurred in only one direction for each method, conducting a large number of observations could not control for this error. Additionally, error remained large even when intervals lasted only 30 s and was not directly related to either the frequency or duration of the behavior. The authors suggest that this may lead researchers and clinicians to inaccurately interpret changes in behavior due to treatment. Conversely, momentary time sampling was fairly accurate when observations were conducted at 5, 10, 20, or 60-s intervals. However, when intervals went beyond this length, error began to increase. Finally, momentary time sampling was found superior to both types of interval time sampling for estimating the duration a behavior occurred.

Another study compared momentary time sampling and partial-interval time sampling in measuring behavior change, both absolute and relative (Harrop & Daniels, 1986). Both methods tended to overestimate the absolute rate of behaviors. Additionally, partial-interval time sampling overestimated the absolute duration of behaviors, especially when behaviors occurred at lower rates and shorter durations. Conversely, momentary time sampling did not produce such errors. Based on these findings, the authors suggested that duration, not rate, should be the dependent measure when using momentary time sampling. However, when measuring relative changes, the authors found partial-interval time sampling to be more sensitive than momentary time sampling. Despite this superiority, partial-interval time sampling underestimated the change in a behavior if it was of high frequency and short duration.

One shortcoming of these studies was their use of simulated or computer-simulated behaviors. Therefore, it is unclear to what extent they apply to behavioral observations in naturally settings. Unfortunately, few studies have been conducted that examine these methods with naturally occurring challenging behaviors (Matson &

Nebel-Schwalm, 2007). One of the only such studies, by Gardenier, MacDonald, and Green (2004), compared partial-interval time sampling and momentary time sampling for recording stereotypies in children with autism spectrum disorders. In this study, partial-interval time sampling was found to consistently overestimate the duration of stereotypies. Momentary time sampling was found to both overestimate and underestimate duration, but to a lesser extent than partial-interval time sampling. Across all samples, partial-interval time sampling overestimated the duration by an average of 164%, whereas momentary time sampling over- and underestimated the duration by an average of 12–28% (depending on the interval length). The authors concluded that momentary time sampling should, therefore, be used for duration recording of stereotypy. There is clearly a need for additional research examining the use of these methods with challenging behaviors.

As a whole, these studies suggest a number of strengths and limitations inherent in each method of time sampling. It does not appear that any form of time sampling provides a true representation of the frequency at which behaviors occur, although partial-interval may be more representative for behaviors that do not occur at high frequencies (Harrop & Daniels, 1986; Repp et al., 1976). Conversely, momentary time sampling may be less susceptible to error when recording the duration of behaviors (Gardenier et al., 2004; Harrop & Daniels, 1986; Powell et al., 1975, 1977). The limitations of these methods must be taken into account when considering how data will be collected.

Electronic Data Collection

Although most data are collected by hand (i.e., using pen and paper), electronic equipment is being increasingly used to collect real-time data (Tarbox, Wilke, Findel-Pyles, Bergstrom, & Granpeesheh, 2010). Potential advantages of electronic data collection include simplicity, electronic storage of data, the ability to electronically analyze data, and simpler recording (Tarbox

et al., 2010). Kahng and Iwata (1998) conducted a review of 15 computerized systems for collecting real-time data. Although the reviewers were unable to systematically analyze these systems, they provided descriptive reports of the various systems. Most of the systems reviewed included software for analyzing data and many could be used on handheld devices. Systems ranged from free in price to over $1,500.

Unfortunately, there has been little empirical research comparing electronic data collection with hand-collected data. One such study compared the two methods for recording responses of children with autism during discrete trial training (Tarbox et al., 2010). Results found that electronic data collection required more time than pen and paper collection for all four participants. Accuracy of data was similar for both methods, with the average accuracy of electronic data ranging from 83.75% to 95% and the average accuracy of pen and paper data ranging from 98.13% to 100%. Graphing data was accomplished faster via electronic data collection for all participants. Although this study employed a small sample size, it is one of the only to empirically examine electronic data collection. The researchers summarize that although electronic data collection may save time outside of therapy sessions, it may require more time during actual sessions.

General Problems with Data Collection

In addition to the problems discussed thus far, there are additional problems general to all in vivo data collection procedures. In vivo data collection procedures can be very time consuming, especially if narrative accounts are required (Arndorfer & Miltenberger, 1993; Iwata et al., 1990). This decreases the likelihood of compliance with data collection procedures. For example, teachers may not have time to complete ABC or time-sampling data, which require their frequent attention (Arndorfer & Miltenberger, 1993). On the other hand, they may be much more likely to complete interviews and indirect assessments, which can be conducted in one session. An additional problem is that most of these techniques require extensive training (Gardner, 2000; Hartmann et al., 2004; Tarbox et al., 2009). Inadequate training may lead to decreases in the reliability of collected data, as will be discussed later (Bijou et al., 1968).

It is important that the data collected be representative of the individual's typical behavior. However, how does one determine when enough data has been collected? How does one know that the data is now representative? If the behavior frequently occurs, one may need to collect many observations in many settings to get a full picture (Lipinski & Nelson, 1974). Unfortunately, there is no objective criterion for making this determination (Lipinski & Nelson, 1974). This is especially problematic, considering the time and training needed to implement these techniques.

In order for accurate in vivo data collection to occur, the observer must maintain contact with the subject of data collection. A number of factors, such as movement during the observation session, may interfere with this contact or make observation of the target behavior more difficult (Johnston & Pennypacker, 1993). For example, if the target behavior is biting one's hands, the observer must be able to see the individual's hands and mouth. If the individual moves during the observation so that these are no longer visible, the observation can no longer occur. Other behaviors by the individual, or other individuals in the environment, may similarly make data collection difficult, if not impossible (Barrios, 1993; Johnston & Pennypacker, 1993). For example, a noisy environment may make it difficult to record instances of cursing. To counter such problems, one may need to manipulate the environment to restrict these possibilities (Johnston & Pennypacker, 1993). However, this adds a possible confounding variable, as the setting is no longer truly the natural setting in which the behavior typically occurs.

Another problem with in vivo data collection is the presence of frequent variables unrelated to the target behavior. These unrelated events might overshadow or mask relevant variables that occur less frequently (Iwata et al., 1990). Consider an observation in which another individual is constantly yelling and screaming next to the subject of the observation. This variable (i.e., others yelling)

may have no relationship to the target behavior; however, its presence may deter the observer from detecting other important, but less frequently occurring, antecedents.

A final problem is that some behaviors and stimuli are difficult, if not impossible, to quantify (Bijou et al., 1968). This is especially true of biological or internal stimuli. For example, how does one quantify feelings of anxiousness through observation? Challenging behaviors may serve physical functions (Paclawskyj, Matson, Rush, Smalls, & Vollmer, 2000), such as being uncomfortable or feeling ill. However, how can one record the frequency, duration, or intensity of these feelings through in vivo data collection? Similarly, social stimuli can be very difficult to objectively quantify. However, Bijou et al. (1968) stress that such specific biological and social variables must be assessed for a thorough functional assessment to take place. Additional problems that may occur while collecting data, such as reactivity and observer effects will be discussed more in depth below.

Reliability of Data

One of the most important factors to consider when examining real-time data is the reliability of the data. It is extremely important that the data that is collected be both consistent and accurate. It should be noted that agreement and accuracy are not synonymous (Kazdin, 1977). Agreement exists when multiple raters make similar recordings, regardless of if these recordings are correct. For example, if both raters record that a behavior occurs 10 times, agreement is 100%. This is true regardless of how often the behavior actually occurred. In contrast, accuracy reflects if raters record how often the behavior truly occurs. Typically, interobserver agreement is calculated and agreement is assumed to reflect accuracy (Kazdin, 1977). However, agreement alone may not be enough to ensure the quality of data; accuracy and generalizability should also be reported when possible (Mitchell, 1979).

While on the surface it seems that reliability should be easy to achieve, there are a number of factors that can affect the achieved reliability. Firstly, as discussed above, the definition of the behavior itself can affect reliability (Bijou et al., 1968). If there is room for subjective interpretation, two observers may define the behavior differently. The two observers may, therefore, be recording two different behaviors, thereby affecting the reliability of the data. Additional factors that will be discussed below include the method of calculating reliability, the coding system employed, inadequate training, reactivity to the reliability assessment, observer drift, and characteristics of the observers (Bijou et al., 1968; Kazdin, 1977; Lipinski & Nelson, 1974).

Calculating Reliability

There are a number of methods for calculating the reliability of data, each with its advantages and disadvantages. While a full discussion of reliability techniques is beyond the scope of this chapter, a brief discussion about the importance of selecting an appropriate technique is given. This is extremely important, as selecting an inappropriate method for calculating reliability may be one reason that inadequate reliability of data is found (Bijou et al., 1968).

Interobserver agreement is one of the most common methods by which researchers calculate reliability of data (Hartmann, 1977). Interobserver agreement refers to the extent to which data between observers agree with one another (Mudford, Martin, Hui, & Taylor, 2009). There are a number of ways to calculate interobserver agreement, and the limitations of each method should be known before selecting one for use. For example, one can divide the number of sessions in which the two observers agreed by the number of total sessions and multiply by 100. This method, while commonly used, is very stringent and does not use all of the information available (Hartmann, 1977). For a more detailed review of methods of calculating interobserver agreement, the reader is directed elsewhere in the literature (e.g., Hopkins & Hermann, 1977; House, House, & Campbell, 1981; Mudford et al., 2009). For the purposes of this chapter, it is merely important to understand that there is more than one method for calculating the reliability of data. It is important to understand the advantages and disadvantages of each, so that the results can be interpreted correctly. Incorrectly used methods may inflate or deflate the perceived reliability of the data, leading to incorrect interpretations.

Coding Systems

There are many different ways to code behavior, each of which can impact the reliability. As discussed previously, one decision that must be made is whether to use specific or general codes (Bijou et al., 1968). General codes allow for more complex behavioral patterns to be recorded; however, general codes allow more room for interpretation. This, in turn, can lead to a decrease in reliability. The more comprehensive and specific the code is, the higher reliability will be (Bijou et al., 1968).

A second reliability factor related to coding is the complexity of the coding system. Complexity can be defined as the number of categories in the coding system, the number of behaviors being observed, or the number of individuals being observed (Kazdin, 1977). As these numbers increase, the complexity of the coding system increases. The question then becomes what impact does increasing complexity have on reliability? A number of researchers have sought to answer this question. Mash and McElwee (1974) examined the effects of complexity, defined as the number of categories, on both accuracy and agreement. They compared the use of two coding systems, one with four behavior categories and the other with eight. Additionally, the eight-category system required the observer to make more complex discriminations between categories. The authors found an inverse relationship between complexity and reliability. They found that agreement increased over time in the more complex group, to the point that significant differences were no longer found after the fourth trial. Accuracy similarly increased over time, although it remained significantly lower in the more complex group throughout the study. This was despite the fact that both groups showed mastery of the coding systems during training. The predictability of the behavior did not have any effect on accuracy.

Taplin and Reid (1973) conducted a study on the effects of instructions and experimenters on observer reliability. While not the primary aim of the study, the researchers also examined the effect of complexity, defined as the number of different codes used, on reliability. They found a moderate negative correlation ($r=-0.52$) between complexity and reliability.

Kazdin (1977) provides a number of implications of these findings. Firstly, estimates of reliability must be interpreted with respect to complexity. Additionally, the complexity of the data collection system may change over time. For example, if interventions are successful, the number of behaviors being recorded may decrease. Therefore, calculations of reliability may not be comparable across different phases.

Barrios (1993) calls for a rational appraisal of the demands of the coding system. This involves having the system evaluated by those creating the system, colleagues, and potential observers. If the demands are found to be too high, one may need to decrease the number of behaviors being tracked, simplify the nature of the behavior being tracked, or decrease the duration of observations.

Training

Another factor that can influence the reliability of data is the training of observers. If observers are not properly trained, they may inaccurately collect data and fail to control their own behaviors (Bijou et al., 1968). Bijou et al., (1968) provide some recommendations for ensuring adequate training, such as familiarizing observers with recording tools and employing a second observer during training.

Barrios (1993) provides a six-step model for training and monitoring observers. The first step is orientation. This involves conveying the importance of objective data collection to observers. In this step, observers are also told what they will be doing and what is expected of them. This includes

warnings against potential sources of error, including biases, observer drift, and reactivity (as discussed below). The second step is to educate observers about the operational definition that will be used and how data will be recorded. This may be accomplished through written materials, filmed instructions, or in-person demonstrations. The third step is to evaluate the observer's training. Observers are assessed to ensure that they have an adequate understanding of the operational definition and coding system. Feedback and corrections are given at this step, until the observer has mastered the system. Additionally, the operational definition and coding system may be altered at this step if they are found to be inadequate. The fourth step is application; observers begin using the data collection system, first in analog situations and then in real situations. Observers must attain sufficient agreement and accuracy to progress. This ensures that observers have mastered the system before collecting data in the situation of interest. Observers are gradually introduced to data collection in the setting of interest, as mastery in analog sessions does not ensure mastery in actual sessions (as discussed further below). Additionally, observers are continually provided feedback concerning their reliability and reminded that reliability will be periodically checked. The fifth step is recalibration. This is where reliability of data collection is assessed in the actual situation of interest. The final step in training and monitoring is termination. After data collection is completed, observers are asked for feedback on the data collection system, provided information on what was found and how it will be used, reminded of confidentiality, and thanked for their assistance. Hartmann and Wood (1982) provide a similar seven-step model.

An additional aspect of training is the type of behavior that is trained. Mash and McElwee (1974) found that observers who were trained to code unpredictable behavior had better accuracy in novel situations than those trained to code predictable behavior sequences. This is critical as in vivo data collection necessitates that observations occur in varying settings and situations.

As mentioned above, even if observers achieve mastery in training, this does not necessarily mean that they have been adequately trained. Mash and McElwee (1974) found that the reliability of data collected by observers using a complex coding system was inadequate, despite the fact that they had achieved mastery of the coding system during training. Similarly, Taplin and Reid (1973) found that observers never attained the same level of performance during data collection that they achieved in training. In fact, reliability decreased, on average, 15% once training was completed and data collection began. Thus, the reliability achieved during training is likely to be an overestimate of the reliability that will be achieved during actual data collection. The steps outlined above by Barrios (1993) are intended to help protect against this drop in reliability.

Reactivity to the Assessment of Reliability

As reliability of data is crucial, researchers and clinicians will often compute reliability as data are being collected. However, knowledge of this reliability assessment can, in and of itself, affect reliability. Reid (1970) conducted an experiment in an analog setting to examine this effect. Participants were instructed to code behavioral data in a lab, believing that the reliability was being assessed only during the first two sessions (reliability was covertly assessed during the remaining three sessions). The reliability of observers significantly decreased when they did not believe that reliability as being checked. Reliability dropped by an average of approximately 25% when reliability was covertly checked. This change was not gradual, occurring immediately upon switching conditions. Although a complex coding system was used in this study, it should be noted that in the previously discussed study by Mash and McElwee (1974), reliability increased over time in the complex condition. The opposite was found in the current study due to the covert reliability assessment.

A follow-up study by Taplin and Reid (1973) compared three conditions: covert reliability assessment, random overt reliability assessment, and spot-check assessment. That is to say participants

believed that no reliability assessment would take place, that about 20% of their data would randomly be checked for reliability after observations were completed, or that periodic overt checks would take place. Results showed that reliability during spot-checks was significantly higher than both before and after the checks. No significant differences were found between the groups with respect to reliability. This is likely because reliability for all groups dropped significantly after training.

Romanczyk, Kent, Diament, and O'Leary, (1973) conducted a similar experiment to examine the differential affects of overt and covert reliability assessment. Two assessors accompanied observers during all observations. In the overt condition, observers were led to believe that either one assessor was computing reliability or both were computing reliability. In reality, both assessors were computing reliability in all conditions each using a unique code. This allowed the researchers to compare reliability with an identified assessor and reliability with an unidentified assessor. In the covert condition, observers were not told that reliability was being assessed. Reliability during covert assessment was consistently lower than reliability during overt assessment. Disruptive behaviors were reported at lower rates (approximately 25% lower) when observers did not believe that reliability was being checked. Additionally, reliability was consistently higher with the identified assessor than with the unidentified assessor. This suggested that, when observers knew who was computing reliability, they shifted their observational criteria to be more like the assessor.

These findings strongly suggest that observers are reactive to knowledge of reliability assessments. Observers are more likely to record reliable data when they believe that reliability is being assessed. Unfortunately, it is not typically possible to continuously assess for reliability. Similarly, it may be difficult to convince observers that their reliability is constantly being checked (Kazdin, 1977). Taplin and Reid (1973) suggest that it may be necessary to overtrain observers, so that reliability remains adequate even if it decreases after training.

Observer Drift

One possible explanation for decreases in reliability after training is known as observer drift. While different researchers have defined the term observer drift differently, the term chiefly refers to changes in an observer's definition of a behavior over time (Kazdin, 1977; Smith, 1986). For example, observers may be trained to collect data on physical aggression, defined as hitting, pushing, and pinching. If pinching is low in frequency or intensity, the observer may no longer include this in their definition of physical aggression. So while data would include pinching at first, later data would no longer include this aspect of the behavior. As pinching should be recorded based on the behavior's definition, reliability will decrease over time.

Kent, O'Leary, Diament, and Dietz (1974) examined the variance in behavioral recordings accounted for by observer. Observer pairs accounted for a total of about 17% of the variance in recordings of disruptive behavior, with about 5% representing consistent differences between pairs of observers throughout the experiment. Additionally, about 12% of the total variance in disruptive behavior recordings were accounted for by interactions of observer pair with other factors.

Observer drift may be difficult to detect, as agreement between observers may remain high, while accuracy decreases (Kazdin, 1977). Observers who work together closely may make similar changes to their definitions, thereby maintaining agreement and losing accuracy. This effect is known as consensual observer drift (Johnson & Bolstad, 1973; Power, Paul, Licht, & Engel, 1982; Smith, 1986). Observer drift may also affect within subjects research designs, as the observer may change his or her definition over the course of the study (Lipinski & Nelson, 1974). Taking the above example of pinching, data might show a decrease in physical aggression over time. However, this decrease would be confounded by the observer's modification of the definition of physical aggression. The best way to combat this problem is likely to periodically retrain observers, ensuring they are applying the definition correctly (Hartmann et al., 2004;

Kazdin, 1977). Observer drift is, therefore, another reason that in vivo data assessment can require extensive training and costs.

Observer Bias, Distraction, and Discontent

Characteristics of the observer can also threaten the reliability of real-time data. Both implicit and explicit biases by the observer, distractions to the observer, and discontent can all affect the reliability of collected data. Additionally, the manner in which data is presented by observers can affect the way in which the data is interpreted.

Observer expectancies and biases can influence the reliability of collected data. Such biases include hypotheses about the purpose of the data collection, hypotheses as to how the subject of data collection should behave, and beliefs about what the data should look like (Hartmann & Wood, 1982). Biases can also be developed based on subject characteristics and information expressed by the primary investigator (Hartmann & Wood, 1982).

A study by Kent et al. (1974) examined the effect of expectation biases on behavior recording. Observers were either told to predict changes in behavior or to predict no change. They found that the evaluations of the treatment effects were significantly affected by predictions. Those told to predict changes in behavior reported seeing a global change in behavior. However, actual behavior recordings did not significantly differ between the groups. Those who believed the behavior would change were just as accurate as those who did not believe the behavior [would] change. This would seem to suggest that expectancies do not bias in vivo data collection, although they may affect global evaluations.

A follow-up study (O'Leary, Kent, & Kanowitz, 1975) examined the influence of both instructions and feedback on data collection. Observers were told that two behaviors were expected to decrease, whereas two other behaviors would experience no change. Positive feedback was given when observers reported decreases in the behavior that was expected to change, whereas negative feedback was provided when they reported no change or increases in the target behaviors. After feedback, observers recorded the target behaviors significantly less frequently, suggesting that significant bias had occurred. No changes were found with respect to the control behaviors. These findings suggest that while expectancies may not bias data collection, a combination of both expectancies and feedback can have a significant impact.

Another possible source of bias involves the presentation and analysis of data. Although often overlooked as a source of bias, inappropriate analysis and misleading presentation of data can be another form of bias (Mcnamara & MacDonough, 1972). For example, data may be biased if no statistical analyses are conducted. Similarly, graphical data can be misleading if not displayed accurately. It is critical that data be reported as unambiguously as possible, so that anyone who uses the data can come to similar conclusions (Mcnamara & MacDonough, 1972).

If observers are distracted, either externally or internally, collected data may not be reliable (Barrios, 1993). For example, if there is a lot of noise in the environment, the observer may be unfocused and unable to record all relevant behaviors. Similarly, worries or preoccupations by the observer may distract him or her from accurately recording data. Barrios (1993) also discusses discontent as a type of internal distractor that may be especially problematic. If observers are treated in a disrespectful or harsh manner, discontent may arise. Discontent may also arise from unpleasant interactions between observers and others involved in the data collection process. While steps can be taken to reduce possible external distractors, they are likely to reduce the external validity of data. Barrios (1993) suggests monitoring observers for signs of internal distractions and intervening if necessary. However, it may not be possible to detect all internal distractions.

Validity of Data

In addition to ensuring accuracy and agreement, it is critical that data collection remain valid. One of the main advantages of in vivo data collection is that it can occur in the natural environment, increasing the external validity of data. Unfortunately, there are still a number of extraneous factors that may influence in vivo data collection, threatening the validity of the data. In vivo data collection is often used to measure the frequency, intensity, and duration of a target challenging behavior. Extraneous variables, such as observer effects and reactivity, can alter these target variables during data collection sessions, making the data no longer representative of the behavior.

Observer Effects and Reactivity

As discussed, one of the primary advantages of in vivo data collection is that it can be conducted in the natural environment in which the behavior occurs (Gardner, 2000). This assumes, however, that the presence of an observer does not affect this environment. Research has shown that this is not necessarily the case (Hartmann & Wood, 1982; Lipinski & Nelson, 1974; Repp, Nieminen, Olinger, & Brusca, 1988). Those being observed may even be hostile about the fact that they are being observed (Lipinski & Nelson, 1974). Conversely, they may try to impress observers or reduce challenging behaviors in the presence of observers (Lipinski & Nelson, 1974). Such changes in behavior during observations are often termed reactive effects or reactivity (Hartmann & Wood, 1982). A number of factors can contribute to reactive effects, such the child's gender and age, the gender of the observer, the familiarity of the participant with the observer, and the observation setting (Gardner, 2000).

The issue of reactivity is a complex one and its effects on the validity of data are unclear (Goldfried, 1982; Hartmann & Wood, 1982). Hartmann and Wood (1982) outlined five factors that may contribute to reactivity: social desirability, subject characteristics, conspicuousness of observation, observer attributes, and the rational for observation. Individuals may try to suppress undesirable behaviors or engage in more socially appropriate behaviors when being observed. Therefore, an individual may be less likely to engage in the challenging behavior during observations, as they are not socially desirable behaviors. Characteristics of those being observed may also contribute to reactivity. Hartmann and Wood (1982) suggest that those who are more sensitive, less confident, and older than 6 years old may be more reactive than others during observations. Additionally, the more obtrusive the data collection is, the more likely reactive effects will occur. However, findings on obtrusiveness are not consistent and do not guarantee that the data will be invalid. The fourth factor outlined by Hartmann and Wood, 1982 is characteristics of the observer. Attributes of the observer, such as race and gender, may influence reactive effects. Finally, the rationale for observation is potentially influential factor. If there is not a good rationale for the presence of the observer, reactive effects may be more likely.

Unfortunately, there is a general lack of research on the effects of such characteristics, particularly with respect to challenging behaviors (Goldfried, 1982; Harris & Lahey, 1982). If substantial changes in behavior occur, reactivity can affect the external and internal validity of collected data. It is not possible to separate the effects of reactivity and one cannot be sure the data are similar to what would be found without the effect of reactivity (Repp et al., 1988).

Researchers have also found that children can be reactive to parents' behavior during observations (Harris & Lahey, 1982). Lobitz and Johnson (1975) examined the effects of parental manipulation on their children's behaviors. Parents were asked to present their child as bad, good, or normal. Significantly more challenging behaviors were found under the bad condition, when compared with the other two. This was true for both children with a history of challenging behaviors and those without such a history. No significant differences were found between the good and normal conditions, suggesting that parents could not make their children look better, only worse.

In a similar study examining compliance, parents were asked to make their children appear obedient and later disobedient in a clinic playroom (Green, Forehand, & McMahon, 1979). Significant changes in compliance were found in children with a history of challenging behaviors and those without such a history. Parental behaviors, such as use of rewards and questioning versus commanding, differed between the two

conditions, likely accounting for the changes in compliance.

Taken together, these findings are quite significant. Suppose parents wants to ensure that their children will receive treatment. Parents could manipulate their behavior to make the children's behavior appear worse than it typically is during an observation. The data collected in this observation would not be representative of the true behavior and thus no longer valid (Harris & Lahey, 1982). However, it may be difficult to detect if this is occurring. While certain parental behaviors were associated with changes in behavior (e.g., commanding), it is unlikely that the observer will know if this behavior is typical of the parent.

Interpretation and Use

The use of real-time data for functional assessment is described in greater detail elsewhere in this text. However, a brief consideration should be given to how in vivo data is used and interpreted. When in vivo data is used to examine the maintaining variable of a challenging behavior, it is often termed descriptive analysis (Iwata et al., 1990; Lerman & Iwata, 1993). There are many ways to conduct descriptive analyses, many of which are slight adaptations of others. A brief description of two of the more basic methods will be given, along with associated problems. The reader is directed to Chap. 8 for a more in-depth discussion of these methods.

The first method, as discussed above, is the use of ABC cards, also known as sequential analysis (Bijou et al., 1968; Sulzer-Azaroff & Mayer, 1977). As data are quantified, one can calculate the probability that a target behavior will follow a specific antecedent or be followed by a specific consequence (Iwata et al., 1990). However, as mentioned previously, there are no standards for interpreting this data (Tarbox et al., 2009). Additionally, the results from such an analysis are often inconsistent; the function suggested by the antecedent may be inconsistent with the function suggested by the consequence (Tarbox et al., 2009).

A second method, developed by Touchette, MacDonald, and Langer (1985), is known as a scatter plot analysis. Data is graphed on a scatter plot, with levels of a behavior observed during specified time intervals being recorded throughout the day. The main purpose of this method is to see if there is a pattern of distribution of behaviors throughout the day. Thus the scatter plot shows when a behavior typically occurs and when it rarely occurs. This allows for identification of possible temporal variables that may be affecting the target variable. The authors suggest that the scatter plot analysis be used when a behavior is frequently occurring, as informal observation may not suggest a reliable functional relationship. The main problem with scatter plot analyses is that the scatter plot only provides information on environmental variables related to the time of day (Axelrod, 1987; Iwata et al., 1990). For example, suppose an individual engages in self-injury when he or she sees another individual with a preferred item. As this could occur at any point during the day, the scatter plot is unlikely to reveal information about this relationship. Thus, the scatter plot will only identify antecedents and consequences that are relate to the behavior on a fixed, regular basis (Axelrod, 1987).

A major problem for all methods of descriptive analyses is that established relationships are correlational (Bijou et al., 1968; Iwata et al., 1990; Lerman & Iwata, 1993; Tarbox et al., 2009). Just because a relationship has been established, it does not necessarily reflect a functional relationship. For example, as described above, the target behavior may be highly correlated with frequently occurring, but unrelated events (Iwata et al., 1990). Conversely, the true functional variable may be one that is only reinforced intermittently. For example, take a child who engages in tantrums in an attempt to escape hygiene-related tasks. This may serve as the function even if the probability of escape is very low. Therefore, a very low correlation would be found between the behavior and the consequence of escaping. Conversely, if the mother of the child provides the child with attention during the tantrum, there would be a high correlation found between the behavior and the consequence of attention. Thus descriptive analysis may incorrectly identify attention as the maintaining variable, when it is, in fact, escape.

Conclusions

The collection of data is one of the primary aspects of conducting a functional assessment. Data are used to help understand the nature of the challenging behavior, including characteristics such as the frequency, duration, intensity, and function of the behavior. The primary method in which this data is collected in vivo. In vivo data has its primary advantage in that it is collected in the natural environment in which the behavior occurs, bypassing the sources of bias and error that may come from indirect data.

While in vivo data no doubt has its advantages, many potential problems with such data have been discussed. There are a number of factors that can influence the reliability and validity of in vivo data. Careful consideration should be given to these factors at each stage of data collection, from defining the behavior to using the data. While the problems of in vivo data have been discussed at length in this chapter, in vivo data are not without utility. Several researchers have provided recommendations on how to minimize many of these sources of error (e.g., Barrios, 1993; Repp et al., 1988). Additionally, while research does not support conducting functional assessments based solely on in vivo data (Iwata et al., 1990; Lerman & Iwata, 1993; Tarbox et al., 2009), there may be value in combining this approach with others.

While a great deal of research has been conducted on this subject matter, there is still a need for more. Much of the research that has been conducted on in vivo data collection predates the popularization of modern functional assessment. Thus little research has been conducted on these sources of error with respect to their use in the functional assessment process. While much of the findings are likely to hold true, there is a need for more research examining this empirically. Additional research in this area will help to ensure the reliability and validity of data, so that more meaningful interpretations can be made.

References

Arndorfer, R. E., & Miltenberger, R. G. (1993). Functional assessment and treatment of challenging behavior: A review with implications for early childhood. *Topics in Early Childhood Special Education, 13*, 82–105.

Axelrod, S. (1987). Functional and structural analyses of behavior: Approaches leading to reduced use of punishment procedures? *Research in Developmental Disabilities, 8*, 165–178.

Barrios, B. A. (1993). Direct observation. In T. H. Ollendick & M. Hersen (Eds.), *Handbook of child and adolescent assessment* (pp. 140–164). Boston: Allyn & Bacon.

Bijou, S. W., Peterson, R. F., & Ault, M. H. (1968). A method to integrate descriptive and experimental field studies at the level of data and empirical concepts. *Journal of Applied Behavior Analysis, 1*, 175–191.

Eddy, J. M., Dishion, T., & Stoolmiller, M. (1998). The analysis of intervention change in children and families: Methodological and conceptual issues embedded in intervention studies. *Journal of Abnormal Child Psychology, 26*, 53–69.

Fergusson, D., Lynskey, M., & Horwood, L. (1993). The effect of maternal depression on maternal ratings of child behavior. *Journal of Abnormal Child Psychology, 21*, 245–269.

Gardenier, N. C., MacDonald, R., & Green, G. (2004). Comparison of direct observational methods for measuring stereotypic behavior in children with autism spectrum disorders. *Research in Developmental Disabilities, 25*, 99–118.

Gardner, F. (2000). Methodological issues in the direct observation of parent-child interaction: Do observational findings reflect the natural behavior of participants? *Clinical Child and Family Psychology Review, 3*, 185–198.

Goldfried, M. R. (1982). Behavioral assessment. In A. S. Bellack, M. Hersen, & A. E. Kazdin (Eds.), *International handbook of behavior modification and therapy*. New York: Plenum.

Green, K. D., Forehand, R., & McMahon, R. J. (1979). Parental manipulation of compliance and noncompliance in normal and deviant children. *Behavior Modification, 3*, 245–266.

Harris, F. C., & Lahey, B. B. (1982). Subject reactivity in direct observational assessment: A review and critical analysis. *Clinical Psychology Review, 2*, 523–538.

Harrop, A., & Daniels, M. (1986). Methods of time sampling: A reappraisal of momentary time sampling and partial interval recording. *Journal of Applied Behavior Analysis, 19*, 73–77.

Hartmann, D. P. (1977). Considerations in the choice of interobserver reliability estimates. *Journal of Applied Behavior Analysis, 10*, 103–116.

Hartmann, D. P., Barrios, B. A., & Wood, D. D. (2004). Principles of behavioral observation. In S. N. Haynes & E. M. Heiby (Eds.), *Comprehensive handbook of psychological assessment: Behavioral assessment* (Vol. 3, pp. 108–127). Hoboken: Wiley.

Hartmann, D. P., & Wood, D. D. (1982). Observational methods. In A. S. Bellack, M. Hersen, & A. E. Kazdin (Eds.), *International handbook of behavior modification and therapy* (pp. 109–138). New York: Plenum.

Hawkins, R. P., & Dobes, W. (1977). Behavioral definitions in applied behavior analysis. In B. C. Etzel, J. M. LeBlanc, & D. M. Baer (Eds.), *New developments in behavioral research: Theory, method and application*. Hillsdale: Erlbaum.

Hopkins, B. L., & Hermann, J. A. (1977). Evaluating interobserver reliability of interval data. *Journal of Applied Behavior Analysis, 10*, 121–126.

House, A. E., House, B. J., & Campbell, M. B. (1981). Measures of interobserver agreement: Calculation formulas and distribution effects. *Journal of Psychopathology and Behavioral Assessment, 3*, 37–57.

Iwata, B. A., Vollmer, T. R., & Zarcone, J. R. (1990). The experimental (functional) analysis of behavior disorders: Methodology, applications, and limitations. In A. C. Repp & N. N. Singh (Eds.), *Perspectives on the use of nonaversive and aversive interventions for persons with developmental disabilities* (pp. 301–330). Sycamore: Sycamore Publishing.

Johnson, S. M., & Bolstad, O. D. (1973). Methodological issues in naturalistic observation: Some problems and solutions for field research. In L. A. Hamerlynck, L. C. Handy, & E. J. Mash (Eds.), *Behavior change: Methodology, concepts, and practice*. Champaign: Research Press.

Johnston, J. M., & Pennypacker, H. S. (1993). *Strategies and tactics of behavioral research* (2nd ed.). Hillsdale: Erlbaum.

Kahng, S. W., & Iwata, B. A. (1998). Computerized systems for collecting real-time observational data. *Journal of Applied Behavior Analysis, 31*, 253–261.

Kazdin, A. E. (1977). Artifact, bias, and complexity of assessment: The ABCs of reliability. *Journal of Applied Behavior Analysis, 10*, 141–150.

Kent, R. N., O'Leary, K. D., Diament, C., & Dietz, A. (1974). Expectation biases in observational evaluation of therapeutic change. *Journal of Consulting and Clinical Psychology, 42*, 774–780.

Lerman, D. C., & Iwata, B. A. (1993). Descriptive and experimental analyses of variables maintaining self-injurious behavior. *Journal of Applied Behavior Analysis, 26*, 293–319.

Lipinski, D., & Nelson, R. (1974). Problems in the use of naturalistic observation as a means of behavioral assessment. *Behavior Therapy, 5*, 341–351.

Lobitz, W. C., & Johnson, S. M. (1975). Parental manipulation of the behavior of normal and deviant children. *Child Development, 46*, 719–726.

Martens, B. K., DiGennaro, F. D., Reed, D. D., Szczech, F. M., & Rosenthal, B. D. (2008). Contingency space analysis: An alternative method for identifying contingent relations from observational data. *Journal of Applied Behavior Analysis, 41*, 69–81.

Mash, E. J., & McElwee, J. D. (1974). Situational effects on observer accuracy: Behavioral predictability, prior experience, and complexity of coding categories. *Child Development, 45,* 367–377.

Matson, J. L., & Nebel-Schwalm, M. (2007). Assessing challenging behaviors in children with autism spectrum disorders: A review. *Research in Developmental Disabilities, 28,* 567–579.

McNamara, J. R., & MacDonough, T. S. (1972). Some methodological considerations in the design and implementation of behavior therapy research. *Behavior Therapy, 3,* 361–378.

Mitchell, S. (1979). Interobserver agreement, reliability, and generalizability of data collected in observational studies. *Psychological Bulletin, 86,* 376–390.

Mudford, O. C., Martin, N. T., Hui, J. K. Y., & Taylor, S. A. (2009). Assessing observer accuracy in continuous recording of rate and duration: Three algorithms compared. *Journal of Applied Behavior Analysis, 42,* 527–539.

O'Leary, K. D., Kent, R. N., & Kanowitz, J. (1975). Shaping data collection congruent with experimental hypotheses. *Journal of Applied Behavior Analysis, 8,* 43–51.

Paclawskyj, T. R., Matson, J. L., Rush, K. S., Smalls, Y., & Vollmer, T. R. (2000). Questions about behavioral function (QABF): A behavioral checklist for functional assessment of aberrant behavior. *Research in Developmental Disabilities, 21,* 223–229.

Powell, J., Martindale, A., & Kulp, S. (1975). An evaluation of time-sample measures of behavior. *Journal of Applied Behavioral Analysis, 8,* 463–469.

Powell, J., Martindale, B., Kulp, S., Martindale, A., & Bauman, R. (1977). Taking a closer look: Time sampling and measurement error. *Journal of Applied Behavior Analysis, 10,* 325–332.

Power, C. T., Paul, G. L., Licht, M. H., & Engel, K. L. (1982). Evaluation of self-contained training procedures for the Time-Sample Behavioral Checklist. *Journal of Psychopathology and Behavioral Assessment, 4,* 223–261.

Reid, J. B. (1970). Reliability assessment of observation data: A possible methodological problem. *Child Development, 41,* 1143–1150.

Repp, A. C., Nieminen, G. S., Olinger, E., & Brusca, R. (1988). Direct observations: Factors affecting the accuracy of observers. *Exceptional Children, 55,* 29–36.

Repp, A. C., Roberts, D. M., Slack, D. J., Repp, C. F., & Berkler, M. S. (1976). A comparison of frequency, interval and time-sampling methods of data collection. *Journal of Applied Behavior Analysis, 9,* 501–508.

Romanczyk, R. G., Kent, R. N., Diament, C., & O'Leary, K. D. (1973). Measuring the reliability of observational data: A reactive process. *Journal of Applied Behavior Analysis, 6,* 175–184.

Singh, N. N., Matson, J. L., Lancioni, G. E., Singh, A. N., Adkins, A. D., McKeegan, G. F., et al. (2006). Questions about behavioral function in mental illness (QABF-MI): A behavior checklist for functional assessment of maladaptive behavior exhibited by individuals with mental illness. *Behavior Modification, 30,* 739–751.

Smith, G. A. (1986). Observer drift—A drifting definition. *Behavior Analyst, 9,* 127–128.

Sulzer-Azaroff, B., & Mayer, G. R. (1977). *Applying behavior analysis procedures with children and youth.* New York: Holt, Rinehart and Winston.

Taplin, P. S., & Reid, J. B. (1973). Effects of instructional set and experimenter influence on observer reliability. *Child Development, 44,* 547–554.

Tarbox, J., Wilke, A. E., Findel-Pyles, R. S., Bergstrom, R. M., & Granpeesheh, D. (2010). A comparison of electronic to traditional pen-and-paper data collection in discrete trial training for children with autism. *Research in Autism Spectrum Disorders, 4,* 65–75.

Tarbox, J., Wilke, A. E., Najdowski, A. C., Findel-Pyles, R. S., Balasanyan, S., Caveney, A. C., et al. (2009). Comparing indirect, descriptive, and experimental functional assessments of challenging behavior in children with autism. *Journal of Developmental and Physical Disabilities, 21,* 493–514.

Touchette, P. E., MacDonald, R. F., & Langer, S. N. (1985). A scatter plot for identifying stimulus control of problem behavior. *Journal of Applied Behavior Analysis, 18,* 343–351.

Scaling Methods of Functional Assessment

10

Megan Sipes and Johnny L. Matson

Challenging behaviors are common in those with developmental disabilities (DD) and intellectual disabilities (ID) (Matson, Cooper, Malone, & Moskow, 2008; Matson, Kiely, & Bamburg, 1997; Murphy et al., 2005) and also in typically developing children with emotional and behavioral problems (Brestan & Eyberg, 1998). Estimates suggest that in those with DD, such as Autism Spectrum Disorders (ASD), 8–17% of individuals exhibit challenging behaviors (Emerson & Bromley, 1995; Kiernan et al., 1997; Lowe et al., 2007). These behaviors range from physical aggression (i.e., hitting, kicking, and biting others) to self-injurious behavior (SIB; i.e., hitting self, head banging, skin picking) to property destruction. While severe challenging behaviors are common in those with DD and ID, a similar number of typically developing children also exhibit challenging behaviors that may lead to emotional and behavioral disorders later on (Webster-Stratton, 1997). It has been well established in the literature that the most effective treatments are interventions based on the functions of the behavior (DuPaul & Ervin, 1996;

Gettinger & Callan Stoiber, 2006). As such, functional assessments have grown in popularity. One review found that previous to 1985, approximately 35% of studies which used behavioral intervention for aggressive behavior in those with DD or ID used some form of functional assessment. However, this percentage increased to 71% for more recent studies which used functional assessment (Hile & Desrochers, 1993). Functional assessments allow for the identification of the maintaining factor of the behavior so that prevention and intervention strategies can be added to a treatment program, as well as replacement behaviors which allow the person to achieve the goal of the challenging behavior by more appropriate means. Furthermore, functional assessment for each challenging behavior is required as topographically similar behaviors may serve drastically different functions (Iwata et al., 1994).

Functional Assessment Methods

A variety of methods of functional assessment are commonly used in the literature. Just some of the methods include direct observation (i.e., scatter plots and ABC charts), analogue methodologies (i.e., experimental functional analysis; EFA), and indirect methods (i.e., scales and interviews). Conroy, Davis, Fox, and Brown (2002) proposed a three-tier model which suggests the path for functional assessments. The first tier includes environmental assessment and intervention.

M. Sipes(✉)
Louisiana State University, Baton Rouge, LA 70803, USA
e-mail: msipes1@gmail.com

J.L. Matson
Department of Psychology, Louisiana State University,
Baton Rouge, LA 70803, USA
e-mail: johnmatson@aol.com

J.L. Matson (ed.), *Functional Assessment for Challenging Behaviors*,
Autism and Child Psychopathology Series, DOI 10.1007/978-1-4614-3037-7_10,
© Springer Science+Business Media, LLC 2012

These changes are global and are put in place for everyone in that particular setting. For example, there may be physical changes to the environment which may include the seating arrangement or materials available. The first tier also includes instructional changes, such as how individuals are directed and expectations. The second tier is used for children who are at a higher risk for developing problem behaviors. During this level of assessment, children might require behavioral observation or interviews with teachers to gain more information about the behavior. At the final level of assessment, tier three, assessment and intervention is individualized. For this level, techniques may include use of scaling methods or EFAs to gain information about antecedents and consequences of behavior. The scaling methods which are in tier three will be the main focus of this chapter.

However, to fully evaluate the functional assessment scales, it is important to consider other methods of determining the functions of behaviors to examine the pros and cons of these methods. Different methods of functional assessment are briefly described here and the strengths and weaknesses of each method are highlighted. Then, specific scaling methods are reviewed in greater detail.

Direct Methods

The first set of functional assessment methods are referred to as the direct methods. This is because the behaviors are observed in their natural environment and no manipulation of the behavior is typically taking place. Due to the natural observations which are used in direct methods, this form of functional assessment possesses the benefit of higher ecological validity (Hall, 2005). This allows for greater generalization of the results into real-world settings. While direct assessment of challenging behaviors is advantageous because the observer does not need to rely on secondary information from a caregiver or teacher, one can only glean correlational data (Hall). This is because the environment is not controlled, and thus, no causation can be implied

about the function of the problematic behavior. One other possible problem with direct assessment methods may occur when the problem behaviors occur at low frequencies. As a result, many hours of direct observation could be needed to gain the needed information and this may not be feasible. Examples of direct functional assessment methods include scatter plots and ABC charts.

Scatter plots

Originally developed by Touchette, MacDonald, and Langer (1985), the scatter plot method aims to correlate events in the natural environment with certain times of day. The data is collected by defining a specific interval and then obtaining information on the frequency and duration of behaviors. For example, the time interval may be defined as 1 min and then the observer is to record if the targeted challenging behavior occurred at any time during that interval. The percent of intervals that the behavior occurred can be calculated and patterns about when throughout the day the behavior is most likely to occur can be deduced. However, this information is limited because little can be gathered about the antecedents and consequences, though some have suggested that this data can also be collected (Bosma & Mulick, 1990). Furthermore, a benefit of using scatter plots is that data is relatively simple to collect, and as a result, it is easily used in applied settings. Because of the simplicity of this method, scatter plots have been used often in schools and inpatient facilities for those with ID and DD. Unfortunately, a lack of research exists which actually examines the psychometric properties of this method (Matson & Minshawi, 2007).

ABC Charts

A second functional assessment method that uses direct observation is ABC charting. In this method, the observer collects data on A (the antecedent), B (the behavior), and C (the consequence). The antecedent includes events that occurred before the target behavior, while the behavior is the target action of concern. The consequence includes anything that happens after the behavior occurs, whether they are an action of the individual or other people in the environment. The more detailed this information will be, the more helpful it will be in hypothesizing the function of the behavior (Joyce, 2006). Unlike the scatter plot, the ABC charting method provides much information about events occurring around the behavior of interest, but less temporal information is gained (Sulzer-Azaroff & Mayer, 1977). In addition, this method can be more time consuming, especially if detailed information is recorded. Finally, some subjective information may be included in the reports which can contaminate the findings.

Analogue Methods

A second class of functional assessments is referred to as analogue assessments. The most common method of analogue assessment is referred to as EFA. EFA is considered an analogue assessment because the assessments are conducted in a controlled environment in which trained staff serve as therapist. The experiments consist of a multielement design in which several conditions, including social positive reinforcement (attention condition), social negative reinforcement (demand/escape condition), and automatic reinforcement (alone condition) as well as a control condition (play), are presented in a random order (Iwata, Dorsey, Slifer, Bauman, & Richman, 1982; Iwata et al., 1994). Each of the conditions may require several trials which can lead to a relatively high number of total trails. Some studies report 30–50 trials for one child (Derby et al., 2000) with one to eight trials occurring per day (Rojahn, Whittaker, Hoch, & Gonzalez, 2007). The behavioral responses in these trials are then analyzed to hypothesize the maintaining function(s). When compared with the other methods of functional assessment, EFAs offer a greater ability to infer causation about the function of the behavior because of the controlled, experimental nature of the design (Anderson, Freeman, & Scotti, 1999). However, while this method reaps the benefits of being able to imply causality, ecological validity and generalizability are compromised due to the highly

controlled environments which are very different than the individuals' typical environment (Hall, 2005). Furthermore, several other shortcomings of EFAs exist. For example, the nature of this method requires the behavior to be elicited. This brings up ethical considerations when dealing with behaviors that are harmful to the individual as is often the case with SIB. On a similar note, new functions of the behaviors may develop through the manipulations that occur during trails which could make treatment more difficult and complex (Matson & Minshawi, 2007). In addition, certain conditions may be difficult to replicate in the assessment trials. Overall, it has been noted that while EFAs are useful in research settings, these assessments are not often feasible in applied settings (Matson & Minshawi).

Indirect Methods

The final class of functional assessments is indirect assessments. These methods are referred to as indirect because no direct observation or interaction with the behavior of interest occurs. Instead information is obtained through a third party such as a parent, caregiver, or teacher. These indirect methods have several benefits. First, because there is no direct contact with the individual, these methods offer a less intrusive way to gain information about the problem behavior (Floyd, Phaneuf, & Wilczynski, 2005). Secondly, respondents can report about behaviors over a longer period of time, which could be helpful for less frequent behaviors. This is opposed to the direct and EFA methods which only take into account the behaviors that are being exhibited in the moment. In addition, indirect methods may be preferable when it may be unethical to recreate the behavior in an analogue setting (O'Neill et al., 1997). However when EFAs are required, indirect methods can be used previous to EFAs to limit the number of conditions that need to be included and thereby making the EFA more efficient (Floyd et al.). While this class of measures presents many benefits, there are several limitations. For example, the interviewer must depend on the third party to report accurately which can become problematic if there is over- or underreporting (Durand & Crimmins, 1990). Furthermore, as was the case with direct functional assessment methods, the cause of the function cannot be determine and only correlational information can be obtained (Hall, 2005). The two more common types of indirect functional assessments include interviews and rating scales.

Functional Assessment Interviews

Functional assessment interviews collect information on a number of variables that could affect the targeted problematic behavior. For example, information is often collected on the topography of the behavior, setting events, other events surrounding the behaviors, communication skills, previous treatment attempts, etc. One of the most commonly used and most comprehensive interviews is the Functional Assessment Interview (FAI; O'Neill et al., 1997). The FAI requires approximately 45–90 min to administer (Cunningham & O'Neill, 2000). The open-ended questions in these interviews allow for further probing when additional information is needed. Unfortunately, these types of interviews have not been studied thoroughly and thus, their psychometric properties can be questioned (Floyd et al., 2005).

Informant-Based Scales

The second type of indirect functional assessment is informant-based scales. These measures typically have respondents answer questions regarding the functions of behavior on a Likert-type scale. Two of the most common functional assessment scales that are used include the Questions About Behavior Function (QABF; Matson & Vollmer, 1995) and the Motivation Assessment Scale (MAS; Durand, 1988). One of the main benefits of scales compared to the other functional assessment methods is its short administration time. This is important as functions of behaviors can change over time (Bodfish, 2004; Guess & Carr, 1991). Therefore, scaling methods are beneficial because they can easily be administered at regular intervals or when the function of the behavior is thought to have changed. In addition, scales are easily scored and interpreted so that many professionals can be trained and utilize them.

The remainder of this chapter reviews several of the informant-based functional assessment scales which are commonly used in the literature. Reviews include studies available on reliability, validity, factor structure, and other notable research. The two most commonly used scales, the MAS and QABF, are reviewed first, then other less commonly used and researched scales are discussed. Finally, several studies are discussed which compare different scales and methods.

Scaling Methods

Motivation Assessment Scale (Durand, 1988)

Description

The MAS is one of the more highly cited and used informant-based functional assessment scales available in the literature (Sigafoos, Kerr, & Roberts, 1994; Toogood & Timlin, 1996). This measure is composed of 16 items which are rated by the informant on a seven-point Likert scale. As with all informant-based measures, the respondent should know the individual well and should also have experience with the behavior of interest. The most common informants are teachers and parents, and these respondents should answer questions based on the setting in which they know the individual best. The four subscales which represent motivating factors/functions were created based on face validity by the scale's developers, but have since been investigated statistically. The original four factors included escape from aversive events, gaining access to social attention, gaining access to tangible rewards, and sensory reinforcement. Items on each of the subscales are totaled and ranked.

Reliability
Inter-rater Reliability

The first examination of the reliability for the MAS was conducted by Durand and Crimmins (1988), the developers of the scale. In this study, teachers of 50 children with DD who exhibited SIB were administered the MAS. In addition, assistant teachers were administered the MAS to obtain inter-rater reliability. The authors first examined the correlations between informants on each item of the MAS. All items were reported to be significant with Pearson correlations ranging from 0.66 to 0.92. Similarly, the authors looked at function categories and found all correlations to be significant at $p < 0.001$ (range 0.80–0.95). Finally, the rank of functions was compared between respondents, meaning looking at if the two respondents had a specific function, such as escape, ranked first, then looking at the second, third, etc., ranks. Spearman rank-order correlations were all found to be significant at $p < 0.001$ with a range from 0.66 to 0.81. Based on the results from this sample, it can be concluded that the MAS as good inter-rater reliability.

While the developers of the scale found inter-rater reliability to be good, other researchers have not replicated these results. Zarcone, Rodgers, Iwata, Rourke, and Dorsey (1991) found the measure to be less reliable with their samples. In this study, two different samples were examined: one composed of direct care staff for individuals with severe to profound ID who lived at a residential and another of teachers of students who attended a school for those with autism and moderate to severe ID who also exhibited severe behavior problems. Once again, second raters, either a secondary teacher or second direct care staff, were obtained for each individual. The same correlations as in the Durand and Crimmins (1988) study were calculated. Item-by-item correlations ranged from -0.30 to 0.81 ($M = 0.27$). Correlations for the mean scores of each function were -0.80 to 0.99 ($M = 0.41$), and when using Spearman rank order correlations the range was from -0.80 to 1.0 ($M = 0.41$). As can be seen by comparing these correlations to the numbers above, there is certainly a discrepancy. In addition to correlations, Zarcone et al. used percent agreement, both exact and adjacent, for each item. Exact agreement was achieved when the Likert ranking on an item was identical across informants. On the other hand, adjacent agreement, which is less restrictive, was achieved if the ranking between informants was within one Likert rank. With the exact agreement method, agreement on items ranged from 0 to 63% ($M = 20\%$) and as expected adjacent agreement was somewhat higher with a range from 0 to 88% ($M = 48\%$). Exact agreement

for the main function determined was only found for 29.1% of participants. These percentages were similar in both samples. The authors stated that with these findings being so different from Durand and Crimmins' study that the utility of the MAS is brought into question. Zarcone and colleagues hypothesized several reasons for the discrepancies in findings. These reasons included sample characteristics, ambiguity of items (e.g., "Does it seem that he/she enjoys performing the behavior?"), and training of informant (e.g., master's level psychologist versus high-school education). Other characteristics of the behavior, such as behavior frequency, may also contribute to the differences in reliability found.

In addition to the study by Zarcone et al. (1991), Sigafoos and colleagues (1994) found inter-rater reliability that differed from the original study for the MAS. Their sample was smaller and was composed of 18 adolescents and adults with severe to profound ID who also exhibited challenging behaviors. Using Pearson correlations for the overall score on the measure, agreement between two raters ranged from -0.667 to 0.722 with an overall correlation of 0.034. Correlations were significant for 12 of the 18 pairs of raters. Conversely, when examining individual items, none of the correlations were significant with the range from -0.337 to 0.425, and none of the correlations for each of the subscales was significant with a range from -0.093 to 0.168. Similar findings were gained when using percent agreement as opposed to the Pearson correlations. For 8 of the 18 rater pairs (44.4%), agreement on the top-ranked function was achieved. Sigafoos et al. also bring into question the reliability and utility of the MAS, even though this measure is used often in applied settings.

In 1996, Conroy, Fox, Bucklin, and Good administered the MAS to 14 teachers of adolescents and 6 caregivers for adult men in a residential setting all of whom had ID and a challenging behavior. Each person was rated by two people as in the previously discussed studies. The exact match agreement was calculated for each item and was found to be 0.27 (range = 0.06–0.56). Using the adjacent method, the mean percent agreement was 0.56 (range = 0.25–0.78). The reliability of the function identified was also examined, but results were not particularly strong. Overall, the correlation between informant-rated functions was $r=0.66$ and only 28% of the correlations between raters were significant.

The next study by Duker and Sigafoos (1998) added to the previous literature on the MAS be examining the reliability of the individual factors which make up the scale. In this sample, which consisted of caregivers of 86 individuals with ID who exhibited 90 challenging behaviors in all, Pearson correlations for items averaged 0.415 with a range from 0.225 to 0.62, which is similar to the previous three studies discussed. In regard to the subscales, the Pearson correlations for items were 0.510 for Sensory, 0.369 for Escape, 0.115 for Attention, and 0.494 for Tangible. All of these correlations were significant accept for the Attention subscale. Percent agreements, exact and adjacent, were also calculated to examine inter-rater reliability. For exact agreement, the average agreement was 0.31 (range from 0.23 to 0.40). As expected, adjacent agreement was higher with the average being 0.63 (range 0.54–0.71). Percent agreement for the individual subscales was 0.16 for Sensory, 0.89 for Escape, 0.12 for Attention, and 0.12 for Tangible when using the exact agreement and 0.33 for Sensory, 0.30 for Escape, 0.25 for Attention, and 0.25 for Tangible. As can be seen by the reported numbers on the subscales, certain factors seem to have greater inter-rater reliability. One final study to note was conducted by Shogren and Rojahn (2003) which briefly examined several types of reliability for the MAS. This study found inter-rater reliability to be good based on the guidelines from Cicchetti (1994) with a range from 0.35 to 0.73.

As can be seen from the studies reviewed, the inter-rater reliability of the MAS has been examined quite extensively, but mixed results have been found. By far, the highest inter-rater reliability was found by the developers of the measures who found reliability to be in the fair to excellent range based on Cicchetti (1994) definitions (Durand & Crimmins, 1988). However, when looking at the studies in total, it is difficult to get a good picture of the inter-rater reliability.

Test–Retest Reliability

Some of the studies discussed above also examined test–retest reliability to examine the stability of MAS scores across time. The first study of this type of reliability was by the developers of the test, Durand and Crimmins (1988). By administering the MAS to the teachers 30 days apart, the researchers calculated the correlations between items, functional categories, and also examined the Spearman rank-order coefficients. Based on their sample, the item correlations ranged from 0.89 to 0.99, the function categories ranged from 0.92 to 0.98, and the Spearman coefficient was 0.82–0.89. All of these were found to be significant at the 0.001 level.

Other researchers have also examined test–retest reliability over a 1-month interval. Conroy and colleagues (1996) administered the MAS four times over a 1-month period. Percent agreement for items requiring an exact match had a large range from 0.0 to 0.88 with a mean of 0.40. In addition, the adjacent agreement, or what the authors referred to as plus/minus-one agreement was higher and ranged from 0.12 to 1.0 with a mean of 0.76.

In a similar study, Barton-Arwood, Wehby, Gunter, and Lane (2003) examined test–retest reliability of the MAS using 10 teachers who rated 30 students with challenging behaviors at three different times: the first administration, 1 week later, and 4 weeks after that. On the MAS over all three administrations, item-by-item correlations were significant for 88% of items across all three administrations. Seventy percent of functions were stable from time 1 to time 2, 1 week later, but this percentage dropped during the last administration. For the one-third of cases which the function was not consistently determined, 63% of cases had the top-ranked function and second-ranked function switched. Additionally, the authors noted that the primary function of behavior remained fairly consistent even if item-by-item was not consistent which may indicate that the item by item reliability is not as important. Also in 2003, Shogren and Rojahn (2003) also reported good test–retest reliability of 0.71–0.89.

In sum, it seems that the MAS demonstrates good test–retest reliability. However, it is important to remember that the function of a challenging behavior can fluctuate over time (Joyce, 2006). And thus, if assessments are not consistent over a period of time, it may be a product of a newly developed behavioral function as opposed to a flaw in the test.

Internal Consistency

The final type of reliability which has been examined for the MAS is internal consistency of the items within each factor of the MAS. The first of two studies found that the internal consistency to be 0.684 for Sensory, 0.738 for Escape, 0.759 for Attention, and 0.867 for Tangible (Duker & Sigafoos, 1998). Shogren and Rojahn (2003) found comparable results with Cronbach's alpha ranging from 0.80 to 0.96 on each of the subscales. Overall, the internal consistencies of the subscales which make up the MAS are fair to excellent (Cicchetti, 1994).

Validity

While a larger amount of research exists regarding the reliability of the MAS, less research has examined the validity of this measure. The developers of the MAS were the first to examine the validity by comparing results of functional assessments using the MAS to the results of experimental analyses (Durand & Crimmins, 1988). Using a sample of eight children with DD, five experimental conditions (i.e., baseline, attention, escape, tangible, and unstructured) were conducted and results were compared to those of the MAS. The authors examined the correlation of ranks of certain functions and found that there was high agreement between the two measures ($r = 0.99$ and $p < 0.001$).

A second study by Paclawskyj, Matson, Rush, Smalls, and Vollmer (2001) also examined the convergent validity of the MAS with EFAs (as described by Iwata et al., 1982). The percent agreement between the two methods was 43.8%. In addition to examining the agreement of the MAS with the EFA, the authors also investigated the agreement was between the MAS and

the QABF, another informant-based functional assessment measure. The agreement between these two informant-based measures was even higher than what was found for the EFA method with agreement in 61.5% of the cases.

Factor Structure

While the developers of the MAS created the subscales of the MAS based on face validity, other researchers have examined statistically if these factors are appropriate. Among these studies, there have been mixed results regarding the factor structure of the MAS. The first of these studies was conducted by Singh and colleagues (1993) who used two separate samples. The first included direct care staff of individuals with DD and high-frequency (>15 times per hour) SIB in residential facilities, while the second sample was teachers of students with mild to moderate ID who exhibited lower rates (<15 times per hour) of SIB. For the residential sample, a factor structure was found that was consistent with the factors based on face validity. However, the authors found no meaningful factor structure for the sample of students, even though they examined structures with three to five factors. The authors cite the differences in frequency of the challenging behavior, the level of ID, and training of the informants as possible reasons that the results of the factor analyses differed. They conclude that the MAS may be a useful clinical tool for those with more severe ID who exhibit higher frequency problem behaviors as opposed to higher functioning individuals with lower rates of challenging behaviors.

The second attempt analyze the factors of the MAS was by Bihm, Kienlen, Ness, and Poindexter (1991). These researchers used principle axis factoring analysis with varimax rotation to determine the factors of the MAS. Their findings more closely supported the original subscale proposed by the authors of the MAS. There were, however, two items that different. The first "Does the behavior occur when you stop attending?" was originally on the attention scale, but may be more appropriate on the sensory scales. And the second item "Does the person seem to do the behavior to upset or annoy you when you are getting him to do something else?" might fit better with the attention scale though it was originally on the escape subscale. In sum, Bihm and colleagues found support for the factors proposed by Durand and Crimmins (1988).

A third study by Duker and Sigafoos (1998), however, did not find statistical support for the four factors of the MAS. Using a sample of care-givers of individuals with mental retardation and challenging behaviors, the MAS was adminis-tered and principal components analysis with varimax rotation was conducted. In addition to the previously conducted factor analysis, Duker and Sigafoos also divided behavior into three dif-ferent topographies, maladaptive, destructive, and disruptive, to see if the factors found differed. For maladaptive, disruptive, and destructive behaviors, the four factors found explained 69.6, 83.5, and 76.4% of the variance, respectively. However, while each of the behavior topogra-phies indicated four factors, the individual items that loaded onto each scale were not consistent with the original proposed factor structure.

Interestingly, these factor structure studies used exploratory methods as opposed to confirmatory methods, even though factors for measure were already proposed. Therefore, Kearney, Cook, Chapman, and Bensaheb (2006) chose to use confirmatory methods to see if the face valid scales would be supported. Using a sample of adults with severe to profound ID who exhibited moderate levels of maladaptive behav-ior, the authors examined three indices for good-ness of fit which is recommended in the literature (Kline, 2005). When examining all of the items, the original factor structure found by Durand and Crimmins (1988) was not supported by all of the indices. However, the authors then deleted sev-eral of the items which lowered the internal con-sistency (four out of seven of these items were in the sensory reinforcement function). Once sev-eral items were deleted, the new CFA with the select items did support the proposed factor analysis.

In the most recent examination of the factor structure of the MAS, Joosten and Bundy (2008) examined if the MAS was actually measuring a unidimensional construct since previous studies on factor analysis were inconsistent. Their findings neither supported the unidimensional hypothesis or the four factors as described by Durand (1988). However, this study only exam-ined the behaviors of stereotypies and other repetitive behaviors. The authors suggest that these types of behaviors may be different from some of the other maladaptive behaviors such as aggression.

As can be seen from the results above, there has not been a consensus from research about the factors of the MAS. While a handful of studies have been conducted, researchers have not yet suggested what to do regarding the measure and if the original factors should continue to be used or if the factors should be revised somehow. This would be helpful to increase the confidence that can be put behind the MAS.

Questions About Behavior Function (Matson & Vollmer, 1995)

Description

The (QABF) is a functional assessment scale designed to aid in determining the function of challenging behaviors in those with DD by gain-ing information from informants, such as parents or caregivers. The 25-items are rated by infor-mants on a four-point Likert scale as Never, Rarely, Some, or Often. Total administration time is approximately 20 min and the measure is eas-ily scored and interpreted. When interpreting results, a clear function is considered an endorse-ment of four or five of the items endorsed within one subscale with no other subscales containing significant endorsements. Since behaviors may have multiple or secondary functions, elevations of one or more scales need to be interpreted accordingly.

Reliability
Inter-rater Reliability

The first study which examined the inter-rater reliability of the QABF used a sample of 57 adults with severe to profound ID and challeng-ing behaviors (Paclawskyj, Matson, Rush, Smalls,

& Vollmer, 2000). Inter-rater reliability was found to be good with Spearman rank-order correlations for the primary function ranging from −0.095 to 1.0 with 52% of the items exceeding 0.80. Total percent agreement for each of the items ranged from 69.57 to 95.65% with 56% of the items exceeding 80% agreement. Finally, Pearson product-moment for each subscale and the total score between the two informants were 0.79–0.98, $p < 0.01$.

To replicate these results, Shogren and Rojahn (2003) examined the reliability of the QABF with a sample of 20 adults diagnosed with mental retardation who required a behavior treatment plan to target challenging behaviors such as aggression, self-injury, and property destruction. The results demonstrated the inter-rater reliability to be fair to good ($r = 0.46$–0.60) which was lower than what Paclawskyj and colleagues (2000) found. The authors cite the smaller sample size as a possible reason for the difference in findings.

In another study, Nicholson, Konstantinidi, and Furniss (2006) looked at inter-rater reliability for items, scales, and overall total with both exact and adjacent agreement as was done with the MAS. Exact agreement for items ranged from 32.2 to 61.86% with a mean agreement of 43.22%. As expected, adjacent agreement was higher with a range from 69.49 to 84.75% with a mean of 77.97%. Pearson correlations for each of the subscales ranged from 0.421 to 0.623.

While the previous three studies examined inter-rater reliability for the measure generally, others have looked at other variables which may affect psychometrics such as number of maintaining variables and low- versus high-frequency behaviors. Matson and Boisjoli (2007) examined inter-rater reliability for behaviors that had more than one function. Agreement was achieved when both raters ranked the functions of the same severity. For example, if rater 1 found attention to be the strongest maintaining variable and tangible as the second, then to be considered agreement rater 2 would have to have both function severities ranked the same as well. For those challenging behaviors only maintained by one variable (i.e., four or five of the items endorsed within one

subscale with no other subscales containing significant endorsements), agreement was achieved on 63.6% of participants with aggression, and 50% of those exhibiting SIB. For behaviors with multiple functions, reliability decreased as the rank of the function decreased, with the agreement ranging from 57.7% for the first ranked function down to 0% for the fifth ranked function. While the lower functions did not demonstrate good inter-rater reliability, this may be less important in relation to having good reliability for the stronger maintaining functions.

A second variable that has been explored with the QABF is the effect of frequency of the challenging behavior. Matson and Wilkins (2009) examined how reliability varied with low- and high-frequency behaviors. They defined low-frequency behaviors as those that occurred only on a monthly or weekly basis, while those that occurred daily or hourly were defined as high frequency. For low-frequency behaviors, Spearman correlations ranged from 0.162 to 0.429 with four of the scales having significant correlations (i.e., attention, nonsocial, physical, and tangible) and for high-frequency behaviors Spearman correlations ranged from 0.069 to 0.477 and three of the subscales reached significance (i.e., escape, physical, and tangible). Overall, while both low- and high-frequency behaviors were reliability identified, high-frequency behaviors had higher reliability on average. This may be because informants are more familiar with the behavior since it happens more often and there have been more experiences to based responses on.

Based on the studies that have been conducted with the QABF, the measure seems to exhibit adequate inter-rater reliability. Furthermore, the findings seem to more consistent and favorable when compared with the inter-rater reliability of the MAS. It should be noted that the samples from these studies have been limited to primarily caregivers of adults with ID; thus, it would be useful to expand the samples examined to see if the inter-rater reliability remains strong.

Test–Retest Reliability

Several studies have also examined the test–retest reliability of the QABF. In the first study by

Paclawskyj and colleagues (2000), the QABF was administered to the caregiver two times with an interval of 3 weeks. Spearman rank-order correlations were high with 76% of the item statistics exceeding 0.80. Total percent agreement was also good with 96% of items exceeding 80% agreement. The only other study noted to examine test–retest reliability also found test–retest reliability to be good with Pearson-r for the subscales ranging from 0.62 to 0.93 (Shogren & Rojahn, 2003).

Internal Consistency

Three studies have reported investigated the internal consistency of the QABF. The first by Paclawskyj and colleagues (2000) found high internal consistency with Cronbach's alpha on the subscales ranging from 0.900 to 0.928. The second study, while still finding good internal consistency, did not find coefficient alphas quite as high (Shogren & Rojahn, 2003). The authors point out that for the subscales that have equivalents on the MAS, the alphas ranged from 0.82 to 0.88; however, for the physical subscale which has no MAS equivalent the Cronbach's alpha was only 0.24.

The last study by Nicholson and colleagues (2006) replicated previous results, and also took their examination of internal consistency a step further. Similar to previous findings, the alphas for the subscales ranged from 0.785 to 0.922. Next the authors looked at internal consistency in regards to how it varied with high- and low-frequency behaviors as well as different behavioral topographies such as disruptive, maladaptive, and destructive behaviors. Internal consistency remained high regardless of these variables.

Validity

While the QABF has been shown to have good reliability, in order for it to be a strong measure, its validity must also be established. Matson, Bamburg, Cherry, and Paclawskyj (1999) examined the predictive validity of the QABF by examining outcomes of functional based treatment plans which used the QABF to determine the function. For example, if the behavior was determined to be maintained by a nonsocial

function, environmental enrichment, and social skills training would be included in the treatment plan. These functional assessment-based plans were compared to general plans which used techniques such as blocking, redirecting and interrupting, not based on the outcome of the QABF. For the behavior examined, SIB, aggression, and stereotypies, significant decreases were seen when using the function-based treatment plan. For example, using the QABF-based plan, SIB decreased 66%, whereas it only decreased by 21% with the generic plan. These findings speak to the validity and utility of the QABF, especially in applied setting in which the findings from the functional assessment would be used to determine a treatment plan.

In a second study, Pacwalskyj and colleagues (2001) examined the convergent validity of the QABF with EFA (Iwata et al., 1982) just as they had compared to the MAS to EFA. The QABF and experimental method showed an agreement on the maintaining function 56.3% of the time. This was slightly higher than what was found when examining the MAS and EFA. In addition to examining the agreement of the QABF with the EFA, the authors also investigated the agreement between the QABF and MAS. Sixty-one percent of the time the MAS and QABF exhibited agreement which was an improvement when compared with their agreements with the EFA method.

Factor Structure

Matson and colleagues (1996) presented data from exploratory factor analysis which used a sample of 462 individuals, ages 13–86 years with ID who exhibited the challenging behaviors of SIB, aggression, or property destruction. These data, which were later published by Paclawskyj and colleagues (2000), supported five factors to the measure including Attention, Escape, Physical, Tangible, and Nonsocial. These factors were found to explain 74.5% of the variance. More recently, Nicholson and colleagues (2006) replicated factor analysis on the severity scores of the QABF using a younger sample ($N=40$) with ID who exhibited a total of 118 challenging behaviors. Their finding also highly supported the original factors proposed by the authors of the measure. The first four factors were commensurate with the physical, attention, tangible, and escape subscales. The fifth factor found included four of the five nonsocial items, but the last of these nonsocial items (i.e., engages in the behavior in a highly repetitive manner, ignoring his/her surroundings) loaded onto a separate sixth factor. Overall, their factor structure explained 73% of the variance. A last study by Singh and colleagues (2009) also replicated the factor analysis of the QABF when the attempted to shorten the measure (to be discussed later). Their findings were similar to the previous studies in which five factors were found which explained 73.9% of the total variance. With these three studies, there is good evidence that the five factors of the QABF are supported statistically as well as rationally.

Profiles of Challenging Behaviors

While there is a wide range of challenging behaviors that can be investigated using functional assessment, certain behaviors are fairly common in the literature, such as physical aggression, SIB, and stereotypies (Poppes, van der Putten, & Vlaskamp, 2010). Because some of these behaviors are common, especially in those with ID or DD, researchers have begun to study if certain functions are more likely to maintain certain behaviors. That is, are there common functional profiles for specific problematic behaviors?

Several studies have examined the results of QABF to look for trends in functions. One such study by Dawson, Matson, and Cherry (1998) examined the three challenging behaviors of SIB, aggression, and stereotypies to determine if certain functions were more commonly identified based on behavior topography. The findings supported possible function profiles for certain behaviors. For example, aggression was most likely maintained by attention, while stereotypies were more likely maintained by a nonsocial function. SIB was not supported by a particular function. In a similar study, Applegate, Matson, and Cherry (1999) examined the behaviors of SIB, stereotypies, aggression, pica, or rumination in adults with ID. In this case, aggression was once again found to be maintained by more environmental variables

such as attention, while the other behaviors served more of a nonsocial function. Other studies have revealed similar trends in the maintaining functions of certain challenging behaviors. Matson and colleagues (1999) found that with the QABF as the tool for functional assessment, SIB was most often the function of nonsocial and also escape. Aggression most often served the function of gaining access to attention and escape from demands, while stereotypies were once again found to serve a nonsocial function. Matson and Boisjoli (2007) also found aggression was most often maintained by escape and SIB by nonsocial.

Based on these results, there are implications for treatment. While each individual needs a functional assessment, in certain circumstances knowing the typical functions of challenging behaviors could aid in developing a treatment plan. In addition, prevention strategies may want to be included for certain behaviors even if that particular function was not found to be the primary-maintaining function (Tarbox et al., 2009). For example, even though aggression may be found to be maintained by gaining access to a tangible, it may be worthwhile to include prevention strategies that target attention. This may decrease the chances that this behavior would later be maintained by attention because the person could be getting attention through appropriate means.

Multiple Functions

The QABF has been shown to be able to clearly identify at least one function in 84% of cases (Matson et al., 1999). However, as mentioned previously, some challenging behaviors are maintained by more than one function (Matson & Boisjoli, 2007). Matson and Boisjoli, using the QABF, discovered that multiple functions of behavior are fairly common with approximately half of the behaviors examined being maintained by multiple functions. Multiple functions were defined by having a severity of score that was greater than six. Twenty-two percent were maintained by two functions, 18% by three functions, 7% by four functions, and 7% met criteria for being maintained by all five functions.

These findings have implications for treatment planning specifically, so that all maintain functions are being addressed properly. However, as noted in the reliability section for the QABF, the reliability decreases for the lower-rank functions and this should be considered when examining lower-rank functions (Matson & Boisjoli).

Questions About Behavior Function—Short Form (Singh et al., 2009)

The original QABF consisted of 25 items. However, if the number of items was decreased, the efficiency of the functional assessment would be increased. Singh and colleagues (2009) conducted exploratory and confirmatory factor analysis to determine if the full QABF could be shortened to create a briefer measure which still possessed adequate psychometrics. First, the authors attempted to replicate the factor structure that Paclawskyj and colleagues (2000) found for the full-length measure. Using exploratory factor analysis with varimax rotation, the same five factors (i.e., Attention, Escape, Physical, Tangible, and Nonsocial) were found which explained 73.9% of the total item variance. Secondly, to determine which items should be retained for the shortened version of the QABF, a priori calculations of reliability and validity (see Singh et al., 2009 for full description of criteria to maintain or eliminate items) were examined. Based on these calculations, ten items from the original measure were eliminated. Thus, the new Questions About Behavior Function—Short Form (QABF-SF) consisted of 15 items. A second factor analysis was used to confirm that the factor structure of the original measure was retained for the new version. Results showed that the five factors in the original full-length QABF were also found in the QABF-SF. The authors also examined the reliability of the QABF-SF. Cronbach's alpha showed high-internal consistency for each of the subscales: 0.92 for attention, 0.91 for escape, 0.84 for nonsocial, 0.94 for physical, and 0.80 for tangible. To examine test–retest reliability, Pearson product moment correlations were examined.

Results showed the correlations ranged from 0.098 to 0.836, $p < 0.01$, for each of the subscales. Finally, inter-rater reliabilities for each of the subscales were all significant at the 0.01 level with correlations of 0.932 for attention, 0.933 for escape, 0.955 for nonsocial, 0.927 for physical, and 0.815 for tangible. Based on this primary study of the QABF-SF, it seems that this measure would be useful as a functional assessment measure; however, to further prove the utility of this measure, validity studies need to also be conducted.

Questions About Behavior Function—Mental Illness (Singh et al., 2006)

While the original QABF was developed for those with developmental disabilities, this measure has been extended for those with severe mental illness as well as challenging behaviors are also observed with this population (Serper et al., 2005). Thus far, limited information is available on this measure. However, Singh et al. (2006) did examine the factors of the newly adapted measure by administering the Questions About Behavior Function—Mental Illness (QABF-MI) to 135 adults with serious mental illness from three inpatient psychiatric hospitals. Their finding supported the factor structure which was found by Paclawskyj et al. (2000). Across the five factors of physical discomfort, social attention, tangible reinforcement, escape, and nonsocial, inter-rater reliability ranged from 0.96 to 0.98, and Pearson r test–retest reliability ranged from 0.86 to 0.99. Coefficient alpha suggested acceptable internal consistency ranging from 0.84 to 0.92 for the target behaviors of aggression and property destruction. The authors also pointed out that while analogue functional analyses have considerable utility for persons with developmental disabilities, it would not be possible to use this method for individuals with normal intellectual functioning and mental illness on practical grounds. Thus, a measure such as the QABF-MI would be beneficial for this population so that functions of challenging behaviors can be identified and appropriate treatments can be put in place. Additionally, by using functional assessment for challenging behaviors in a typical population, environmental causes could be identified which could reduce the chance of unwarranted psychotropic medications.

Problem Behavior Questionnaire

While some of the other scaling methods discussed in this chapter were created for those with more severe behavior problems and impairments, the Problem Behavior Questionnaire (PBQ) was developed out of a need to functional-based assessment for those with milder behavior problems in a general education setting (Barton-Arwood et al., 2003). The PBQ consists of 15 items which describe situations in which the behavior is likely to occur. For example, "Does the problem behavior occur in the presence of specific peers?" These items are then rated based on how often each situation occurs by the informant on a seven-point Likert scale with the anchors of never, 10, 25, 50, 75, 90%, or always. Within the 15 items, there are five main functions being addressed: access to peer attention, access to teacher attention, escape from peer attention, escape from teacher attention, and setting events. Those items with a score of three or above (i.e., occurring 50% or more of the time) are considered as a potential hypothesis for problem behavior and those functions with two or more items scored at a three or above are considered to be primary hypotheses.

In terms of psychometrics, only one study was found which examined reliability of this measure (Barton-Arwood et al., 2003). In this study, which also examined the MAS, there were 10 teachers who rated 30 students' behaviors across three separate times: the first administration, 1 week later, and 4 weeks after that. The results showed that the percent of significant item-by-item correlations between any of the two administration periods ranged from 47% to 74%. As might be expected, the lowest amount of significant correlations occurred from the first and third administration periods. When examining the percent of

significant item-by-item correlations across all three administrations of the PBQ, only 20% were significant. In addition to item-by-item consistency, the consistency of the function identified was also explored. When examining exact agreement, the functions remained stable 59–81% of the time across administration periods. In 50% of cases when the function was not stable, the first and second ranked function switched some time during the three administrations. The authors noted that while item-by-item consistent may not have been high, the primary function of behaviors remained fairly over time which may be more meaningful.

Functional Assessment for Multiple CausaliTy (Matson et al., 2003)

The purpose of the Functional Assessment for Multiple CausaliTy (FACT) is to determine the hierarchy of functions for challenging behaviors that have multiple functions. Researchers have noted that approximately up to half of challenging behaviors may serve multiple functions (Matson & Boisjoli, 2007). Therefore, in some cases, it would be beneficial to determine which function is more prominent to aid in treatment development. While other measures rank functions, the FACT more directly tests the different functions against one another.

The FACT is composed of 35 items that are presented in a forced-choice format in which two possible functions are presented and the respondent must decide which is more applicable to the individual. While the original measure was composed of 50 items each with three possible responses, due to the lengthy time to administer the measure, some items were eliminated and only two response options were used to result in a 35-item measure. An example item from the FACT is "Engages in the behavior more (A) to get attention, or more (P) because he/she is in pain, or (N) neither?" Based on a factor analysis which was conducted, a five-factor model was suggested (Matson et al., 2003). The five factors found were consistent with the five subscales of the QABF: Tangible, Physical, Attention,

Escape, and Nonsocial. In regard to reliability, the internal consistency was computed with the Kuder-Richardson formula 20 (KR-20). All sub-scales of the FACT yielded good to high esti-mates of reliability (0.88–0.92). At this time, no other psychometric studies have been completed. More research is needed to determine the validity and general utility of the FACT.

Motivation Analysis Rating Scale (Wieseler, Hanson, Chamberlain, & Thompson, 1985)

The Motivation Analysis Rating Scale (MARS), also referred to as the Contingency Analysis Questionnaire (CAQ) was one of the first func-tional assessment scales developed. The measure assessed the following functions of behavior: social and tangible positive reinforcement, social and situational escape, and self-stimulation. The six items that make up the scale are answered on a five-point Likert scale ranging from "never" to "almost always." While this measure was one of the first to be developed, little research has been conducted to investigate its psychometric proper-ties. As a result, little can be said about the utility of this measure.

Functional Analysis Screening Tool (Iwata & DeLeon, 1995)

The Functional Analysis Screening Tool (FAST) is a 27-item informant-based functional assess-ment measure. This measure is composed of three factors: (1) social influences on behavior, (2) social reinforcement, and (3) nonsocial (auto-matic) reinforcement. Once again there has been very limited research on this measure in terms of psychometric properties. The only information found reported that the inter-rater reliability was found to be 67%. As a result of the limited research on this measure, it is not reportedly used in the literature and requires more investi-gation into its psychometrics if it is going to be used.

Comparison of Functional Assessment Methods

With such a variety of methods available to con-duct functional assessments, the question arises as to which of these methods may be the best or even if these methods are comparable. While the strengths and weaknesses of these different meth-ods, including ABC charts, scatter plots, EFAs, interviews, and rating scales, were reviewed at the beginning of this chapter, some researchers have compared methods in more controlled settings.

One study conducted by Lerman and Iwata (1993) compared experimental and descriptive methods of functional assessment in six adults with ID, all of whom exhibited the challenging behavior of SIB. Descriptive analysis used par-tial-interval recording in which the occurrence of the behavior, as well as subject and staff responses and other environmental factors were recorded in 10-s intervals. EFA methods were similar to those in Iwata et al. (1982). On five of six trials, results on the functions obtained using descriptive meth-ods were not consistent with those using the experimental methods. The authors concluded that due to the correlational nature of descriptive methods that these methods are not sufficient and may not be necessary in determining the function of challenging behaviors.

While Lerman and Iwata (1993) only exam-ined experimental and descriptive methods, sev-eral other studies have also included scaling methods to compare results. One of the first was by Crawford, Brockel, Schauss, and Miltenberger (1992). In their study, the authors first completed the MAS, then the EFA followed by the ABC charts for two men and two women with severe to profound ID who exhibited high rates of stereo-typic behaviors. The MAS and ABC charts were conducted with both home and vocational staff. However, there were some discrepancies between these informants which may have been due to behaviors actually differing in various settings. The findings showed that the MAS reliability identified the function of behaviors as being sen-sory most often. The next assessment, the EFA, reportedly obtained inconsistent results. On the other hand, of all three assessment methods, the ABC chart most clearly determined the function of the challenging behaviors to be sensory. The authors note that the ABC charting and MAS are most useful in applied settings due to their relative accuracy and brevity. In addition, in analyzing the structure of the study, one should consider that the ABC chart was completed after the EFA was conducted. This is a concern as some researchers have noted that EFAs can change and create new functions to challenging behaviors (Matson & Minshawi, 2007).

In a similar study, Toogood and Timlin (1996) examined 92 individuals with severe ID and challenging behaviors. The methods compared in this study included informant-based interview, informant-based rating scale (MAS), ABC chart, scatter plot analysis, and EFA. It should be noted that two versions of the MAS were used. The first was the original version and the second had four additional items added to differentiate between social avoidance and task avoidance. Authors examined the percent of behaviors that were ascribed functions. The method that predicted clear functions the most often was clinical interview, followed by the MAS (both versions), scatter plot analysis, EFA, and ABC charts. The agreement rate overall five methods was extremely low at only 2.5% (i.e., 3 of the 121 behaviors assessed). When including all assessed behaviors (i.e., including those behaviors that no function was determined), agreement rates between any two methods ranged from 10 to 62%. When only behaviors for which a function was determined was included, agreement rates rose to 44–89%. In either case, the methods which resulted in the highest agreement were between MAS and interview. When examining these results, the reader should note that the function rank was not examined, and thus, behaviors which identified multiple functions, it did not matter if the function was first or second ranked. If the level of agreement had been considered, these rates would have been much lower.

While Toogood and Timlin (1996) found the MAS to have good concordance with informant-based interview, the QABF has been shown to have good agreement with EFA methods (Hall, 2005). In this study, the sample consisted of four individuals with severe to profound ID and who also exhibited a challenging behavior. The three methods examined were descriptive methods (i.e., time-based lag sequential analysis (Sackett, 1987), Iwata and colleagues (1994) experimental methods, and the QABF (Matson & Vollmer, 1995). Each of these methods was conducted for the sample and their challenging behavior so that agreement rates on the determined function of the behavior could be compared. Based on the authors' findings, experimental and informant-based assessments were concordant for three of four participants, whereas the descriptive assessment was only concordant with the experimental results in one of four trials. Furthermore, descriptive methods took approximately 10 h, the experimental method took 2 h, and while the QAFB took 15 min. Thus, the time benefits of certain methods are evident. Clearly, a limitation of this study is the very small sample size which makes it difficult to put forth strong conclusions based on these results.

One study by Paclawskyj et al. (2001) compared the QABF and MAS more directly by administering both measures and also conducting an EFA. Between the three types of functional assessment, the QABF and MAS demonstrated the greatest concordance rate by identifying the same function 61.5% of the time. This would make sense since both measures use the same format of asking informants to provide information about the behavior and each is composed of similar subscales. However, when compared with the EFA, the QABF had greater agreement than the MAS with agreement rates being 56.3 and 43.8%, respectively. However, as can be seen by the percentage, the QABF and MAS seem to be quite comparable.

The next more recent study by Tarbox and colleagues (2009) compared different functional assessment methods for seven children with autism diagnoses. The three methods examined included ABC data and specific coding for antecedents and consequences as the descriptive method, the QABF as indirect method, and Iwata and colleagues' (1982) EFA method as the analogue method. Once again, each method was conducted for each child's challenging behavior so that concordance rates could be obtained. The results indicated that the QABF (indirect method) and EFA (experimental method) had the greatest concordance rates. Exact agreement was achieved for three of seven participants, and partial agreement (at least one of the same functions were concordant) was achieved on six of the seven participants. On the other hand, partial and/or exact agreement was only obtained for two of seven between indirect and descriptive and one of seven between descriptive and EFA. Interestingly, when examining the concordance across all three methods, exact agreement was only found for one of the seven cases examined. While this study used a small sample size, it highlights the discrepancies in results across different functional assessment methods. In the discussion, the authors state that the QABF identified all of the same functions as the EFA except on one occasion, but in addition the QABF also identified some functions of behavior that were not found with EFA. The authors state that the QABF found "false positives." However, this statement assumes that the EFA is correct in its functions identified and that the QABF is identifying functions that are not valid. However, one could also argue that the QABF is more sensitive because it samples a large range of behavior that the EFA was actually missing secondary functions of the challenging behavior. In either case, the authors state that it may not be detrimental to obtain false positives on the assessment. If functions were identified that are not actually maintaining the challenging behavior, then the treatment plan would have extra prevention and intervention strategies. This would be preferable to a functional assessment which did not detect a maintaining function and resulted in an inadequate treatment plan that could worsen behaviors.

When examining the studies above, one can see that there is not always good agreement between different methods of functional assessment. However, it is also important to remember that each method has its own strengths and weaknesses, and these should be considered when choosing a method. In many cases, a clinician may want to progress from one method to another until they feel an accurate function has been

determined. For example, one may begin with a scaling method, such as the QABF or MAS, because these methods are time and cost efficient. At this point, no further assessment may be needed. However, if it was felt necessary, other more time-consuming methods, such as ABC charts or EFA, could be used to glean additional information.

General Conclusions

When working with individuals with challenging behaviors, specifically those individuals with ID or DD, completing a functional assessment for challenging behaviors is of the utmost importance to develop appropriate behavior treatment plans. As can be seen from the review above, there are several methods of functional assessment which each offer their own strengths and weaknesses. It can be argued that each of these methods has its place in certain situations.

Scaling methods are beneficial because a larger amount of information can be gathered from caregivers or direct care staff in a short amount of time. These measures are also easy to score and interpret. This allows for the readministration of the measure over periods of time which is important as new behaviors may develop or functions of behaviors may change. While there are a handful of scaling measures that have been created, many have not been thoroughly research. However, the QABF and MAS have been investigated thoroughly enough to state that they have adequate psychometric properties and should be top choices for applied settings. These scales, along with other forms of functional assessment, should be used often to ensure the best treatment of individuals with challenging behaviors.

References

Anderson, C. M., Freeman, K. A., & Scotti, S. R. (1999). Evaluation of the generalizability (reliability and validity) of analog functional assessment methodology. *Behavior Therapy, 30*, 31–50.

Applegate, H., Matson, J. L., & Cherry, K. E. (1999). An evaluation of functional variables affecting severe problem behaviors in adults with mental retardation using the Questions About Behavioral Function Scale (QABF). *Research in Developmental Disabilities, 20,* 229–238.

Barton-Arwood, S. M., Wehby, J. H., Gunter, P. L., & Lane, K. L. (2003). Functional behavior assessment rating scales: Intrarater reliability with students with emotional or behavioral disorders. *Behavioral Disorders, 28,* 386–400.

Bihm, E. M., Kienlen, T. L., Ness, M. E., & Poindexter, A. R. (1991). Factor structure of the Motivation Assessment Scale for persons with mental retardation. *Psychological Reports, 68,* 1235–1238.

Bodfish, J. W. (2004). Treating the core features of autism: Are we there yet? *Mental Retardation and Developmental Disabilities Research Reviews, 10,* 318–326.

Bosma, A., & Mulick, J. A. (1990). Brief report: Ecobehavioral assessment using transparent scatter plots. *Behavioral Residential Treatment, 5,* 137–140.

Brestan, E. V., & Eyberg, S. M. (1998). Effective psychosocial treatments of conduct disordered children and adolescents: 29 years, 82 studies, and 5,272 kids. *Journal of Clinical Child Psychology, 27,* 180–189.

Cicchetti, D. V. (1994). Guidelines, criteria, and rules of thumb for evaluating normed and standardized assessment instruments in psychology. *Psychological Assessment, 6,* 284–290.

Conroy, M. A., Davis, C. A., Fox, J. J., & Brown, W. H. (2002). Functional assessment of behavior and effective supports for young children with challenging behaviors. *Assessment for Effective Intervention, 27,* 35–47.

Conroy, M. A., Fox, J. J., Bucklin, A., & Good, W. (1996). An analysis of the reliability and stability of the Motivation Assessment Scale in assessing the challenging behaviors of persons with developmental disabilities. *Education & Training in Mental Retardation & Developmental Disabilities, 31,* 243–250.

Crawford, J., Brockel, B., Schauss, S., & Miltenberger, R. G. (1992). A comparison of methods for the functional assessment of stereotypic behavior in persons with mental retardation. *Journal of the Association for Persons with Severe Handicaps, 17,* 77–86.

Cunningham, E., & O'Neill, R. (2000). Comparison of results of functional assessment and analysis methods with young children with autism. *Education and Training in Mental Retardation and Developmental Disabilities, 35,* 406–414.

Dawson, J. E., Matson, J. L., & Cherry, K. E. (1998). An analysis of maladaptive behaviors in persons with autism, PDD-NOS, and mental retardation. *Research in Developmental Disabilities, 19,* 439–448.

Derby, K. M., Hagopian, L., Fisher, W. W., Richman, D., Augustine, M., Fahs, A., et al. (2000). Functional analysis of aberrant behavior through measurement of separate response topographies. *Journal of Applied Behavior Analysis, 33,* 113–117.

Duker, P. C., & Sigafoos, J. (1998). The Motivation Assessment Scale: Reliability and construct validity across three topographies of behaviour. *Research in Developmental Disabilities, 19,* 131–141.

DuPaul, G. J., & Ervin, R. A. (1996). Functional assessment of behavior related to attention deficit/hyperactivity disorder: Linking assessment to intervention design. *Behavior Therapy, 27,* 601–622.

Durand, V. M. (1988). The motivation assessment scale. In M. Hersen & A. Bellack (Eds.), *Dictionary of behavioral assessment techniques* (pp. 309–310). Tarrytown: Pergamon.

Durand, V. M., & Crimmins, D. B. (1988). Identifying the variables maintaining self-injurious behavior. *Journal of Autism and Developmental Disabilities, 17,* 17–28.

Durand, V. M., & Crimmins, D. (1990). Chapter 3 Assessment. In V. M. Durand (Ed.), *Severe behaviour problems: A functional communication training approach.* New York: Guilford.

Emerson, E., & Bromley, J. (1995). The form and function of challenging behaviours. *Journal of Intellectual Disability Research, 39,* 388–398.

Floyd, R. G., Phaneuf, R. L., & Wilczynski, S. M. (2005). Measurement properties of indirect assessment methods for functional behavioral assessment: A review of research. *School Psychology Review, 34,* 58–73.

Gettinger, M., & Callan Stoiber, K. (2006). Functional assessment, collaboration, and evidence-based treatment: Analysis of a team approach for addressing challenging behaviors in young children. *Journal of School Psychology, 44,* 231–252.

Guess, D., & Carr, E. G. (1991). Emergence and maintenance of stereotypy and self-injury. *American Journal on Mental Retardation, 96,* 299–319.

Hall, S. S. (2005). Comparing descriptive, experimental and informant-based assessments of problem behaviors. *Research in Developmental Disabilities, 26,* 514–526.

Hile, M. G., & Desrochers, M. N. (1993). The relationship between functional assessment and treatment selection for aggressive behaviors. *Research in Developmental Disabilities, 14,* 265–274.

Iwata, B. A. & DeLeon, I. G. (1995). The functional analysis screening tool (FAST). Unpublished manuscript, Gainesville: University of Florida.

Iwata, B. A., Dorsey, M. F., Slifer, K. E., Bauman, K. E., & Richman, G. S. (1982). Towards a functional analysis of self-injury. *Analysis and Intervention in Developmental Disabilities, 2,* 3–20.

Iwata, B. A., Pace, G. M., Dorsey, M. F., Zarcone, J. R., Vollmer, T. R., Smith, R., et al. (1994). The functions of self-injurious behavior: An experimental-epidemiological analysis. *Journal of Applied Behavior Analysis, 27,* 215–240.

Joosten, A. V., & Bundy, A. C. (2008). The motivation of stereotypic and repetitive behavior: Examination of construct validity of the Motivation Assessment Scale. *Journal of Autism and Developmental Disorders, 38,* 1341–1348.

Joyce, T. (2006). Functional assessment and challenging behaviour. *Psychiatry, 5,* 312–315.

Kearney, C. A., Cook, L. C., Chapman, G., & Bensaheb, A. (2006). Exploratory and confirmatory factor analyses of the Motivation Assessment Scale and Resident Choice Assessment Scale. *Journal of Developmental and Physical Disabilities, 18,* 1–11.

Kiernan, C., Reeves, D., Hatton, C., Alborz, A., Emerson, E., Mason, H., et al. (1997). *The HARC challenging behavior project report 1: Persistence and change in the challenging behavior of people with a learning disability.* Manchester: Hester Adrian Research Centre, University of Manchester.

Kline, R. B. (2005). *Principles and practice of structural equation modeling* (2nd ed.). New York: Guilford.

Lerman, D. C., & Iwata, B. A. (1993). Descriptive and experimental analyses of variables maintaining self injurious behavior. *Journal of Applied Behavior Analysis, 26,* 293–319.

Lowe, K., Allen, D., Jones, E., Brophy, S., Moore, K., & James, W. (2007). Challenging behaviours: Prevalence and topographies. *Journal of Intellectual Disability Research, 51,* 625–636.

Matson, J. L., Bamburg, J. W., Cherry, K. E., & Paclawskyj, T. R. (1999). A validity study on the Questions About Behavioral Function (QABF) Scale: Predicting treatment success for self-injury, aggression, and stereotypies. *Research in Developmental Disabilities, 20,* 163–176.

Matson, J. L., & Boisjoli, J. (2007). Multiple versus single maintaining factors of challenging behaviors as assessed by the QABF for adults with intellectual disability (ID). *Journal of Intellectual and Developmental Disability, 32,* 39–44.

Matson, J. L., Cooper, C., Malone, C. J., & Moskow, S. L. (2008). The relationship of self-injurious behaviors and other maladaptive behaviors among individuals with severe and profound intellectual disability. *Research in Developmental Disabilities, 29,* 141–148.

Matson, J. L., Kiely, S. L., & Bamburg, J. W. (1997). The effect of stereotypies on adaptive skills as assessed with the DASH-II and Vineland Adaptive Behavior Scales. *Research in Developmental Disabilities, 18,* 471–476.

Matson, J. L., Kuhn, D. E., Dixon, D. R., Mayville, S. B., Laud, R. B., Cooper, C. L., et al. (2003). The development and factor structure of the functional assessment for multiple causaliTy (FACT). *Research in Developmental Disabilities, 24,* 485–495.

Matson, J. L., & Minshawi, N. F. (2007). Functional assessment of challenging behavior: Toward a strategy for applied settings. *Research in Developmental Disabilities, 28,* 353–361.

Matson, J. L., & Vollmer, T. (1995). *Questions About Behavioral Function (QABF).* Baton Rouge: Disability Consultants, LLC.. Translated into Italian, German, and Korean.

Matson, J. L., Vollmer, T. R., Paclawskyj, T. R., Smiroldo, B. B., Applegate, H. R., & Stallings, S. (1996). *Questions About Behavioral Function (QABF): An instrument to assess functional properties of problem behaviors.* Poster presented at the 22nd Annual Convention of the Association for Behavior Analysis, San Francisco, CA.

Matson, J. L., & Wilkins, J. (2009). Factors associated with the QABF for functional assessment of low rate and high rate challenging behaviors in adults with intellectual disability. *Behavior Modification, 33,* 207–219.

Murphy, G., Beadle-Brown, J., Wing, L., Gould, J., Shah, A., & Holmes, N. (2005). Chronicity of challenging behaviors in people with severe intellectual disabilities and/or autism: A total population sample. *Journal of Autism and Developmental Disorders, 35,* 405–418.

Nicholson, J., Konstantinidi, E., & Furniss, F. (2006). On some psychometric properties of the Questions About Behavior Function (QABF). *Research in Developmental Disabilities, 27,* 337–352.

O'Neill, R. E., Homer, R. H., Ablin, R. W., Sprague, J. R., Storey, K., & Newton, J. S. (1997). *Functional assessment and program development for problem behaviors: A practical handbook.* New York: Brooks/Cole.

Paclawskyj, T. R., Matson, J. L., Rush, K. S., Smalls, Y., & Vollmer, T. R. (2000). Questions about Behavioral Function (QABF): A behavioral checklist for functional assessment of aberrant behavior. *Research in Developmental Disabilities, 21,* 223–229.

Paclawskyj, T. R., Matson, J. L., Rush, K. S., Smalls, Y., & Vollmer, T. R. (2001). Assessment of the convergent validity of the Questions about Behavioral Function Scale with analogue functional analysis and the motivation assessment scale. *Journal of Intellectual Disability Research, 45,* 484–494.

Poppes, P., van der Putten, A. J. J., & Vlaskamp, C. (2010). Frequency and severity of challenging behaviour in people with profound intellectual and multiple disabilities. *Research in Developmental Disabilities, 31,* 1269–1275.

Rojahn, J., Whittaker, K., Hoch, T. A., & Gonzalez, M. L. (2007). Assessment of self-injurious and aggressive behavior. *International Review of Research in Mental Retardation, 34,* 281–319.

Sackett, G. P. (1987). Analysis of sequential social interaction data: Some issues, recent developments, and a causal inference model. In J. D. Osofsky (Ed.), *Handbook of infant development* (2nd ed., pp. 855–878). New York: Wiley.

Serper, M. R., Goldberg, B. R., Herman, K. G., Richarme, D., Chou, J., Dill, C. A., et al. (2005). Predictors of aggression on the psychiatric inpatient service. *Comprehensive Psychiatry, 46,* 121–127.

Shogren, K. A., & Rojahn, J. (2003). Convergent reliability and validity of the questions about behavioral function and the motivation assessment scale: A replication study. *Journal of Developmental and Physical Disabilities, 15,* 367–375.

Sigafoos, J., Kerr, M., & Roberts, D. (1994). Inter-rater reliability of the Motivation Assessment Scale: Failure to replicate with aggressive behavior. *Research in Developmental Disabilities, 15,* 333–342.

Singh, N. N., Donatelli, L. S., Best, A., Williams, D. E., Barrera, F. J., Lenz, M. W., et al. (1993). Factor structure of the Motivation Assessment Scale. *Journal of Intellectual Disability Research, 37,* 65–74.

Singh, N. N., Matson, J. L., Lancing, G. E., Singh, A. N., Adkins, A. D., McKeegan, G. F., et al. (2006). Questions

About Behavior Function in Mental Illness (QABF-MI): A behavior checklist for functional assessment of maladaptive behavior exhibited by individuals with mental illness. *Behavior Modification, 30,* 739–751.

Singh, A. N., Matson, J. L., Mouttapa, M., Pella, R. D., Hill, B. D., & Thorson, R. (2009). A critical item analysis of the QABF; Development of a short form assessment instrument. *Research in Developmental Disabilities, 30,* 782–792.

Sulzer-Azaroff, B., & Mayer, G. R. (1977). *Applying behavior-analysis procedures with children and youth.* New York: Holt, Rinehart, & Winston.

Tarbox, J., Wilke, A. E., Najdowski, A. C., Findel-Pyles, R. S., Balasanyan, S., Caveney, A. C., et al. (2009). Comparing indirect, descriptive, and experimental functional assessments of challenging behavior in children with autism. *Journal of Developmental and Physical Disabilities, 21,* 493–514.

Toogood, S., & Timlin, K. (1996). The functional assessment of challenging behaviour: A comparison of informant-based, experimental and descriptive methods. *Journal of Applied Research in Intellectual Disabilities, 9,* 206–222.

Touchette, P. E., MacDonald, R. F., & Langer, S. N. (1985). A scatter plot for identifying stimulus control of problem behavior. *Journal of Applied Behavior Analysis, 18,* 343–351.

Webster-Stratton, C. (1997). Early intervention for families of preschool children with conduct problems. In M. J. Guralnick (Ed.), *The effectiveness of early intervention* (pp. 429–453). Baltimore: Paul H. Brookes.

Wieseler, N. A., Hanson, R. H., Chamberlain, T. P., & Thompson, T. (1985). Functional taxonomy of stereotypic and self-injurious behavior. *Mental Retardation, 23,* 230–234.

Zarcone, J. R., Rodgers, T. A., Iwata, B. A., Rourke, D. A., & Dorsey, M. F. (1991). Reliability analysis of the Motivation Assessment Scale: A failure to replicate. *Research in Developmental Disabilities, 12,* 349–360.

Nicole M. Rodriguez, Wayne W. Fisher, and Michael E. Kelley

Treatment Methods Commonly Used in Conjunction with Functional Assessment

Treatments designed to address the function of behavior have become a hallmark of behavior analysis. To identify environmental variables maintaining problem behavior, a functional analysis is typically conducted prior to developing treatment. This process allows the clinician or researcher to understand why the problem behavior occurs such that the treatment can be tailored to address those variables (e.g., by rearranging reinforcement contingencies or addressing the motivating operation).

Environmental variables responsible for maintaining operant behavior fall into three broad categories: social-positive reinforcement, social-negative reinforcement, and automatic reinforcement. It was not until Iwata, Dorsey, Slifer, Bauman, and Richman (1982/1994) that behavioral sensitivity to reinforcers falling within each of these categories was assessed within one comprehensive functional analysis.

N.M. Rodriguez (✉) • W.W. Fisher • M.E. Kelley
Center for Autism Spectrum Disorders,
Munroe-Meyer Institute, University of Nebraska
Medical Center, 985450 Nebraska Medical Center,
Omaha, NE 68198-5450, USA
e-mail: nicole.rodriguez@unmc.edu; wfisher@unmc.edu;
michael.kelley@unmc.edu

Prior to this point, behavioral interventions more commonly involved the application of potential reinforcers and punishers generally based on reports in the literature or the clinician's experience with prior cases. In some cases, these alternative reinforcers and punishers were sufficient to override existing contingencies of reinforcement for problem behavior (Carr, Taylor, Carlson, & Robinson, 1989; Cataldo, 1989). Functional analysis has provided a means of taking into account the variables responsible for the maintenance of problem behavior when developing a treatment, and this methodology has been demonstrated to have strong predictive validity of successful treatment outcomes. Further, treatments based on the results of a functional analysis are less likely to involve punishment or contain superfluous treatment components (Pelios, Morren, Tesch, & Axelrod, 1999).

This chapter focuses on function-based treatments for challenging behavior such as self-injurious behavior (SIB), aggression, or disruptive behavior. Because procedures may vary depending on the function of behavior, treatments for social-positive reinforcement, social-negative reinforcement, and automatic reinforcement are discussed separately. When discussing reinforcement-based procedures, we refer to the use of the functional reinforcer identified via a functional analysis. We refer the reader to Chap. 7 in this book for a discussion of how to identify the function of behavior.

Operant Mechanisms of Reinforcement Contingencies

Iwata and colleagues (Iwata, Pace, Cowdery, & Miltenberger, 1994; Iwata, Pace, & Dorsey et al., 1994) described three operant mechanisms related to the function of problem behavior—reinforcer, motivating operation, and discriminative stimulus. Because of their relevance to the arrangement of the conditions of a functional analysis and the development of function-based treatments, we will review the components of a reinforcement contingency briefly here.

One functional component of a reinforcement contingency is the reinforcing consequence delivered after emission of the target response. A reinforcer is defined by the effect it has on behavior; when applied contingent on a response class, the probability of responses that belong to that class occurring again in the future increases (Catania, 1992). The reinforcer can either involve the presentation of an appetitive event (positive reinforcement) or the prevention or termination of an aversive event (negative reinforcement).[1] In addition, the reinforcer can be social in that its delivery is mediated by another person or automatic in that the behavior directly produces the reinforcer (e.g., rubbing one's own temple to alleviate a headache; scratching an itch). An understanding of the reinforcers responsible for the maintenance of behavior is integral for developing function-based treatments. In fact, several studies have shown that in many cases it may be necessary to disrupt the response-reinforcer relation (i.e., extinction) to ensure successful treatment outcomes (e.g., Iwata, Pace, & Cowdery et al., 1994; Mazaleski, Iwata,

Vollmer, Zarcone, & Smith, 1993; Shirley, Iwata, Kahng, Mazaleski, & Lerman, 1997; Zarcone, Iwata, Hughes, & Vollmer, 1993).

A second functional component of a reinforcement contingency is its motivating operation. A motivating operation is an environmental variable that alters the efficacy of a reinforcer as well as the current frequency of all behavior under control of that reinforcer (Laraway, Snycerski, Michael, & Poling, 2003). In social-positive reinforcement contingencies, periods of time without access to the reinforcer (e.g., caregiver attention and preferred materials) *establish* or increase the value of the reinforcer, whereas periods of time with access to the reinforcer *abolish* or decrease the value of the reinforcer. In social-negative reinforcement contingencies, the presentation of the aversive stimulus (e.g., academic tasks and medical procedures) establishes or increases the value of avoidance or escape (the reinforcer), whereas the absence of the aversive stimuli abolishes or decreases the value of avoidance or escape. Other variables, such as the delivery of appetitive stimuli (e.g., time-based delivery of highly preferred edibles) during aversive events can also serve to reduce the aversive nature of an event and abolish the effectiveness of escape as a reinforcer (Lomas, Fisher, & Kelley, 2010). An understanding of how motivating operations influence the probability of a target response facilitates the use and manipulation of those motivating operations during treatment of problem behavior. In fact, one of the advantages of reinforcement-based procedures (e.g., differential reinforcement of alternative behavior [DRA], differential reinforcement of other behavior [DRO], noncontingent reinforcement [NCR]) is that the functional reinforcer continues to be available, which can serve to reduce the establishing operation for problem behavior.

A third functional component of a reinforcement contingency is its discriminative stimulus. A discriminative stimulus is an antecedent stimulus whose presence signals the availability of a particular reinforcer. A discriminative stimulus enters a reinforcement contingency through repeated exposure to a functional stimulus–behavior–consequence relation, which can vary depending on an individual's history of

---

[1] Whereas some researchers have proposed that the distinction between positive and negative reinforcement should be abandoned on account that the distinction is ambiguous and without functional significance (e.g. Baron & Galizio, 2005; Michael, 1975), others argue that the distinction is both useful and sufficiently engrained in our terminology (e.g., Iwata, 2006; Lattal & Lattal, 2006; Sidman, 2006). We maintain the distinction here to describe whether the stimulus change involved the introduction or withdrawal of a stimulus following the target behavior and stress the importance of describing and analyzing both sides of the stimulus change, including the relevant motivating operations and discriminative stimuli.

reinforcement. For example, under naturally occurring conditions, it is possible for a reinforcement history to develop in which the presence of a child's mother but not the father may signal the availability of physical attention (e.g., hugging and rocking the child) following SIB if the mother frequently delivered this consequence for SIB in the past and the father did not. In a functional analysis, discriminative stimuli help to signal the consequence that is available within each condition. Such discriminative stimuli can be naturalistic like the presence of academic materials signaling the availability of escape for SIB, contrived like different colored t-shirts or poster boards being associated with different conditions, or both. Conners et al. (2000) demonstrated that associating salient discriminative stimuli with each condition of the functional analysis can reduce carry-over effects between conditions, thereby improving the efficiency or clarity of a functional analysis.

An understanding of the relation between a target response and these three operant mechanisms is important not only for understanding the principles that underlie a functional analysis but also for developing effective function-based interventions for problem behaviors. That is, function-based treatments for problem behavior generally involve manipulation of one or more of these mechanisms (i.e., the consequence for problem behavior, the motivating operation that establishes the effectiveness of that consequence as a reinforcer for problem behavior, and/or the discriminative stimulus that signals that problem behavior will produce that reinforcer). When developing function-based treatments, a fruitful place to start is to ask a series of questions related to these three components: (1) How can the reinforcing consequence maintaining problem behavior be altered to decrease problem behavior and increase appropriate behavior? (2) How can the relevant motivating operation be altered to decrease the probability of problem behavior? and (3) How can discriminative stimuli be arranged to signal changes in the availability of reinforcement for appropriate behavior and the continued unavailability of reinforcement for problem behavior?

The relevance of the three operant mechanisms of reinforcement contingencies to the development of function-based treatments will be discussed further in the remainder of this chapter.

Functioned-Based Treatments for Behavior Maintained by Social-Positive Reinforcement

A wide variety of problem behavior (e.g., SIB, aggression, property destruction, elopement, and pica) has been shown to be maintained by social-positive reinforcement. For example, in their review of 152 single-subject functional analyses, Iwata, Pace, & Dorsey, et al. (1994) found that the SIB of 26.3% (40) of the participants included in their analysis was maintained by social-positive reinforcement. Examples of potential social-positive reinforcers that may be responsible for the maintenance of problem behavior include caregiver attention such as verbal reprimands, physical consoling (e.g., rubbing back), physical restraint or access to preferred items such as food, toys, or TV.

Extinction

When contingencies are arranged such that problem behavior no longer produces reinforcement, extinction is in effect. For social-positive contingencies, this involves withholding delivery of the reinforcer following problem behavior (e.g., Fisher et al., 1993). For example, if problem behavior is maintained by caregiver attention, then extinction would involve assuring that attention is no longer provided contingent on the undesirable behavior (i.e., planned ignoring; Iwata, Pace, & Cowdery et al., 1994).

As previously noted, results of several studies (e.g., Mazaleski et al., 1993; Shirley et al., 1997) suggest that extinction is an integral component of successful treatment packages. That is, problem behavior may not decrease if it continues to produce reinforcement, even if the functional reinforcer is also provided contingent on, for example, an appropriate alternative response. For this reason, extinction is commonly included as at least one component of a larger treatment package (e.g., functional communication training [FCT] plus extinction).

Despite the role extinction plays in ensuring successful treatment outcomes, however, extinction is rarely prescribed in isolation. This recommendation is due in large part to the negative side effects sometimes associated with extinction (e.g., extinction bursts, aggression, or emotional behavior) as well as the dangers associated with implementing extinction at less than perfect integrity (thereby producing an intermittent schedule of reinforcement that strengthens the behavior). Ensuring the continued availability of the functional reinforcer but independent of problem behavior is thought to attenuate some of the negative side effects associated with extinction (Lerman & Iwata, 1995; Vollmer, Iwata, Zarcone, Smith, & Mazaleski, 1993; Vollmer et al., 1998). Combining extinction with reinforcement-based procedures allows for both the response–reinforcer relation and the motivating operation to be addressed.

Functional Communication Training

FCT, a form of DRA, is one of the most commonly used function-based treatments for problem behavior (Tiger, Hanley, & Bruzek, 2008). In FCT, the reinforcer found to maintain problem behavior is provided contingent on an alternative communicative response. If problem behavior is found to be maintained by access to preferred materials, then FCT would involve teaching the individual an appropriate means of obtaining that reinforcer (e.g., handing over a card that says, "snack, please."). The aim is to teach and reinforce an alternate means of obtaining the functional reinforcer. This allows the individual control over when the reinforcer is obtained, which may also serve to reduce the motivating operation that evokes problem behavior. However, because contact with the new reinforcement contingency (i.e., reinforcement for the functional communication response) may not be sufficient to shift responding from problem behavior to appropriate behavior, extinction is often used during FCT to assure that problem behavior no longer produces reinforcement.

Based on their review of the literature on FCT, Tiger et al. (2008) provided several guidelines for selecting and teaching a functional communication response. Because individuals with developmental disabilities may have limited verbal repertoires, the target topography of the communicative response may include any one of a variety of modalities such as vocal responses, picture exchanges, sign language or gestures, or use of voice or text output devices. Tiger et al. identified three areas for consideration when selecting the topography of the communicative response: (a) the effort associated with emitting the response should be less than that of emitting problem behavior (Horner & Day, 1991), (b) the response should be easily recognizable by others, including adults that are not familiar with the individual's behavioral treatment (to increase the likelihood that novel individuals will provide reinforcement contingent on the response; Durand, 1999; Durand & Carr, 1992), and (c) the response should be simple enough (based on the individual's current repertoire) to be acquired quickly. For example, for children with limited vocal repertoires (e.g., who can speak in one- to two-word sentences), teaching the vocal response, "play" would be more appropriate than, "play with me please." In general, vocal responses may be better than nonvocal responses as they are more likely to recruit reinforcement from others but would not be ideal if the response was not recognizable (e.g., due to poor enunciation). In this case or in the case of an individual who does not speak, exchanging a card (e.g., that has a picture of two people playing and/or that has the words "please play with me" written on it) may be appropriate as it is simple and easily recognizable by others.

Despite the fact that FCT is one of the most researched function-based treatments, few studies have provided clear, replicable procedural details for the training of a functional communication response (e.g., Carr & Durand, 1985; Fisher et al., 1993; Shirley et al., 1997; Wacker et al., 1990). There are two general strategies that have been reported: graduated prompts (e.g., most-to-least prompts, least-to-most promps) and time-delay prompts. In most-to-least prompting procedures, a physical or vocal prompt to engage in the target communicative response is provided immediately upon the removal of the reinforcer and then gradually faded in intensity (e.g., after a number of trials involving full physical guidance, the therapist might guide the individual' hand such that it is hovering over the card). Prompted responses are reinforced to ensure contact with the contingencies and to prevent exposure to deprivation from the functional reinforcer (e.g., attention), which helps to decrease the probability of evoking problem behavior during training. The intensity of the prompt is faded, generally according to some predetermined criteria (e.g., two consecutive sessions without problem behavior) until the response is being emitted consistently in the absence of any prompts. With least-to-most prompting, the therapist proceeds from the least intense to the most intense prompt sequentially within each trial (e.g., progressing from vocal, model, to physical prompts, as necessary).

In time-delay prompting procedures, the relevant establishing operation is provided (e.g., attention is removed or a demand is presented) and then the individual is provided with a short period of time (e.g., 1 s) to respond before being vocally or physically prompted to engage in the communicative response. The period of time before the prompt is delivered is gradually extended (e.g., in 1-s intervals) to transfer control from the therapist's prompt to the evocative event. Regardless of the strategy used to train the response, reinforcement should be delivered immediately and following each occurrence of the communicative response (i.e., an FR 1 schedule; Horner & Day, 1991). We refer the reader to Tiger et al. (2008) for additional guidelines for developing FCT interventions.

One criticism of FCT as a treatment for problem behavior is that the communicative response often requires an FR 1 schedule of reinforcement to assure that problem behavior decreases to near-zero levels of responding. However, it is often impractical or even impossible for caregivers to maintain such a dense schedule of reinforcement in the natural environment (Fisher et al., 1993). One approach to addressing this issue is to bring the functional communicative response under stimulus control such that it occurs at times when

reinforcement is available and does not occur at times when reinforcement is not available (Fisher, Kuhn, & Thompson, 1998; Hanley, Iwata, & Thompson, 2001). The use of schedule-correlated stimuli (multiple schedules) can help ensure that the communicative response is not weakened via extinction during those periods in which reinforcement is not available. To teach discriminate responding, the individual is typically provided with repeated exposure to the schedule-correlated stimuli (e.g., different-colored cards for reinforcement and extinction periods) and the respective contingencies operating when those stimuli are present. Hanley et al. (2001) began with brief periods of extinction (S−) and then gradually increased the length of the time that the S− was present and decreased the length of the time the S+ (indicating reinforcement was available) was present. When the communicative response involves a picture exchange card system, restricting access to the picture card may serve as a practical approach to reinforcer-schedule thinning (Roane, Fisher, Sgro, Falcomata, & Pabico, 2004). In addition to the absence of the FCT, card serving as a discriminative stimulus that signals the unavailability of reinforcement, restricting access to the materials necessary to emit the response makes it impossible for the individual to emit the response at times when it will not produce reinforcement (e.g., when the parent is occupied changing the diaper of an infant sibling).

Differential Reinforcement of Other Behavior

Reinforcement can also be provided contingent on the nonoccurrence of the problem behavior (DRO). This can involve programming the delivery of the reinforcer based on the absence of problem behavior either (a) throughout the duration of the DRO interval (e.g., 30 s; whole-interval DRO; see Repp, Barton, & Brulle, 1983) or (b) during a brief momentary observation at the end of the DRO interval (momentary DRO; Lindberg, Iwata, Kahng, & DeLeon, 1999). This latter procedure serves as a practical alternative to whole-interval DRO schedules as it requires considerably less vigilance on the part of the observer.

Varying the interval lengths of momentary DRO schedules may be important for obscuring the potential discrimination of the point in time at which the individual is being observed (Lindberg, Iwata, & Kahng, et al., 1999). If the end of the DRO interval is signaled (e.g., a timer beeps) or predictable (e.g., occurs at fixed intervals), then it is possible for the individual to engage in inappropriate behavior throughout the remainder of the interval and still receive the reinforcer. Lindberg, Iwata, Kahng, et al. suggested that the predictability of the observation period in momentary DRO schedules when the intervals are fixed may have contributed to the ineffectiveness of such schedules in previous studies comparing whole-interval and momentary DRO schedules (e.g., Repp et al., 1983; cf., Derwas & Jones, 1993).

Another important consideration for DRO schedules is the length of the interval (or in the case of variable schedules, the *average* length of the interval). The interval length should be short enough to prevent periods of deprivation due to low rates of reinforcement. This is particularly important for whole-interval schedules in which the criteria for reinforcement is much more stringent (one instance of problem behavior resets the DRO interval). Based on a formula described by Poling and Ryan (1982), Vollmer et al. (1993) used the mean interresponse time from the prior n sessions as the DRO interval. The interval length increased based on decreases in SIB, but if performance worsened (SIB increased) the interval length was never shortened. In this way, the interval length was gradually extended such that longer periods of time without problem behavior were required for reinforcement to be delivered. Similar procedures for selecting and modifying the DRO interval length were used for other procedural variations of DRO schedules (including the variable-momentary DRO schedule) in Lindberg, Iwata, & Kahng, et al., 1999.

Response-Independent Delivery of Positive Reinforcement

Another reinforcement-based approach to the treatment of problem behavior is to deliver reinforcement independent of all behavior, on a time-based schedule (Fisher, DeLeon, Rodriguez-Catter, & Keeney, 2004; Vollmer et al., 1993). This approach is commonly referred to as NCR.[2] For behavior maintained by attention, this could involve providing a brief form of attention such as verbal praise every 10 s or more extended forms of attention wherein attention is provided continuously within a play context (e.g., 15 min of play).

Kahng, Iwata, Thompson, and Hanley (2000) noted that reductions in problem behavior during NCR can be attributed either to a reduction in the establishing operation for problem behavior or the disruption of the response–reinforcer contingency. The large and immediate reduction in problem behavior commonly observed when reinforcement is delivered on a dense schedule or in large magnitudes (e.g., Hagopian, Fisher, & Legacy, 1994; Roscoe, Iwata, & Rand, 2003) suggests that the effects of NCR are largely attributable to a reduction in the establishing operation for problem behavior. This pattern of responding is in contrast to that observed when extinction is implemented in isolation (e.g., Fisher et al., 2004).

One way to assure that the establishing operation for problem behavior has been eliminated or reduced is to provide reinforcement continuously (Vollmer et al., 1993). Alternatively, the schedule of reinforcement can be based on either the mean latency to the first instance of problem behavior during baseline (Lalli, Casey, & Kates, 1997) or the mean interresponse time of problem behavior during baseline (Kahng et al., 2000). In such cases, it is recommended that the density of the reinforcement schedule be accommodated to prevent the development of adventitious reinforcement by making it either noticeably more or less dense

---

[2]The term, NCR, has been criticized because the intended (and often observed) effect is the weakening of the target response; yet, reinforcement is defined as an increase in responding to the contingent delivery of a reinforcer (Poling & Normand, 1999). The term, fixed-time (FT) schedule, has been offered as an alternative but this label does not acknowledge the previous functional relation between the target response and the stimulus delivered on the time-based schedule. We use the term NCR in this chapter to maintain contact with the relevant applied literature.

than the mean interresponse time. Alternatively, a DRO contingency could be added to the NCR schedule in which the delivery of a scheduled reinforcer in the NCR schedule would be delayed (e.g., by 5 s), if problem behavior occurs immediately prior to the scheduled delivery (e.g., Britton, Carr, Kellum, Dozier, & Weil, 2000).

To increase the practicality of NCR schedules, the density of the reinforcement schedule can be gradually thinned (Hagopian et al., 1994). Alternatively, it has been shown that the availability of other, albeit nonfunctional, reinforcers such as toys can increase function-based treatments for behavior maintained by attention, if the items that are made available compete with the attention provided by caregivers (e.g., Hanley, Piazza, & Fisher, 1997). A competing items assessment (described below under treatments for automatically maintained problem behavior; Piazza et al., 1998) can be adapted to identify items likely to compete with problem behavior maintained by attention or other social contingencies (Fisher, O'Connor, Kurtz, DeLeon, & Gotjen, 2000).

Functioned-Based Treatments for Behavior Maintained by Social-Negative Reinforcement

Social-negative reinforcement, particularly escape from demands, is one of the most common maintaining variables for problem behavior. In fact, Iwata, Pace, Dorsey et al. (1994) found that the SIB of 38.1% (58) of the 152 participants in their analysis was maintained by social-negative reinforcement. Social-negative reinforcement can take the form of avoidance or escape from academic demands, medical procedures (Iwata, Pace, Kalsher, Cowdery, & Cataldo, 1990), noise (McCord, Iwata, Galensky, Ellingson, & Thomson, 2001), or social interaction (Hall, DeBernardis, & Reiss, 2006).

Extinction

To assure that the response–reinforcer relation is disrupted in social-negative contingencies, contingencies must be rearranged such that problem behavior no longer results in the prevention or termination of the aversive stimulus or event. To assure the continued presentation of the stimulus, researchers have used instructional sequences such as three-step guided compliance (e.g., Iwata et al., 1990). This procedure involves a series of three types of prompts: verbal, gestural/model, and physical prompt (hand-over-hand guidance), in which the child is provided with approximately 5 s between each prompt to comply before the therapist moves onto the next prompt in the three-step series. If the child complies with the demand following the verbal or gestural/model prompt, verbal praise (e.g., "Nice job!" or "That's right!") is delivered. If problem behavior occurs at any point throughout the three-step sequence, the clinician or researcher either immediately physically guides the correct response (e.g., Iwata et al., 1990) or continues the three-step sequence (e.g., Kuhn, DeLeon, Fisher, & Wilke, 1999). When physical guidance is impossible or near impossible (e.g., due to the size of the individual), a partial physical prompt followed by the representation of the demand may be sufficient to produce an escape extinction effect. Although procedural variations in escape extinction are commonly implemented in clinical practice, additional research is needed on the conditions under which such procedural variations would or would not be effective. Finally, because escape extinction may be difficult to implement (e.g., physical guidance with large, strong clients), it may be necessary to explore other function-based treatments that can be used either in conjunction with or in place of escape extinction.

Differential Negative Reinforcement of Alternative Behavior (DNRA)

Functional Communication Training
FCT for social-negative reinforcement involves training and reinforcing a communicative response that results in breaks from (e.g., Horner & Day, 1991) or assistance with (e.g., Carr & Durand, 1985) nonpreferred or aversive stimuli or tasks (e.g., academic demands). Examples of communicative responses include teaching the individual to say, "Break, please" to receive a

break from the task or "I don't understand" to receive assistance with a task. Other modalities such as sign language, gestures, or the handing over of a picture card with picture and/or textual stimuli depicting the reinforcer can also be used as the communicative response. As previously noted, FCT is commonly combined with extinction (e.g., Durand & Merges, 2001) or punishment (e.g., Hanley, Piazza, Fisher, & Maglieri, 2005) to ensure successful treatment outcomes.

One limitation of FCT for behavior maintained by escape is that the individual can, and usually does, emit the communicative response frequently enough to escape all or almost all the instructional demands. In such circumstances, the individual is not learning or benefiting from the instruction (Fisher et al., 1993). Instructional fading (also known as demand or stimulus fading) involves gradually increasing the number of demands presented per session, and it is one approach that can be used to assure the continued presentation of instructional demands (Pace, Iwata, Cowdery, Andree, & McIntyre, 1993). One of the advantages of instructional fading is that it may increase tolerance of instructional tasks (e.g., through processes akin to that of systematic desensitization).

Differential Reinforcement of Compliance
Another approach to decreasing problem behavior while assuring the continued presentation of academic demands is to provide escape contingent on compliance (e.g., Marcus & Vollmer, 1995; Vollmer, Roane, Ringdahl, & Marcus, 1999). Differential reinforcement of compliance can result in concomitant decreases in problem behavior, even when the consequences for problem behavior remain unchanged (Parrish, Cataldo, Kolko, Neef, & Egel, 1986; Russo, Cataldo, & Cushing, 1981). Similarly, escape extinction can result in concomitant increases in compliance. As suggested by Cataldo and colleagues, it is possible that such indirect effects of treatments are observed when compliance and problem behavior are inverse members of an overarching response class call "instruction following."

Another approach to treating problem behavior maintained by escape is to deliver positive reinforcement (e.g., a highly preferred edible) for compliance. Positive reinforcement for compliance has been shown to be effective even when problem behavior continues to result in escape (e.g., DeLeon, Neidert, Anders, & Rodriguez-Catter, 2001; Kodak, Lerman, Volkert, & Trosclair, 2007; Lalli et al., 1999). Lalli et al. suggested two operant mechanisms that may explain the efficacy of differential positive reinforcement of compliance in treating behavior maintained by negative reinforcement: (a) that the relative value of the positive reinforcer is greater than that of escape (DeLeon et al., 2001) and/or (b) that the availability of the positive reinforcer serves as an abolishing operation that lessens the aversive properties of the demand context. Two recent studies have provided strong support for this latter hypothesized mechanism by demonstrating that the provision of positive reinforcers (i.e., food plus praise), either on a time-based schedule or contingent on compliance, can produce marked reductions in problem behavior reinforced by escape even when the escape contingency remains in effect (Lomas et al., 2010; Lomas, Fisher, Kelley, & Fredrick, in press).

Differential Negative Reinforcement of Other Behavior

Differential negative reinforcement of other behavior (DNRO) involves providing escape contingent on zero levels of responding throughout the DNRO interval (Buckley & Newchok, 2006; Vollmer & Iwata, 1992). Because the timing of reinforcement in DNRO schedules is under control of the clinician or researcher, DNRO may be particularly useful when it is important for the clinician or researcher to maintain control over *when* ongoing activities are disrupted (e.g., during medical procedures). DNRO also involves the continued presentation of the aversive stimulus, which may produce habituation and make their subsequent presentation less aversive.

Response-Independent Delivery of Negative Reinforcement

Like positive reinforcers, escape can be delivered independent of problem behavior, on a time-based schedule (Kodak, Miltenberger, & Romanuik, 2003; Vollmer, Marcus, & Ringdahl, 1995). This procedure has also been referred to as noncontingent escape (NCE). The delivery of escape on a dense fixed-time schedule can produce immediate and large reductions in problem behavior, after which the schedule can be leaned (e.g., from 10 s to 2.5 or 10 min; Vollmer et al., 1995). Further, there is some evidence to suggest that NCE may be effective even when problem behavior continues to result in escape (e.g., Lalli et al., 1997), which is important when escape extinction cannot be implemented with perfect procedural integrity (e.g., the individual is large and difficult to physically guide).

An alternative method of addressing the motivating operation is to identify the specific features of a demand context that makes it aversive and then to modify procedures in ways that lessen those aversive properties. Examples of properties of demand contexts that have been found to establish the efficacy of escape as reinforcement for problem behavior include the inclusion of difficult (Weeks & Gaylord-Ross, 1981), less preferred (Dunlap, Kern-Dunlap, Clarke, & Robbins, 1991), or novel tasks (Mace, Browder, & Lin, 1987; Smith, Iwata, Goh, & Shore, 1995). The duration of an instructional session, the rate of instructions, massed trials, certain prompting strategies, and the cancelation of a planned and preferred activity prior to the instructional session have also been shown to function as motivating operations for escape (Dunlap et al., 1991; Horner, Day, & Day, 1997; Munk & Repp, 1994; Smith et al., 1995). To abolish or lessen the value of escape as reinforcement for problem behavior, researchers have used strategies such as interspersing less aversive tasks (Ebanks & Fisher, 2003; Horner, Day, Sprague, O'Brien, & Heathfield, 1991), gradually increasing the rate or aversiveness of tasks (Pace, Ivancic, & Jefferson, 1994; Pace et al., 1993), and providing choices regarding the order or timing in which tasks are completed (Dyer, Dunlap, & Winterling, 1990).

Functioned-Based Treatments for Behavior Maintained by Automatic Reinforcement

A third potential source of reinforcement for problem behavior has been referred to as automatic reinforcement because the reinforcing consequence is one that is a direct or "automatic" result of the target response (Skinner, 1953; Vaughn & Michael, 1982; Vollmer, 1994). Because the direct consequences of automatically maintained behavior are often difficult to manipulate, automatic reinforcement is inferred in a functional analysis based on the persistence of behavior in the absence of social contingencies (e.g., when the individual is alone). The overwhelming majority of the literature on the assessment and treatment of stereotypy suggests that most stereotypy is maintained by automatic reinforcement (Rapp & Vollmer, 2005). Potential examples of behavior maintained by automatic reinforcement include body rocking that persists due to favorable kinesthetic sensations, or the repeated waving of colorful objects in front of the eyes that persists due to favorable visual sensations.

Extinction

One approach to decreasing automatically maintained problem behavior is to disrupt or attenuate the response–reinforcer relation (also referred to as sensory extinction, e.g., Kuhn et al., 1999; Rincover, Cook, Peoples, & Packard, 1979). Perhaps the most common method for doing so is to block the response from occurring.[3] For example, if self-injury in the form of eye poking is found to be maintained by automatic reinforcement, then one might program extinction by

---

[3] In some cases, the effects of response blocking on problem behavior may be more appropriately attributed to the effects of punishment. We refer the reader to Lerman and Iwata (1996) for an example of a procedure that can be used to identify the processes (automatic extinction versus punishment) responsible for decreased responding when response blocking is applied contingent on problem behavior.

having someone physically block the individual's finger from making contact with his or her eye (e.g., by placing their hand between the individual's hand and eye). Sensory extinction could also take different forms such as having the individual wear eye goggles for eye poking (Kennedy & Souza, 1995), gloves for hand mouthing or self-scratching (Reid, Parsons, Phillips, & Green, 1993; Roscoe, Iwata, & Goh, 1998), or a protective helmet for head hitting (Silverman, Watanabe, Marshall, & Baer, 1984). If, for example, eye poking was maintained by the visual-like sensations it produces, then eye goggles, which prevent the finger from making contact with the eye, would assure that this behavior no longer contacts this form of automatic reinforcement.

In one of the first applications of function-based procedures for automatically reinforced behavior, Rincover et al. (1979) demonstrated the application of sensory extinction and matched stimuli to the assessment and treatment of automatically reinforced problem behavior. Based on teacher interviews and casual observations, Rincover et al. developed hypotheses as to the sensory consequences maintaining each of four participants' problem behavior (object spinning, hand flapping, hand waving, or finger flapping). In the first phase, sensory extinction was applied in a reversal design to isolate the specific source of sensory stimulation. For example, during casual observations, one participant appeared to be listening to the noise produced by a plate spinning. Assuming that auditory stimulation was the reinforcing consequence for object spinning, sensory extinction for this participant was introduced by installing carpet on top of the table, which markedly reduced the volume and quality of the sound produced by object spinning. Sensory extinction decreased levels of problem behavior across all participants, suggesting that the specific source of automatic reinforcement had been identified. Rather than using sensory extinction as the treatment for the problem behavior exhibited by the individuals in their study, Rincover et al. went on to assess the effects of providing noncontingent access to matched stimuli (described below), perhaps due to the practical limitations of using some of their sensory

extinction procedures as a treatment (e.g., extinction for two participants involved limiting the putative visual stimulation by either dimming overhead lights or applying a blindfold).

One potential limitation of sensory extinction procedures that involve innovative manipulations such as the ones described above is that the clinician must first identify the *specific* source of automatic reinforcement, which is often difficult. In contrast, response blocking or interruption (which prevents the completion of the problem behavior) is often sufficient to disrupt the response–reinforcer relation regardless of the specific source of automatic reinforcement. On the other hand, one disadvantage of response blocking is that it often requires constant monitoring to assure that the individual's behavior does not contact the automatic reinforcer on an intermittent reinforcement schedule. If eye-poking is maintained by the visual stimulation it produces, the ability to use goggles to prevent access to this reinforcer (and thereby increase this potentially dangerous form of SIB) serves as a practical alternative to response blocking because the former procedure requires much less monitoring of the individual's behavior than does the latter procedure.

Response-Independent Delivery of Alternate Sources of Automatic Reinforcement

An alternate approach commonly used to treat behavior maintained by automatic reinforcement is to provide alternate sources of stimulation that compete with or substitute for the automatic reinforcer for problem behavior (e.g., Goh et al., 1995; Piazza, Adelinis, Hanley, Goh, & Delia, 2000; Piazza et al., 1998; Rincover et al., 1979; Roscoe et al., 1998; Shore, Iwata, DeLeon, Kahng, & Smith, 1997; Wilder, Draper, Williams, & Higbee, 1997). This approach to intervention has also been referred to as an enriched environment (e.g., Horner, 1980; Vollmer, Marcus, & LeBlanc, 1994).

In the second phase of Rincover et al. (1979), stimuli matching the sensory consequences produced by problem behavior were provided noncontingently and continuously and compared to unmatched stimuli (recall that the specific source of automatic reinforcement was identified through the systematic application of sensory extinction in the first phases of their study). When matched and unmatched stimuli were concurrently available, all participants (a) exclusively or primarily engaged with matched stimuli and (b) engaged in zero or near-zero levels of problem behavior. These results demonstrated that providing access to matched stimuli may produce both an increase in item engagement and a decrease in problem behavior.

Piazza and colleagues presented an alternate method for empirically deriving potentially substitutable or competing stimuli (e.g., Piazza et al., 1998, 2000). Prior to assessing the relative effects of matched versus unmatched stimuli, Piazza et al. conducted a preference assessment to determine stimuli associated with high levels of item engagement and low levels of problem behavior. Stimuli included in the competing-stimulus assessment were selected based on the topography of the behavior (climbing, saliva play, and hand mouthing), observations, and experimenters' hypotheses with respect to the source of automatic reinforcement. For example, for the participant who engaged in dangerous behavior such as climbing on furniture and jumping out of windows, stimuli hypothesized to match the putative automatic reinforcer—kinesthetic stimulation from jumping or bouncing—included a green bouncy ball, an air mattress for bouncing, and a balance board. The preference assessment served as a basis from which to identify stimuli likely to substitute for, or compete with, the automatic reinforcement produced by problem behavior. In addition, Piazza et al. demonstrated that providing access to stimuli hypothesized to match the automatic reinforcement was generally more effective than unmatched stimuli in reducing automatically reinforced problem behavior. However, it should be noted that there are studies that suggest that simply providing access to alternate activities (regardless of whether they are matched) may be sufficient to compete with the reinforcer maintaining problem behavior (Ahearn,

Clark, DeBar, & Florentino, 2005; Vollmer et al., 1994), particularly if the problem behavior primarily occurs when little to no alternate sources of stimulation are available (e.g., an austere institutional environment). For example, Vollmer et al. demonstrated that the use of highly preferred toys or leisure items identified via a paired-choice preference assessment (Fisher et al., 1992) was sufficient to reduce problem behavior, and Ahearn et al. showed that unmatched but highly preferred stimuli were more effective than matched stimuli at producing desirable treatment outcomes.

One of the advantages of providing access to alternate sources of stimulation as treatment for automatically maintained problem behavior is that it provides an opportunity to engage in an appropriate alternative response. However, simply providing access to alternate stimuli may not be sufficient to decrease automatically maintained problem behavior or increase item engagement (Lindberg, Iwata, & Kahng, 1999; e.g., Hanley, Iwata, Thompson, & Lindberg, 2000; Piazza et al., 1998). In such cases, additional strategies such as prompts, response blocking, or reinforcement may be necessary to increase contact with the alternate source of stimulation or prevent access to the stimulation produced by problem behavior.

Differential Reinforcement of Alternative Behavior

Several researchers have shown that access to the opportunity to engage in automatically reinforcing problem behavior (e.g., stereotypy) can be used to increase an alternative response such as appropriate engagement with leisure items or correct responding on academic or prevocational tasks (e.g., Charlop, Kurtz, & Casey, 1990; Charlop-Christy & Haymes, 1996; Hanley et al., 2000; Sugai & White, 1986; Wolery, Kirk, & Gast, 1985). DRA for automatically maintained problem behavior may be desirable, if it is socially acceptable to allow some of the problem behavior to occur (e.g., the target behavior is considered a problem because it occurs at times that interfere with other activities such as work). It should be noted, however, that to arrange problem behavior as a reinforcer other strategies such as response blocking will likely be needed to prevent access to the problem behavior when the contingency for reinforcement has not yet been met.

As an example of the application of contingent access to automatically maintained problem behavior as a reinforcer for alternate behavior, Hanley et al. (2000) measured the additive effects of several treatment components on the effects of the automatically maintained problem behavior (e.g., skin pressing and hand mouthing) and item engagement of three individuals with developmental disabilities. The treatment components that were evaluated were: (a) continuous access to alternate stimulation, (b) prompts to engage with materials, (c) response blocking, and (d) access to stereotypy as reinforcement for item engagement. Prompts to engage with materials were insufficient for decreasing problem behavior or increasing the appropriate alternative for all three participants. When response blocking was added to prompts, stereotypy decreased for all three participants and appropriate item engagement increased for two participants. The addition of contingent access to stereotypy was necessary to increase appropriate item engagement for the third participant.

Concluding Remarks

The process of identifying a treatment based on the results of a functional analysis has been associated with a number of advantages, including increasing the likelihood that the treatment will produce rapid and clinically significant reductions in problem behavior. By identifying the variables that maintain problem behavior, clinicians and researchers can manipulate those variables to shift responding from problem behavior to appropriate behavior. Function-based interventions tend to be more efficient because the results of the functional analysis direct the behavior analyst to focus on a small number of environmental variables that have a large influence on problem behavior, and thus function-based treatments are generally free of superfluous intervention components. Finally, research has shown that interventions based on a

prior functional analysis tend to be more effective and less likely to include a punishment component than ones not based on a functional analysis.

References

Ahearn, W. H., Clark, K. M., DeBar, R., & Florentino, C. (2005). On the role of preference in response competition. *Journal of Applied Behavior Analysis, 38,* 247–250.

Baron, A., & Galizio, M. (2005). Positive and negative reinforcement: Should the distinction be preserved? *The Behavior Analyst, 28,* 85–98.

Britton, L. N., Carr, J. E., Kellum, K. K., Dozier, C. L., & Weil, T. M. (2000). A variation of noncontingent reinforcement in the treatment of aberrant behavior. *Research in Developmental Disabilities, 21,* 425–435.

Buckley, S. D., & Newchok, D. K. (2006). Analysis and treatment of problem behavior evoked by music. *Journal of Applied Behavior Analysis, 39,* 141–144.

Carr, E. G., & Durand, V. M. (1985). Reducing behavior problems through functional communication training. *Journal of Applied Behavior Analysis, 18,* 111–126.

Carr, E. G., Taylor, J. C., Carlson, J. I., & Robinson, S. (1989). *Reinforcement and stimulus-based treatments for severe behavior problems in developmental disabilities.* Background paper prepared for the National Institutes of Health Consensus Development Panel on the Treatment of Destructive Behavior. Bethesda, MD: National Institutes of Health.

Cataldo, M. F. (1989). *The effects of punishment and other behavior reducing procedures on the destructive behaviors of persons with developmental disabilities.* Background paper prepared for the National Institutes of Health Consensus Development Panel on the Treatment of Destructive Behavior. Bethesda, MD: National Institutes of Health.

Catania, A. C. (1992). *Learning.* Englewood Cliffs: Prentice Hall.

Charlop-Christy, M. H., & Haymes, L. K. (1996). Using obsessions as reinforcers with and without mild reductive procedures to decrease inappropriate behaviors of children with autism. *Journal of Autism and Developmental Disorders, 26,* 527–546.

Charlop, M. H., Kurtz, P. F., & Casey, F. G. (1990). Using aberrant behaviors as reinforcers for autistic children. *Journal of Applied Behavior Analysis, 23,* 163–181.

Conners, J., Iwata, B. A., Kahng, S. W., Hanley, G. P., Worsdell, A. S., & Thompson, R. H. (2000). Differential responding in the presence and absence of discriminative stimuli during multielement functional analyses. *Journal of Applied Behavior Analysis, 33,* 299–308.

DeLeon, I. G., Neidert, P. L., Anders, B. M., & Rodriguez-Catter, V. (2001). Choices between positive and negative reinforcement during treatment for escape-maintained behavior. *Journal of Applied Behavior Analysis, 34,* 521–525.

Derwas, H., & Jones, R. S. P. (1993). Reducing stereotyped behavior using momentary DRO: An experimental analysis. *Behavioral Interventions, 8*, 45–53.

Dunlap, G., Kern-Dunlap, L., Clarke, S., & Robbins, F. R. (1991). Functional assessment, curricular revision, and severe behavior problems. *Journal of Applied Behavior Analysis, 24*, 387–397.

Durand, V. M. (1999). Functional communication training using assistive devices: Recruiting natural communities of reinforcement. *Journal of Applied Behavior Analysis, 32*, 247–267.

Durand, V. M., & Carr, E. G. (1992). An analysis of maintenance following functional communication training. *Journal of Applied Behavior Analysis, 25*, 777–794.

Durand, V. M., & Merges, E. (2001). Functional communication training: A contemporary behavior analytic intervention for problem behaviors. *Focus on Autism and Other Developmental Disorders, 16*, 110–119.

Dyer, K., Dunlap, G., & Winterling, V. (1990). Effects of choice making on the serious problem behaviors of students with severe handicaps. *Journal of Applied Behavior Analysis, 23*, 515–524.

Ebanks, M. E., & Fisher, W. W. (2003). Altering the timing of academic prompts to treat destructive behavior maintained by escape. *Journal of Applied Behavior Analysis, 36*, 355–359.

Fisher, W. W., DeLeon, I. G., Rodriguez-Catter, V., & Keeney, K. M. (2004). Enhancing the effects of extinction on attention-maintained behavior through noncontingent delivery of attention or stimuli identified via a competing stimulus assessment. *Journal of Applied Behavior Analysis, 37*, 171–184.

Fisher, W. W., Kuhn, D. E., & Thompson, R. H. (1998). Establishing discriminative control of responding using functional and alternative reinforcers during functional communication training. *Journal of Applied Behavior Analysis, 31*, 543–560.

Fisher, W. W., O'Connor, J. T., Kurtz, P. F., DeLeon, I. G., & Gotjen, D. L. (2000). The effects of noncontingent delivery of high- and low-preference stimuli on attention-maintained destructive behavior. *Journal of Applied Behavior Analysis, 33*, 79–83.

Fisher, W. W., Piazza, C. C., Bowman, L. G., Hagopian, L. P., Owens, J. C., & Slevin, I. (1992). A comparison of two approaches for identifying reinforcers for persons with severe and profound disabilities. *Journal of Applied Behavior Analysis, 25*, 491–498.

Fisher, W. W., Piazza, C. C., Cataldo, M., Harrell, R., Jefferson, G., & Conner, R. (1993). Functional communication training with and without extinction and punishment. *Journal of Applied Behavior Analysis, 26*, 23–36.

Goh, H., Iwata, B. A., Shore, B. A., DeLeon, I. G., Lerman, D. C., Ulrich, S. M., et al. (1995). An analysis of the reinforcing properties of hand mouthing. *Journal of Applied Behavior Analysis, 28*, 269–283.

Hagopian, L. P., Fisher, W. W., & Legacy, S. M. (1994). Schedule effects of noncontingent reinforcement on attention-maintained destructive behavior in identical quadruplets. *Journal of Applied Behavior Analysis, 27*, 317–325.

Hall, S. S., DeBernardis, G. M., & Reiss, A. L. (2006). Social escape behaviors in children with fragile X syndrome. *Journal of Autism and Developmental Disorders, 36*, 935–947.

Hanley, G. P., Iwata, B. A., & Thompson, R. H. (2001). Reinforcement schedule thinning following treatment with functional communication training. *Journal of Applied Behavior Analysis, 34*, 17–38.

Hanley, G. P., Iwata, B. A., Thompson, R. H., & Lindberg, J. S. (2000). A component analysis of "stereotypy as reinforcement" for alternative behavior. *Journal of Applied Behavior Analysis, 33*, 285–297.

Hanley, G. P., Piazza, C. C., & Fisher, W. W. (1997). Noncontingent presentation of attention and alternative stimuli in the treatment of attention-maintained destructive behavior. *Journal of Applied Behavior Analysis, 30*, 229–237.

Hanley, G. P., Piazza, C. C., Fisher, W. W., & Maglieri, K. A. (2005). On the effectiveness of and preference for punishment and extinction components of function-based interventions. *Journal of Applied Behavior Analysis, 38*, 51–65.

Horner, R. D. (1980). The effects of an environmental "enrichment" program on the behavior of institutionalized profoundly retarded children. *Journal of Applied Behavior Analysis, 13*, 473–491.

Horner, R. H., & Day, H. M. (1991). The effects of response efficiency on functionally equivalent competing behaviors. *Journal of Applied Behavior Analysis, 24*, 719–732.

Horner, R. H., Day, H. M., & Day, J. R. (1997). Using neutralizing routines to reduce problem behaviors. *Journal of Applied Behavior Analysis, 30*, 601–614.

Horner, R. H., Day, H. M., Sprague, J. R., O'Brien, M., & Heathfield, L. T. (1991). Interspersed requests: a nonaversive procedure for reducing aggression and self-injury during instruction. *Journal of Applied Behavior Analysis, 24*, 265–278.

Iwata, B. A. (2006). On the distinction between positive and negative reinforcement. *The Behavior Analyst, 29*, 121–123.

Iwata, B. A., Dorsey, M. F., Slifer, K. J., Bauman, K. E., & Richman, G. S. (1994). Toward a functional analysis of self-injury. *Journal of Applied Behavior Analysis, 27*, 197–209 (Reprinted from Analysis and Intervention in Developmental Disabilities, 2, 3–20, 1982).

Iwata, B. A., Pace, G. M., Cowdery, G. E., & Miltenberger, R. G. (1994). What makes extinction work: an analysis of procedural form and function. *Journal of Applied Behavior Analysis, 27*, 131–144.

Iwata, B. A., Pace, G. M., Dorsey, M. F., Zarcone, J. R., Vollmer, T. R., Smith, R. G., et al. (1994). The functions of self-injurious behavior: An experimental-epidemiological analysis. *Journal of Applied Behavior Analysis, 27*, 215–240.

Iwata, B. A., Pace, G. M., Kalsher, M. J., Cowdery, G. E., & Cataldo, M. F. (1990). Experimental analysis and extinction of self-injurious escape behavior. *Journal of Applied Behavior Analysis, 23*, 11–27.

Kahng, S., Iwata, B. A., Thompson, R. H., & Hanley, G. P. (2000). A method for identifying satiation versus extinction effects under noncontingent reinforcement schedules. *Journal of Applied Behavior Analysis, 33,* 419–432.

Kennedy, C. H., & Souza, G. (1995). Functional analysis and treatment of eye poking. *Journal of Applied Behavior Analysis, 28,* 27–37.

Kuhn, D. E., DeLeon, I. G., Fisher, W. W., & Wilke, A. E. (1999). Clarifying an ambiguous functional analysis with matched and mismatched extinction procedures. *Journal of Applied Behavior Analysis, 32,* 99–102.

Kodak, T., Lerman, D. C., Volkert, V. M., & Trosclair, N. (2007). Further examination of factors that influence preference for positive versus negative reinforcement. *Journal of Applied Behavior Analysis, 40,* 25–44.

Kodak, T., Miltenberger, R. G., & Romanuik, C. (2003). The effects of differential negative reinforcement of other behavior and noncontingent escape on compliance. *Journal of Applied Behavior Analysis, 36,* 379–382.

Lalli, J. S., Casey, S. D., & Kates, K. (1997). Noncontingent reinforcement as treatment for severe problem behavior: Some procedural variations. *Journal of Applied Behavior Analysis, 30,* 127–137.

Lalli, J. S., Vollmer, T. R., Progar, P. R., Wright, C., Borrero, J., Daniel, D., et al. (1999). Competition between positive and negative reinforcement in the treatment of escape behavior. *Journal of Applied Behavior Analysis, 32,* 285–296.

Laraway, S., Snycerski, S., Michael, J., & Poling, A. (2003). Motivating operations and terms to describe them: some further refinements. *Journal of Applied Behavior Analysis, 36,* 407–414.

Lattal, A. K., & Lattal, A. D. (2006). And yet …: Further comments on distinguishing between positive and negative reinforcement. *The Behavior Analyst, 29,* 129–134.

Lerman, D. C., & Iwata, B. A. (1995). Prevalence of the extinction burst and its attenuation during treatment. *Journal of Applied Behavior Analysis, 28,* 93–94.

Lerman, D. C., & Iwata, B. A. (1996). A methodology for distinguishing between extinction and punishment effects associated with response blocking. *Journal of Applied Behavior Analysis, 29,* 231–233.

Lindberg, J. S., Iwata, B. A., & Kahng, S. W. (1999). On the relation between object manipulation and stereotypic self-injurious behavior. *Journal of Applied Behavior Analysis, 32,* 51–62.

Lindberg, J. S., Iwata, B. A., Kahng, S.W., & DeLeon, I. G. (1999). DRO contingencies: An analysis of variable-momentary schedules. *Journal of Applied Behavior Analysis, 32,* 123–136.

Lomas, L. E., Fisher, W. W., & Kelley, M. E. (2010). The effects of variable-time delivery of food items and praise on problem behavior reinforced by escape. *Journal of Applied Behavior Analysis, 43,* 425–435.

Lomas-Mevers, J., Fisher, W. W., Kelley, M. E., & Fredrick, L. (in press). The Effects of variable-time versus contingent reinforcement delivery on problem behavior maintained by escape. *Journal of Applied Behavior Analysis.*

Mace, F. C., Browder, D., & Lin, Y. (1987). Analysis of demand conditions associated with stereotypy. *Journal of Behavior Therapy and Experimental Psychiatry, 18,* 25–31.

Marcus, B. A., & Vollmer, T. R. (1995). Effects of differential negative reinforcement on disruption and compliance. *Journal of Applied Behavior Analysis, 28,* 229–230.

Mazaleski, J. L., Iwata, B. A., Vollmer, T. R., Zarcone, J. R., & Smith, R. G. (1993). Analysis of the reinforcement and extinction components in DRO contingencies with self-injury. *Journal of Applied Behavior Analysis, 26,* 143–156.

McCord, B. E., Iwata, B. A., Galensky, T. L., Ellingson, S. A., & Thomson, R. J. (2001). Functional analysis and treatment of problem behavior evoked by noise. *Journal of Applied Behavior Analysis, 34,* 447–462.

Michael, J. (1975). Positive and negative reinforcement: A distinction that is no longer necessary; or a better way to talk about bad things. *Behaviorism, 3,* 33–44.

Munk, D. D., & Repp, A. C. (1994). The relationship between instructional variable and problem behavior: A review. *Exceptional Children, 60,* 390–401.

Pace, G. M., Ivancic, M. T., & Jefferson, G. (1994). Stimulus fading as treatment for obscenity in a brain-injured adult. *Journal of Applied Behavior Analysis, 27,* 301–305.

Pace, G. M., Iwata, B. A., Cowdery, G. E., Andree, P. J., & McIntyre, T. (1993). Stimulus (instructional) fading during extinction of self-injurious escape behavior. *Journal of Applied Behavior Analysis, 26,* 205–212.

Pelios, L., Morren, J., Tesch, D., & Axelrod, S. (1999). The impact of functional analysis methodology on treatment choice for self-injurious and aggressive behavior. *Journal of Applied Behavior Analysis, 32,* 185–195.

Piazza, C. C., Adelinis, J. D., Hanley, G. P., Goh, H. L., & Delia, M. D. (2000). An evaluation of the effects of matched stimuli on behaviors maintained by automatic reinforcement. *Journal of Applied Behavior Analysis, 33,* 13–27.

Piazza, C. C., Fisher, W. W., Hanley, G. P., LeBlanc, L. A., Worsdell, A. S., Lindauer, S. E., et al. (1998). Treatment of pica through multiple analyses of its reinforcing functions. *Journal of Applied Behavior Analysis, 31,* 165–189.

Parrish, J. M., Cataldo, M. F., Kolko, D. J., Neef, N. A., & Egel, A. L. (1986). Experimental analysis of response covariation among compliant and inappropriate behaviors. *Journal of Applied Behavior Analysis, 19,* 241–254.

Poling, A., & Normand, M. (1999). Noncontingent reinforcement: An inappropriate description of time-based schedules that reduce behavior. *Journal of Applied Behavior Analysis, 32,* 237–238.

Poling, A., & Ryan, C. (1982). Differential-reinforcement-of-other-behavior schedules. *Behavior Modification, 6,* 3–21.

Rapp, J. T., & Vollmer, T. R. (2005). Stereotypy I: A review of behavioral assessment and treatment. *Research in Developmental Disabilities, 26,* 527–547.

Reid, D. H., Parsons, M. B., Phillips, J. F., & Green, C. W. (1993). Reduction of self-injurious hand mouthing using response blocking. *Journal of Applied Behavior Analysis, 26*, 139–140.

Repp, A. C., Barton, L. E., & Brulle, A. R. (1983). A comparison of two procedures for programming the differential reinforcement of other behaviors. *Journal of Applied Behavior Analysis, 16*, 435–445.

Rincover, A., Cook, R., Peoples, A., & Packard, D. (1979). Sensory extinction and sensory reinforcement principles for programming multiple adaptive behavior change. *Journal of Applied Behavior Analysis, 12*, 221–233.

Roane, H. S., Fisher, W. W., Sgro, G. M., Falcomata, T. S., & Pabico, R. R. (2004). An alternative method of thinning reinforcer delivery during differential reinforcement. *Journal of Applied Behavior Analysis, 37*, 213–218.

Roscoe, E. M., Iwata, B. A., & Goh, H. (1998). A comparison of noncontingent reinforcement and sensory extinction as treatments for self-injurious behavior. *Journal of Applied Behavior Analysis, 31*, 635–646.

Roscoe, E. M., Iwata, B. A., & Rand, M. S. (2003). Effects of reinforcer consumption and magnitude on response rates during noncontingent reinforcement. *Journal of Applied Behavior Analysis, 36*, 525–539.

Russo, D. C., Cataldo, M. F., & Cushing, P. J. (1981). Compliance training and behavioral covariation in the treatment of multiple behavior problems. *Journal of Applied Behavior Analysis, 14*, 209–222.

Shirley, M. J., Iwata, B. A., Kahng, S., Mazaleski, J. L., & Lerman, D. C. (1997). Does functional communication training compete with ongoing contingencies of reinforcement? An analysis during response acquisition and maintenance. *Journal of Applied Behavior Analysis, 30*, 93–104.

Shore, B. A., Iwata, B. A., DeLeon, I. G., Kahng, S., & Smith, R. G. (1997). An analysis of reinforcer substitutability using object manipulation and self-injury as competing responses. *Journal of Applied Behavior Analysis, 30*, 21–40.

Sidman, M. (2006). The distinction between positive and negative reinforcement: Some additional considerations. *The Behavior Analyst, 29*, 135–139.

Silverman, K., Watanabe, K., Marshall, A. M., & Baer, D. M. (1984). Reducing self-injury and corresponding self-restraint through the strategic use of protective clothing. *Journal of Applied Behavior Analysis, 17*, 545–552.

Skinner, B. F. (1953). *Science and human behavior*. New York: The Free Press.

Smith, R. G., Iwata, B. A., Goh, H., & Shore, B. A. (1995). Analysis of establishing operations for self-injury maintained by escape. *Journal of Applied Behavior Analysis, 28*, 515–535.

Sugai, G., & White, W. J. (1986). Effects of using object self-stimulation as a reinforcer on the prevocational work rates of an autistic child. *Journal of Autism and Developmental Disorders, 16*, 459–470.

Tiger, J. H., Hanley, G. P., & Bruzek, J. (2008). Functional communication training: A review and practical guide. *Behavior Analysis in Practice, 1*, 16–23.

Vaughn, M. E., & Michael, J. L. (1982). Automatic reinforcement: An important but ignored concept. *Behaviorism, 10*, 217–228.

Vollmer, T. R. (1994). The concept of automatic reinforcement: Implications for behavioral research in developmental disabilities. *Research in Developmental Disabilities, 15*, 187–207.

Vollmer, T. R., & Iwata, B. A. (1992). Differential reinforcement as treatment for severe behavior disorders: Procedural and functional variations. *Research in Developmental Disabilities, 13*, 393–417.

Vollmer, T. R., Iwata, B. A., Zarcone, J. R., Smith, R. G., & Mazaleski, J. L. (1993). The role of attention in the treatment of attention-maintained self-injurious behavior: noncontingent reinforcement and differential reinforcement of other behavior. *Journal of Applied Behavior Analysis, 26*, 9–21.

Vollmer, T. R., Progar, P. R., Lalli, J. S., Van Camp, C. M., Sierp, B. J., Wright, C. S., et al. (1998). Fixed-time schedules attenuate extinction-induced phenomena in the treatment of severe aberrant behavior. *Journal of Applied Behavior Analysis, 31*, 529–542.

Vollmer, T. R., Marcus, B. A., & LeBlanc, L. (1994). Treatment of self-injury and hand mouthing following inconclusive functional analyses. *Journal of Applied Behavior Analysis, 27*, 331–344.

Vollmer, T. R., Marcus, B. A., & Ringdahl, J. E. (1995). Noncontingent escape as treatment for self-injurious behavior maintained by negative reinforcement. *Journal of Applied Behavior Analysis, 28*, 15–26.

Vollmer, T. R., Roane, H. S., Ringdahl, J. E., & Marcus, B. A. (1999). Evaluating treatment challenges with differential reinforcement of alternative behavior. *Journal of Applied Behavior Analysis, 32*, 9–23.

Wacker, D. P., Steege, M. W., Northup, J., Sasso, G., Berg, W., Reimers, T., et al. (1990). A component analysis of functional communication training across three topographies of severe behavior problems. *Journal of Applied Behavior Analysis, 23*, 417–429.

Weeks, M., & Gaylord-Ross, R. (1981). Task difficulty and aberrant behavior in severely handicapped students. *Journal of Applied Behavior Analysis, 14*, 449–463.

Wilder, D. A., Draper, R., Williams, W. L., & Higbee, T. S. (1997). A comparison of noncontingent reinforcement, other competing stimulation, and liquid rescheduling for the treatment of rumination. *Behavioral Interventions, 12*, 55–64.

Wolery, M., Kirk, K., & Gast, D. L. (1985). Stereotypic behavior as a reinforcer: Effects and side-effects. *Journal of Autism and Developmental Disorders, 15*, 149–161.

Zarcone, J. R., Iwata, B. A., Hughes, C. E., & Vollmer, T. R. (1993). Momentum versus extinction effects in the treatment of self-injurious escape behavior. *Journal of Applied Behavior Analysis, 26*, 135–136.

The Role of Functional Assessment in Treatment Planning

12

Deborah A. Napolitano, Vicki Madaus Knapp, Elizabeth Speares, David B. McAdam, and Holly Brown

Functional Assessment and the Treatment Planning Process

Treatment planning to reduce challenging behavior (e.g., aggression and property destruction) can be complex and requires a prescriptive inter-professional team-based approach. As with other problems that interfere with an individual's quality of life, such as health issues, the best course of treatment is one that accurately assesses the problem, leads to effective treatment for the issue of

concern, and is empirically supported. This is especially important when treating individuals who display challenging behavior which frequently interfere with their opportunities to learn and to live and be educated in less-restrictive settings (Matson, Mayville, & Laud, 2003). The utility of functional behavior assessments (FBAs) and functional analyses (FAs) in the identification of the specific function or purpose of challenging behavior has been embraced commonly by persons charged with supporting individuals who display challenging behavior (e.g., behavior analysts and educators). This is demonstrated by the laws requiring FBAs be conducted when individuals are struggling in educational environments (Individuals with Disabilities Education Improvement Act, 2004) and the belief that the assessments conducted should result in the development of interventions that help preserve the child's placement in the least restrictive appropriate educational setting. The utility of these assessments has been repeatedly demonstrated in the published literature (e.g., Derby et al., 1992; Iwata, Dorsey, Slifer, Bauman, & Richman, 1994; Kennedy & Souza, 1995; Kern, Childs, Dunlap, Clarke & Falk, 1994; McCord, Thompson, & Iwata, 2001; Ellingson, Miltenberger, Stricker, Galensky, & Garlinghouse, 2000). Several excellent reviews of this extensive literature have been conducted and have independently identified functional analysis and assessment as best practice (e.g., Carr, 1994; Hanley, Iwata, & McCord, 2003).

D.A. Napolitano (✉) • D.B. McAdam
University of Rochester School of Medicine,
601 Elmwood Avenue, Box 671, Rochester,
NY 14642, USA
e-mail: deborah_napolitano@urmc.rochester.edu;
david_mcadam@urmc.rochester.edu

V.M. Knapp
Summit Educational Resources, 150 Stahl Road,
Getzville, NY 14068, USA
e-mail: vmknapp@summited.org

E. Speares
Hillside Children's Center, 1183 Monroe Avenue,
Rochester, NY 14620, USA
e-mail: espeares@hillside.com

H. Brown
Hillside Children's Center, 1183 Monroe Avenue,
Rochester, NY 14620, USA

University of Rochester School of Nursing,
601 Elmwood Avenue, Box SON,
Rochester, NY 14642, USA
e-mail: holly_brown@urmc.rochester.edu

J.L. Matson (ed.), *Functional Assessment for Challenging Behaviors*,
Autism and Child Psychopathology Series, DOI 10.1007/978-1-4614-3037-7_12,
© Springer Science+Business Media, LLC 2012

Research using functional analyses and assessments has demonstrated that challenging behavior is maintained by both social and nonsocial factors (Hanley et al., 2003). In the majority of cases, the challenging behavior of persons have proven functional for the individual by allowing them to obtain desired social reinforcers (positive reinforcement) such as toys or attention (e.g., Kodak, Northup, & Kelly, 2007), to avoid or eliminate aversive events (negative reinforcement) such as instructional demands or proximity to other people (e.g., Moore & Edwards, 2003), and to identify internally occurring (automatic) reinforcers (e.g., Kuhn, DeLeon, Fisher, & Wilke, 1999). Thus, an assessment process that successfully identifies these factors is a powerful tool in providing the members of an individual's treatment team with the necessary information to choose among potentially effective evidence-based strategies to reduce the individual's challenging behavior (Horner, 1994).

Why Choose a Function-Based Intervention?

There have been many demonstrations that the identification of function of a person's challenging behavior can help researchers develop an effective function-based intervention (Kurtz et al., 2003). In addition to functional assessment, federal law (Individuals with Disabilities Education Improvement Act, 2004) also mandates that for individuals demonstrating challenging behavior, the results should be used to identify potentially effective, function-based interventions [e.g., functional communication training (FCT), differential reinforcement of other behavior (DRO), or extinction]. This seems logical given that researchers have demonstrated that function-based interventions are more effective than nonfunction-based or generic interventions. Ingram, Lewis-Palmer, and Sugai (2005), for example, conducted a comprehensive functional assessment for two boys in sixth grade. Based on the results of the FBA, they then compared the effectiveness of a function-based and a nonfunction-based intervention plan. The function-based intervention plan included setting event manipulations, preventative antecedent

strategies, behavior teaching, and consequence strategies such as DRO. Whereas, the nonfunction-based plan included strategies not linked to the function of a participant's challenging behavior. Both plans were then implemented by the student's teachers within the framework of an ABCBC reversal design. Results showed that the function-based plans produced decreases in challenging behavior, whereas the implementation of the nonfunction-based plans did not result in a clinically significant change in behavior.

In a related study, Newcomer and Lewis (2004) compared function-based interventions to general classroom procedures. Using a multiple baseline across three participants, the researchers demonstrated that function-based interventions produced significant reductions in challenging behavior when compared to baseline and nonfunction-based interventions. Although teachers expressed some concern about the time involved in the assessment process, they rated the use of function-based interventions very positively. Other researchers have demonstrated high-social acceptability (social validity) of and a clear preference by practitioners (e.g., school teachers) for function-based interventions (Ervin, DuPaul, Kern, & Friman, 1998; McLaren & Nelson, 2009; Nahgahgwon, Umbreit, Liaupsin, & Turton, 2010). Given this information, it seems that the use of functional assessment and function-based intervention is the key component in successful treatment planning for the reduction of challenging behavior.

Despite the superiority of function-based interventions to nonfunction-based interventions, the understanding of the necessity and/or the skill of how to move from functional assessment to function-based treatment is still lacking. Several researchers have examined whether function-based interventions are typically used by nonresearchers. They also have examined whether practitioners who routinely develop and write behavioral intervention and support plans know how to correctly develop and implement function-based interventions. Two published studies have examined whether, given the correct function of challenging behavior, teachers would choose function-based strategies (Scott et al., 2005; Sugai, Lewis-Palmer, & Hagan, 1998). In both cases, teachers tended to choose nonfunction-based, contraindicated interventions, such as time-out when behavior was described as being maintained by escape or avoidance of low-preference activities (e.g., math and activities of daily living). In an interesting study, Scott et al. (2005) trained key school team members (e.g., school psychologists and teachers) to rigorous criteria on functional assessment and function-based intervention planning. Areas trained included restructuring antecedent conditions, instructional techniques, consequences for positive behavior, and consequences for negative behavior. Thirty-one students were chosen of those referred to the school treatment team due to the display of recurring challenging behavior. With the guidance of a trained facilitator, the school teams determined the function of the challenging behavior based on available assessment information. The teams then created behavior intervention plans based on the hypothesized function of problem behavior for all 31 students. Experts (i.e., persons who had published in the area of functional assessment and intervention) also chose interventions based on the same hypothesized functions. Experts were more likely to identify teaching strategies (e.g., teaching an alternative communication response) and were less likely to identify the need to use reductive strategies (e.g., response cost). School teams included an exclusionary strategy such as time-out in 70% of the interventions developed. In contrast, the experts identified no students who required the use of exclusionary strategies. Despite being trained to rigorous criteria, school personnel continued to select nonfunction-based reductive interventions. There were some limitations to this study such as discrepancy between choices of interventions by the experts. Despite these limitations, however, this study highlights the concern over FBAs leading to well-designed, function-based interventions in the "real world." These results provide strong support for the need to increase practitioner's skills in developing and implementing function-based interventions.

Umbreit and his colleagues provide several examples of the use of a decision model (see Umbreit, Ferro, Liaupsin, & Lane, 2007 for complete description of the model) for developing function-based interventions across several populations (e.g., Nahgahgwon, et al., 2010; Underwood, Umbreit, & Liaupsin, 2009; Wood, Ferro, Umbreit, & Liaupsin, 2011). The model is designed to facilitate the correct identification of function-based replacement behaviors (e.g., appropriately requesting a break), antecedent arrangements (e.g., visual supports such as a picture activity schedule), and extinction. Underwood et al. (2009) for example, examined the efficacy of the model for the development of a function-based intervention for three adults with intellectual disabilities. The function-based interventions selected using the decision model was effective in reducing the challenging behavior of all three participants. Wood et al. (2011) examined the efficacy of the decision model for three preschool students with intellectual and developmental disabilities. In this study, the student's teachers actively participated in the development of the intervention; however, the researchers took the lead on the development. For all three participants, interventions chosen using the decision model were very effective in reducing the targeted challenging behavior. Despite the demonstrated effectiveness of the decision model, teachers and family members did not take the lead in the development of the interventions. This, combined with the results of the Scott et al. (2005) study, suggests the further need for increased education and training for practitioners in function-based intervention planning.

The Need for Interprofessional Team Planning

In addition to training, effective treatment planning begins with the selection of key team members or stakeholders. In an editorial in the *Journal of Intellectual Disability Research*, Holland (2011) described a changing landscape in the development of interventions for individuals with intellectual disabilities. Practitioners and researchers are increasingly recognizing the need for assessment and intervention that are designed by teams which include professionals from multiple disciplines. Although Holland states that there is a great need for multidisciplinary evaluations, he also acknowledges the challenges involved. Given that both biological and environmental variables may contribute to an individual's challenging behavior, an appropriate, interprofessional team should include experts from the fields of behavior analysis, education (both general and special education teachers), medicine (e.g., nursing, physician, and psychiatry), psychology, support staff (e.g., one-to-one paraprofessionals), family members, and the individual whose challenging behavior is being targeted for reduction whenever possible.

An interprofessional team approach to treatment planning can lead to improved outcomes through systematic evaluation of all variables impacting the individual and a coordinated delivery of care. The work of an interprofessional team is focused on the individual and there is a sense of shared responsibility in the decision-making process. This opportunity for shared decision making allows for increased focus on the integration of disciplines and can lead to innovative interventions for complex problems (Patel, Pratt, & Patel, 2008).

An interprofessional team is in a unique position to evaluate and interpret assessment results and to use the information obtained to develop function-based interventions. All decisions regarding intervention should be based on the most comprehensive data available (Matson et al., 2003). After all contributing factors have been identified, the team can start problem solving to identify an appropriate function-based intervention. Generally, the team begins by identifying effective interventions for setting events or establishing operations. That is, the events which increase the likelihood that the reinforcer for challenging behavior will either be more or less desirable or potent to the individual.

Treatment Planning

In considering how to develop a function-based intervention, it is important to consider all the factors serving to maintain the challenging behavior as well as factors that may make the reinforcer more or less potent (establishing operations/setting events). Additionally, a thorough understanding of positive and negative reinforcement is critical to the designing of an effective intervention. As a general rule, interventions should target each critical variable.

The competing behavior model (O'Neill et al., 1997) is a helpful tool to guide the interprofessional team in the development of a function-based behavior intervention plan (see http://www.pbis.org/common/pbisresources/tools/BSP_Template.doc).

It provides a nice visual representation of the critical variables related to treatment planning. This model identifies (1) setting events, (2) antecedents, (3) replacement behavior, and (4) consequences as the primary targets for intervention. Interventions should be considered based on the factors contributing to the challenging behavior, both distal events and immediate contingencies. The interprofessional team should consider interventions to (1) minimize the impact of *setting events*, (2) minimize the impact of *antecedents*, (3) teach *replacement skills*, and (4) target the *consequence events* by increasing reinforcement for appropriate behavior (e.g., differential reinforcement) and decreasing reinforcement for targeted challenging behavior (i.e., extinction). By identifying these variables, the interprofessional team can focus on conducting problem solving to identify function-based interventions that matched the function and the contributing variables of the person's challenging behavior. For example, a substitute teacher (setting event) gave the student a worksheet to complete (antecedent stimulus), which resulted in flopping to the floor (problem behavior), which allowed the student to successfully escape from having to do the math (maintaining consequence). From this scenario, the team then determines the desired behavior, or the behavior in which you would prefer this student to engage in and its consequence. For example, the desired behavior is completing a worksheet and the current consequence for that is earning a sticker which is then placed on their sticker chart. Finally, the team identifies a behavior that is an adaptive alternative to the problem behavior that will result in the same maintaining consequence as engaging in the problem behavior. For example, requesting a break from math (alternative adaptive behavior) will result in a brief escape from the instructional demand (maintaining consequence).

Essential to the competing behavior model is to identify strategies that make the challenging behavior "irrelevant, ineffective, and inefficient" (O'Neill et al., 1997, p. 66). Identifying and arranging setting events and antecedents so that the challenging behavior would not occur is key in making the problem behavior *irrelevant*. Any situational and contextual rearrangements might result in a relatively artificial environment for the individual, but helpful in reducing challenging behavior, so it is important to gradually reinstitute any changes that were made gradually and systematically over time. Providing an adaptive alternative to the challenging behavior that is easier to obtain or requires less response effort is key in making the challenging behavior *inefficient*. An adaptive alternative might include one rudimentary task or gesture which immediately results in the same maintaining consequence as the display of the challenging behavior. Over time the adaptive alternative behavior should be systematically shaped to become more complex and effortful. Withholding the maintaining consequence or reinforcer after the display of challenging behavior is key to making the behavior *ineffective*. The challenging behavior is placed on extinction. The challenging behavior should no longer result in the maintaining consequence and the individual should be provided with multiple opportunities to engage in the adaptive alternative behavior, which is easier and more quickly results in gaining access to the maintaining consequence. Strategies to ensure that the challenging behavior becomes irrelevant, inefficient, and ineffective should be listed for each of the four major areas of the competing behavior pathways (setting event, antecedent event, problem behavior, and maintaining consequence).

Choosing a Setting Event Intervention

Setting events may sometimes be as simple as a child having a substitute teacher, as described

above. Setting events, however, are often events that are related to complex situations (e.g., family instability) or medical concerns (e.g., mental health challenges or an illness such as chronic ear infections). When setting events are successfully identified, they may be the most difficult factors for the interprofessional team to address successfully. The primary goal when designing an intervention for a setting event is to minimize the impact it may have on the antecedent and consequence to the challenging behavior. This is often difficult to do (e.g., changing family interaction styles) and is best accomplished when an interprofessional team including members with varying expertise are involved in the problem-solving process related to treatment plan development. For example, in the case of increased family stressors, such as lack of health insurance and a family member with high medical needs, a social worker might be prepared to assist the family to identify solutions. In another example, in the case of a child experiencing mental health concerns, having a psychiatrist on the interprofessional team may be critical given their expertise in understanding the effects of medication and the empirical research which suggests that for some individuals the combination of a medication and a behavioral intervention might be more effective than either alone (Napolitano et al., 1999). Other examples of setting events might be specific genetic conditions (e.g., Prader–Willi syndrome and Smith–Magenis syndrome). For genetic conditions such as these the inclusion of an expert on the specific condition might be invaluable. Additionally related to behavioral needs and educational difficulties, an expert may have particularly important contributions in the assessment of learning needs related the genetic condition (e.g., persons with Down syndrome generally show higher levels of adaptive behavior in comparison to intellectual ability). While we may not be able to totally eliminate a setting event, understanding the impact it may have on challenging behavior is extremely valuable in planning an effective intervention. Additionally, minimizing its impact may make a significant difference in the ability of the interpersonal team to develop an intervention which produces a clinically significant effect.

Many researchers have described or investigated the impact of setting events and establishing operations on challenging behavior and effective interventions to eliminate or reduce the impact on the challenging behavior. Specific examples include constipation (e.g., Christensen et al., 2009), menstrual pain (Carr & Smith, 1995), psychiatric disorders (e.g., Baker, Blumberg, Freeman, & Wieseler, 2002), medication (e.g., DiCesare, McAdam, Toner, & Varrell, 2005; Northup, Fussilier, Swanson & Borrero, 1997), and social reinforcers such as attention (e.g., Edrisinha, O'Reilly, Sigafoos, Lancioni, & Choi, 2010).

O'Reilly, Lacey, and Lancioni (2000) evaluated the degree to which noise affected challenging behavior of a child with Williams Syndrome. The authors evaluated the effects of noise using a functional analysis. Three conditions (noise in the background, no noise, and noise plus earplugs) were tested. During the demand condition, when noise was present but no earplugs, the child engaged in aggression to avoid instructional demands. When there was no background noise or noise was present, but the child wore earplugs, he engaged in no or low rates of aggression. Based on the assessment results, the authors recommended a quiet instructional environment for the child and guidelines for the use of earplugs to attenuate the effect of environmental noise.

Consider the following example:

Matilda, a 9-year-old girl, has always enjoyed school and generally received good grades. Recently, however, she has struggled in most classes and particularly in math. Although she had no history of being "rude" to adults, over the last few months she has been sent to the principal's office (often during math) quite frequently for what teachers describe as being "rude, defiant, and unwilling to listen." Some school personnel are even beginning to wonder if she has Oppositional Defiant Disorder (ODD). She was referred to the school's assessment team to do a functional assessment and develop an intervention. Based on a functional assessment, which included an analysis of the setting events, antecedents, and consequences maintaining the challenging behavior, it was determined that there were several possible setting events. First, Matilda's grandmother, who had lived with her family, recently passed away suddenly. Matilda was very close with her grandmother and her grandmother had been a secondary care giver for her when her mother was away on frequent business trips. Additionally, Matilda's grandmother was a great support for her, especially with school and often supervised her homework completion. She also was able to help provide tutoring of sorts for math, a subject that Matilda has not always been as successful in as her other subjects. Likely related to the recent family stressors with Matilda's grandmother passing away, her parents have decided to divorce. This is an additional loss for Matilda during an already difficult time. Finally, Matilda's father reported that several nights a week Matilda has had difficulty sleeping and has been getting up and watching TV in the middle of the night. On the days she has not slept well, data indicate that she is most likely to engage in the challenging behavior.

The example above highlights how complex challenging behavior can be. The setting events identified by the school team are significant and appear to be very difficult, if not impossible to fully eliminate. This is a great example of when an interprofessional team is necessary to treat challenging behavior. Upon review, the interprofessional team determined the following intervention strategies: The social worker determined that it was appropriate to provide some in-home family therapy. This would focus on minimizing the impact of the stressors and specific ways to support Matilda to better cope when she is experiencing difficulties. Matilda's father said that the family were very interested and in full support of this idea. The psychiatrist determined that it would be appropriate for Matilda to be evaluated for depression and ideally receive counseling focusing on how to better cope with her feelings of loss. The teacher identified opportunities for Matilda to receive tutoring in math at least twice per week from a student teacher. Matilda's father identified several consistent times that she could do her homework completion when he could provide her with encouragement and tutoring. The nurse identified that Matilda may be in need to have a sleep study, but the team determined that the behavior analyst should help the family with develop and evaluate a behavioral sleep intervention first.

While these interventions cannot eliminate all concerns (i.e., grandmother passing away and parents divorcing), they are designed to minimize the impact of these events on Matilda's active participation in her educational program. Through the active participation of a carefully constructed interprofessional team Matilda is much better able to cope and more actively participate in her life.

Choosing an Antecedent Intervention

Similar to the goal for setting event intervention, our goal for antecedent intervention is to minimize their impact, modify them, or eliminate them altogether. They also can provide increased structure in the environment (Kern & Clemens, 2007). It is critical that the event preceding or setting the occasion for the challenging behavior have been correctly identified to develop a successful antecedent intervention. Many researchers have demonstrated methods for identifying effective antecedent interventions to decrease the likelihood that challenging behavior will occur. For example if the antecedent is deprivation from attention, how might a situation in which minimal attention is available be made less problematic for the individual? If the antecedent is academic demands (tasks which require hand writing), is there a way to decrease how aversive these are to the individual? A number of researchers have identified interventions that, when the function of the challenging behavior is correctly identified, can be very successful in minimizing the impact of the antecedent on the challenging behavior.

Much research has been conducted on the efficacy of antecedent manipulations on the reduction of challenging behavior. In one example, Mace and Belfiore (1990) demonstrated the efficacy of *behavioral momentum* to increase compliance and decrease escape-maintained stereotypy in a woman with an intellectual disability. A functional analysis indicated that the stereotypy was maintained by escape from demands. The authors used a high-probability demand sequence followed by a low-probability demand with extinction to increase compliance to demands and decrease stereotypy. This intervention was successful and demonstrated how manipulating antecedent conditions can reduce repetitive escape maintained stereotypic behavior.

Vollmer, Iwata, Zarcone, Smith, and Mazaleski (1993) demonstrated the efficacy of another antecedent intervention, *noncontingent reinforcement (NCR)* on the self-injurious behavior (SIB) (e.g., head hitting and head banging) of three adult women with intellectual disabilities. A pretreatment functional analysis was conducted for each of the participants and identified attention as a factor-maintaining SIB. Two interventions were then compared, attention provided noncontingently (NCR) and attention provided according to a DRO schedule. The results obtained showed that both interventions were equally successful in reducing SIB. However, the authors argue that NCR was the better intervention option due to a reduced likelihood that the individual will have an extinction burst and the potential ease of implementation.

The clinical efficacy of many other antecedent function-based interventions has been demonstrated in the published literature including matched stimuli, demand fading, and choice. Piazza, Adelinis, Hanley, Goh, and Delia, (2000), for example, demonstrated that *matched stimuli* was effective in reducing automatically maintained challenging behavior (climbing, saliva manipulation, and hand mouthing) for three individuals with severe developmental disabilities. In another study, *Demand fading*, an antecedent intervention for escape maintained challenging behavior was demonstrated to be effective in reducing destructive behavior when combined with escape extinction and differential reinforcement (Piazza, Moes, & Fisher, 1996). *Choice* was demonstrated to be an effective intervention on increasing assignment completion and decreasing noncompliance to complete school assignments (Stenhoff, Davey, & Linugaris/Kraft, 2008).

All of these interventions demonstrate that manipulation of the antecedent variables can be an effective interventions both alone and in combination with other interventions in the reduction of challenging behavior. Now consider our example of Matilda, described above. The antecedent condition which routinely set the occasion for her problem behavior was instructional demands to complete academic assignments, particularly math. The function identified by Matilda's interprofessional team was social-negative reinforcement in the form of escape or avoidance of academic demands. Based on this information, several of the antecedent interventions described above might be appropriate for Matilda's interdisciplinary team to evaluate. Demand fading, for example, might be an appropriate intervention to consider. Using this approach, Matilda is initially asked to complete a smaller number of tasks (e.g., single-digit addition problems), then is slowly prompted to complete an increased number of math problems contingent on success. Providing Matilda with the opportunity to choose among several math worksheets might also be effective in providing her with the opportunity to have more control over the aversive instructional situation.

Choosing Replacement/Teaching Strategy/Strategies

While antecedent interventions are very important and effective, they are typically not highly effective in the absence of teaching the individual a new skill. It is important that the new skill taught allows the individual to obtain the same reinforcer which they receive through the display of challenging behavior to promote their long-term success (Carr & Durand, 1985). Additionally, the challenging behavior likely has a history of being extremely functional for the individual. That is, it has served them well to this point; therefore, a replacement behavior that allows the individual to gain access to the same or similar reinforcer has the greatest likelihood of working. For example, a child that throws a pencil at the teacher to get her attention can be reinforced for the absence of throwing pencils; however, what adaptive alternative will the student use to get the teacher's attention now? Without a better option or skill to communicate their need the child may resort to another challenging behavior.

Some important considerations in teaching replacement skills are first that it must require less response effort than the challenging behavior. Most people would not work an additional 40 h in a week unless there was something they were trying to avoid (e.g., missing a big payroll

deadline) or earn (e.g., a monetary bonus). The same concept applies to challenging behavior. An individual who can access what they want through the display of challenging behavior will not typically exert greater effort to use a new skill, despite it yielding the same result as their challenging behavior. Therefore, we must take this into consideration when writing a treatment plan.

Sufficient reinforcement must also be available for the replacement behavior and at a greater rate than for challenging behavior, in the natural environment. An individual may attempt to use a replacement behavior if the reinforcer associated it is more potent than the reinforcer associated with the replacement skill.

Take the following example into consideration:

> A child runs out of the classroom for a break. The child is taught to raise his hand and ask for a break when he wants one. He raises his hand appropriately and asks for a break; however, the teacher rarely calls on him. The child gives up on raising his hand and goes back to running out of the classroom.

Although the replacement behavior may not be available in all situations and at all times, it is important to teach something that will be reinforced frequently during the learning phase of implementation. From there, programming for generalization and thinning of the reinforcement schedule can occur after the individual is using the replacement behavior consistently.

FCT is one of the most common replacement behavior interventions. The alternative behavior that is reinforced during FCT is a communication behavior designed to allow the individual to more efficiently access the reinforcer maintaining their challenging behavior. An individual can communicate using a variety of modulates including sign language, pictures communication system such as The Picture Exchange Communication System (PECS), and vocal statements (e.g., talk to me please). Durand and Carr (1991) evaluated the effects of FCT on reducing the challenging behavior (e.g., aggression and SIB) of three boys between 9 and 12 years of age. All three participants had an intellectual disability and engaged in frequent challenging behavior. For two participants, a functional analysis indicated that the reinforcer was to escape demands, while the results of the analysis for the third participant identified both escape from demands and attention as reinforcers for problem behavior. After baseline observation in the natural environment, participants were taught to either request help or attention, based on the results of the functional analysis. The results indicated clinically significant reductions in challenging behavior for all three participants. Two years post the initial intervention, observation indicated that one participant's challenging behavior had returned to the baseline rate. When a booster session was conducted to help this participant more clearly communicate his requests, challenging behavior again reduced significantly.

Many researchers have examined FCT since the initial studies by Carr and Durand (1985) and Durand and Carr (1991). Fisher, et al. (1993), for example, examined the necessity of extinction and a punishment procedure combined with FCT to reduce challenging behavior. Results were mixed, indicating that some participants were successful with FCT alone, some with FCT+extinction, and for some participants the inclusion of a punishment component was a necessary to produce a clinically significant reduction. More recently, Worsdell, Iwata, Hanley, Thompson, and Kahng (2000) determined that errors in the FCT response might result in its ineffectiveness as an intervention; however, the results also suggested that small errors in the implementation of extinction (e.g., occasional reinforcement of an individual's challenging behavior) may not compromise the effectiveness of FCT.

Consider again our example of Matilda. It was determined that in the context of numerous setting events, given the demand to complete assignments, particularly math, she was likely to engage in inappropriate comments (e.g., being "rude") for negative reinforcement (i.e., to avoid her work). If we were to develop an intervention for this using FCT we might teach her to request help when she is struggling with a particular problem or to request a short break when she is feeling the task is too difficult.

Choosing Consequence Interventions

To complete the treatment, based on the results of the functional assessment or analysis, it is important to consider how to reduce the likelihood the reinforcer for challenging behavior is available and how to motivate the individual to want to engage in the desired and replacement behaviors.

Extinction

After the interprofessional team has identified the function of the individual's challenging behavior, they should include *extinction* in the plan. Extinction is the process of withholding the reinforcer maintaining a student's challenging behavior. To be successfully implemented, this intervention requires an educational team to conduct a comprehensive functional assessment or analysis. If you do not have a clear understanding of *why* the person is displaying challenging behavior, you cannot successfully terminate the relationship between the student's behavior and what he or she gets out of the behavior. For example, if an individual's challenging behavior occurs to obtain attention (positive reinforcement) from their teacher, extinction would involve withholding attention contingent on challenging behavior. In contrast, if a student displays challenging behavior to get out of difficult academic work (negative reinforcement), extinction would involve preventing them from using their challenging behavior to get out of their work. This might involve continuing to prompt a person to engage in work despite his or her continued resistance or attempts to get out of the activity. The main advantage of extinction is that it is an intervention that is based on the specific reason why an individual displays his or her challenging behavior. Extinction also has several possible limitations. First, an individual may experience an extinction burst. These bursts are commonly occurring phenomena in which the rate or intensity of a person's challenging behavior may initially increase before decreasing (Lerman, Iwata, & Wallace, 1999). Such behavior can be very problematic for parents or teachers because they may not be able to successfully work with a student during this difficult time. This may be especially true if the individual's increase in challenging behavior jeopardizes their educational or residential placement or occurs in public places such as the grocery store or on field trips. Additionally, placing one challenging behavior on extinction sometime results in an individual displaying forms of challenging of behavior that they have not typically displayed in the past (i.e., extinction-induced resurgence; Lieving, Hagopian, Long, & O'Connor, 2004). Researchers, for example, have shown that placing SIB such as hand biting on extinction can result in an increase in aggression (Magee & Ellis, 2000). Finally, it might not be realistic to expect people to withhold the reinforcer for a behavior. For example, it might not be possible to physically prompt a child who is very resistant and strong to complete their math and not get out of their chair. The failure to successfully implement extinction can result in a student's challenging behavior being strengthened. This process of accidentally strengthening behavior is referred to as intermittent reinforcement by behavior analysts (Kendall, 1974). Due to the concerns described above, extinction in real-life settings is very seldom used in isolation; instead it should be used in combination with other behavioral treatment strategies often differential reinforcement of other or alternative behavior (Lerman & Iwata, 1995). Iwata, Pace, Cowdery, and Milternberger (1994) conducted a study which illustrated both the clinical usefulness of extinction and the need to match the extinction procedure used to the function of the individual's challenging behavior. Three persons with developmental disabilities who engaged in head banging participated in the study. A pretreatment functional analysis demonstrated that the head banging of the three participants was maintained by different consequences (i.e., social attention from other people, escape or avoidance behavior, or automatic reinforcement). Two forms of extinction were implemented for each participant's head banging and only the form that matched the results of the behavioral function identified in the functional analysis was effective in reducing their SIB.

The use of extinction for our example, Matilda, while difficult, is likely an important component of an effective intervention. The interprofessional team and especially the educational professionals on the team need to determine whether the possible extinction burst from not allowing her to leave the classroom might be able to be tolerated by the educational team members who work with her in the classroom. The implementation of extinction might be necessary to promote Matilda's understanding that making inappropriate statements to her teacher will no longer be effective in allowing her to leave the classroom. Extinction, combined with the initial lessening of demands and communication instruction to obtain help and/or a break should be effective in eliminating the extinction burst. If the team determines that a potential extinction burst cannot be handled safely in the classroom, alternative strategies should be identified prior to implementation of the plan. For example, since math is the primary work task Matilda is trying to avoid, can she go to a room with few distractions (e.g., less people, no materials associated with high-preference activities in clear view) to complete her work contingent on challenging behavior, rather than to the office?

Differential Reinforcement

Differential reinforcement involves providing reinforcement for a functionally alternative behavior or the absence of a challenging behavior for a predetermined interval of time while minimizing reinforcement for the challenging behavior of concern. Clinical experience suggests that differential reinforcement may be particularly useful when people cannot implement extinction perfectly. There are two commonly used differential reinforcement procedures. *Differential reinforcement of other behavior* (DRO) involves the delivery of a positive consequence (reinforcer) contingent on the absence of a challenging behavior during a predetermined period of time (e.g., 15 min, 1 h). *Differential reinforcement of alternative behavior* (DRA) involves the delivery of a positive consequence contingent on the display of an alternative response such as compliance or appropriate communication (e.g., asking your teacher to talk to you about a topic in which you have lots of interest, such as baseball). Differential reinforcement procedures should be designed to address the function of an individual's challenging behavior. That is, the reinforcer identified through the functional assessment process to be maintaining the individual's challenging behavior should be used to reinforce either the absence of challenging behavior or the display of an alternative behavior. For example, in the case of a child who becomes upset when he or she is asked to do their spelling, a low-preference activity, DRA might consist of having his one-on-one paraprofessional staff provide him with token each time he spells a word without throwing his pencil or hitting his desks. After earning the required tokens, the child then would have the opportunity to exchange his tokens for the opportunity for a break and to engage in a high-preference activity, preferably one identified as high-preference by a preference assessment.

Punishment

Punishment involves the contingent delivery of an item or event that a student find to be at least mildly aversive or the removal of a preferred item or event (Cooper, Heron, & Heward, 2007). Punishment procedures such as time out and response cost, while widely used in natural environments (Peterson & Martens, 1995), can be controversial particularly with individuals perceived as being highly vulnerable (e.g., persons with intellectual disabilities). Accurate identification of the function of challenging behavior increases the likelihood that effective, non-punishment-based interventions should be used to decrease the likelihood that a punishment procedure is necessary (Pelios, Morren, Tesch, & Axelrod, 1999). Unfortunately, recent research (i.e., Scott et al., 2005 described above) has indicated that despite identification of function, educators still chose punishment-based strategies. Additionally, these strategies were often contraindicated of the behavioral function (e.g., time out for negatively reinforced challenging behavior).

While caution should be used when considering a punishment-based strategy, they should not be excluded when appropriate. Interprofessional team members should recognize that there may

be instances where the use of punishment-based intervention components may be necessary components of successful interventions (van Houten et al., 1988). Interventions may be more effective with the inclusion of punishment procedures and may even be preferred to non-punishment-based interventions by the individual participating in the intervention (Hanley, Piazza, Fisher, & Maglieri, 2005). Hagopian, Fisher, Sullivan, Acquisito, and LeBlanc (1998) summarized the use of FCT to increase replacement skills for challenging behavior for 21 individuals. Functional analyses were conducted for each participant. Ten participants engaged in challenging behavior for positive reinforcement in the form of attention (nine) or tangible items (one), seven participants engaged in challenging behaviors to escape demands (negative reinforcement), four had mixed results (problem behavior was maintained by both positive and negative reinforcement). While the intervention was very successful for all participants, without the use of extinction or punishment, FCT was not successful for any participant. FCT with extinction was implemented 25 times across 19 participants (some participants challenging behavior was maintained by more than one consequence). FCT combined with extinction initially reduced challenging behavior by 90% for 11 of the 25 participants. The addition of a punishment procedure was necessary for 14 participants to reduce the challenging behavior by 90%. This result was particularly evident when demands were increased and reinforcement was delayed.

When an interprofessional team is considering the use of punishment-based interventions some precautions should be taken. First, the intervention should not be contraindicated to the function of the challenging behavior. That is, if the challenging behavior is maintained by negative reinforcement (e.g., escaping instructional demands) the intervention chosen should not also remove the individual from an environment in which the demands are provided. This would likely compete with the other interventions being implemented. Additionally, adequate reinforcement should be available to maintain the desired or competing behaviors (Lerman & Vorndran, 2002).

Developing a Function-Based Treatment Plan

Once the interprofessional team has determined the interventions to be implemented, a treatment plan must be developed. When developing an intervention plan, the interprofessional team must give careful thought to who will be using the plan and implementing the strategies outlined. Is the plan to be carried out by parents or professionals with training in applied behavior analysis, with little or no training or both? The interprofessional team must carefully tailor the strategies described to match the level of knowledge of the people who will be implementing them to ensure ease of implementation. Functional treatment plans should be easy to read yet include all the key components described above. This includes highlighting important aspects, pointing out details in a concise manner, and using a consistent familiar format (see http://www.pbis.org/common/pbisresources/tools/BSP_Template.doc for one example of a suggested format for a behavior intervention and support plans).

Comprehensive intervention plans should include the following components:

What is contributing to this behavior? (Setting events)

What happens leading up to this behavior, and what can I do to help with that? (Antecedent interventions)

What does the behavior look like? (Behavioral definition)

How do I best respond? (Consequence interventions)

Importance of Clarifying Function and Procedures

Often the function of problem behavior is misunderstood by professionals, parents, and support staff who interact with the person on a daily basis. There are several common misinterpretations of problem behavior. First, people might believe that the individual displaying problem behavior is intentionally attempting to manipulate them (e.g., the individual is displaying problem behavior to make other people mad). This can lead to caregivers wanting to implement nonfunctional, consequence-based interventions to establish "control." Second, people might believe that random events that are correlated with the occurrence of challenging behavior even when the results of functional assessment or analysis has determined there is no relationship between these events and an individual's problem behavior. For example, an individual who displays challenging behavior often receives attention from others in the form of a shocked or angry verbal reaction or reprimand. These forms of contingent verbal attention might result in people believing that challenging behavior that is actually maintained by social-negative reinforcement in the form of escape or avoidance behavior is maintained by social-positive reinforcement in the form of attention from other people (Thompson & Iwata, 2007). Finally, some people might believe in faulty or nonevidence-based conceptualization of problem behavior (e.g., that escape-maintained behavior is due to a child's deficits related to the processing of information, stereotypic behavior is due to sensory disregulation). Understanding *why* the behavior is occurring, or what the function of the behavior is, may help the caregiver intervene more objectively. For example, if a child yells at his teacher to get out of science work specifically, giving the child a math paper to do in place of science will not be appropriate. Understandably, this might be very frustrating for the science teacher though, who might interpret the behavior as aimed at him, rather than occasioned by the class topic. This again is an additional rationale for inclusion of all members of the interprofessional team in assessment and treatment planning.

The professionals and caregivers that implement a plan might not have the same knowledge about variables affecting the challenging behavior as the person writing the plan. This factor illustrates why it is important to state other setting events that may be affecting the behavior, in accordance with the interprofessional team perspectives. Medication side effects, physical pains, trauma, or other nonsocial factors affecting the behavior may provide the caregiver with additional understanding of the factors which set the occasion for a participant's problem behavior. This may lead to decreased frustration and increased compliance with the implementation of the intervention. Stating this briefly in the beginning of the functional treatment plan will set the stage for the rest of the plan, much as the setting events of the individual set the stage for the problem behavior.

Defining and Measuring Behavior

During the assessment process, a definition of the challenging behavior was developed and methods for measurement created (see Chap. 7). The goal of a functional treatment plan is for all caregivers to respond in a standardized way and to modify the behavior. As such, all persons implementing the plan should be able to identify when a behavior is occurring and when it is not. Defining behavior in an observable way assists in reaching this goal of treatment planning. This should be stated clearly in the beginning of the plan to focus the attention of the behavioral intervention.

It is important that data are collected prior to the intervention (baseline) and during the intervention. This is to determine whether the intervention is successfully reducing the challenging behavior. It is also ideal to empirically evaluate the intervention by briefly withdrawing the intervention then reinstating it to determine whether the intervention is what is causing behavior change.

Implementation

It is important in beginning a new plan that the person(s) responsible for the daily implementation have received some training on basic behavioral principles, factors that maintain challenging behavior, and the purpose of function-based intervention. Additionally, clinical experience suggests that the more professionals and stakeholders who can participate in the assessment and treatment planning process, the more likely the interprofessional team will be invested in the success of the plan. Team members, including parents

and teachers, should be encouraged to be active participants in the intervention planning process.

Behavioral Skills Training for Implementation

Following caregiver feedback to the clinician writing the plan, and revising when appropriate, teaching can begin. Plan implementation can be broken down into the steps used in Behavioral Skills Training (BST) (see Miltenberger, 2008 for a complete description). These steps include modeling, instruction, rehearsal, and feedback. BST has been demonstrated to be an effective strategy in teaching others to implement a new skill. Some examples of skills taught using BST include safety skills (Himle, Miltenberger, Gatheridge, & Flessner, 2004), and preventing gun play (Miltenberger et al., 2004), instructional skills at a community setting (Wood, Luiselli, & Harchik, 2007), and discrete trial teaching by staff (Sarakoff & Sturmey, 2004). Using a multiple-baseline design, Sarakoff and Sturmey (2004) demonstrated that BST was a useful strategy for teaching staff to implement discrete trial teaching. Three staff members providing support in the participant's group home were trained to implement ten key components of discrete trial teaching (e.g., eye contact, providing immediate reinforcement for correct responding) to 100% accuracy. All four components of BST were used, and the discrete-trial teaching skills were acquired quickly. Sarakoff and Sturmey note that the components of the BST intervention package have not been evaluated separately to determine whether it is necessary to use all of the components; however, given the data on the effectiveness of the intervention package and responsible costs associated with it makes good sense to use all the components when teaching people how to implement a behavior intervention plan.

To use BST to train staff to implement a behavior intervention plan, the staff should first have an opportunity to read the description of function, the rationale for writing the plan, and the intervention steps. Modeling the intervention components, by the clinician writing the plan, other members of the interprofessional team or another highly trained staff member is the next step. This step is essential to further problem solve any idiosyncratic aspects of the plan. During the modeling phase, it is essential that the learner (caregiver) is fully dedicated to learning the plan and is not distracted by other factors (e.g., work responsibilities). Once the opportunity for initial observational learning has occurred, additional modeling may need to occur numerous times, until the key stakeholders can implement the plan fluently with few errors. The clinician must be aware throughout the modeling process that both correct and incorrect procedures can be learned by the caregiver, and therefore there must be a high degree of consistency and accuracy in implementation.

Continuing to have the written plan to refer to while the modeling is taking place will help with the instruction. By giving the caregiver a visual representation of the intervention while modeling (written instruction), as well as providing instruction and feedback after modeling has occurred, the caregiver will have multiple opportunities to ask questions about how to implement the plan correctly. The caregiver should be encouraged to rehearse implementation of the plan soon after the modeling has occurred. The clinician should be present at the time of rehearsal, to provide feedback immediately. Feedback, including praise for correct implementation and correcting errors, should occur immediately after rehearsal has occurred. Predetermined criteria for successful implementation should be determined prior to BST and all steps should continue to be used until the criteria are met. Finally, BST should also be implemented in the natural environment, whenever possible, to provide opportunities for modeling, instruction, rehearsal, and feedback in the environment in which the challenging behavior routinely occurs.

Additional Caregiver Training

A similar process can be used to train multiple caregivers in implementing behavior intervention plans. Once lead or primary caregivers such as parents and teachers are trained to preestablished criteria, they can use the process of modeling, instruction, rehearsal, and feedback to teach secondary or new caregivers (line staff, grandparents, or support staff). This "train the trainer" model is often necessary when a large number of persons will be implementing the intervention. Consistency of implementation is critical and all persons charged with supporting the individual should be trained to the same criteria. Additionally, it is important to have the primary trainers or clinicians do fidelity checks with all persons implementing the intervention. This may prevent problems with the plan due to lack of fidelity.

Modifications

The need to modify a behavior plan should not be thought of as a setback, but rather an opportunity to clarify the details of intervention components and to conduct additional problem solving by the interprofessional team. First, a check for fidelity of implementation should be conducted. If the plan is being implemented correctly, without anticipated results, the potency of the reinforcers being delivered should be tested (e.g., has the individual become satiated with the reinforcers used?). This is particularly true if a plan initially reduced challenging behavior, but is no longer as effective. In the absence of problems with fidelity and reinforcers, the interprofessional team should problem solve reasons for the lack of success (e.g., has there been a change in important variables, such as change in family situation?) and consider whether additional assessment is necessary.

The published behavioral literature has repeatedly demonstrated the clinical efficacy of a function-based approach to reduce challenging behavior. Crafting a successful, individualized intervention is best accomplished through an interprofessional team problem-solving model which uses function-based intervention planning. Through careful problem solving, the interprofessional team may successfully address the various factors which occasion an individual's problem behavior such as setting events and maintaining consequences.

References

Baker, D. J., Blumberg, E. R., Freeman, R., & Wieseler, N. A. (2002). Can psychiatric disorders be seen as establishing operations? Integrating applied behavior analysis and psychiatry. *Mental Health Aspects of Developmental Disabilities, 5,* 118–124.

Carr, E. G. (1994). Emerging themes in the functional analysis of problem behavior. *Journal of Applied Behavior Analysis, 27,* 393–399.

Carr, E. G., & Durand, V. M. (1985). Reducing behavior problems through functional communication training. *Journal of Applied Behavior Analysis, 18,* 111–126.

Carr, E. G., & Smith, C. E. (1995). Biological setting events for self-injury. *Mental Retardation and Developmental Disabilities Research Reviews, 1,* 94–98.

Christensen, T. J., Ringdahl, J. E., Bosch, J. J., Falcomata, T. S., Luke, J. R., & Andelman, M. S. (2009). Constipaiton associated with self-injurious and aggressive behavior exhibited by a child diagnosed with autism. *Education and Treatment of Children, 32,* 89–103.

Cooper, J0., Heron, T. E., & Heward, W. L. (2007). *Applied behavior analysis* (2nd ed.). Upper Saddle River: Pearson Education.

Derby, K. M., Wacker, D. P., Sasso, G., Steege, M., Northup, J., Cigrand, K., et al. (1992). Brief functional assessment techniques to evaluate aberrant behavior in an outpatient setting: A summary of 79 cases. *Journal of Applied Behavior analysis, 25,* 713–721.

Dicesare, A., McAdam, D. B., Toner, A., & Varrell, J. (2005). The effects of methylphenidate on a functional analysis of disruptive behavior: A replication and extension. *Journal of Applied Behavior Analysis, 38,* 125–128.

Durand, V. M., & Carr, E. G. (1991). Functional communication training to reduce challenging behavior: Maintenance and application in new settings. *Journal of Applied Behavior Analysis, 24,* 251–264.

Edrisinha, C., O'Reilly, M., Sigafoos, J., Lancioni, G., & Choi, H. Y. (2010). Influence of motivating operations and discriminative stimuli on challenging behavior maintained by positive reinforcement. *Research in Developmental Disabilities, 32,* 836–845.

Ellingson, S. A., Miltenberger, R. G., Stricker, J., Galensky, T. L., & Garlinghouse, M. (2000). Functional assessment and intervention for challenging behaviors in the classroom by general classroom teachers. *Journal of Positive Behavior Interventions, 2,* 85–97.

Ervin, R. A., DuPaul, G. J., Kern, L., & Friman, P. C. (1998). Classroom-based functional and adjunctive assessments: Proactive approaches to intervention selection for adolescents with attention deficit hyperactivity disorder. *Journal of Applied Behavior Analysis, 31,* 65–78.

Fisher, W. W., Piazza, C., Cataldo, M., Harrell, R., Jefferson, G., & Conner, R. (1993). Functional communication training with and without extinction and punishment. *Journal of Applied Behavior Analysis, 26,* 23–36.

Hagopian, L. P., Fisher, W. W., Sullivan, M. T., Acquisto, J., & LeBlanc, L. A. (1998). Effectiveness of functional communication training with and without extinction and punishment. *Journal of Applied Behavior Analysis, 31,* 211–235.

Hanley, G. P., Iwata, B. A., & McCord, B. E. (2003). Functional analysis of problem behavior: A review. *Journal of Applied Behavior Analysis, 36,* 147–185.

Hanley, G. P., Piazza, C. C., Fisher, W. W., & Maglieri, K. A. (2005). On the effectiveness of and preference for punishment and extinction components of function-based interventions. *Journal of Applied Behavior Analysis, 38,* 51–65.

Himle, M. B., Miltenberger, R. G., Flessner, C., & Gatheridge, B. (2004). Teaching safety skills to children to prevent gun play. *Journal of Applied Behavior Analysis, 37,* 1–9.

Holland, T. (2011). The future for research in intellectual disabilities. *Journal of Intellectual Disability Research, 55,* 1–3.

Horner, R. H. (1994). Functional assessment: Contributions and future directions. *Journal of Applied Behavior Analysis, 27,* 401–404.

Ingram, K., Lewis-Palmer, T., & Sugai, G. (2005). Function-based intervention planning: Comparing the effectiveness of FBA function-based and non-function-based intervention plans. *Journal of Positive Behavior Interventions, 7,* 224–236.

Iwata, B. A., Dorsey, M. F., Slifer, K. J., Bauman, K. E., & Richman, G. S. (1994). Toward a functional analysis of self-injury. *Journal of Applied Behavior Analysis, 27,* 197–209 (Reprinted from *Analysis and Intervention in Developmental Disabilities, 2,* 3–20, 1982).

Iwata, B. A., Pace, G. M., Cowdery, G. E., & Miltenberger, R. G. (1994). What makes extinction work: An analysis of procedural form and function. *Journal of Applied Behavior Analysis, 27,* 131–144.

Individuals with Disabilities Education Improvement Act of 2004, Pub. L. No. 108-446 (2004).

Kendall, S. B. (1974). Preference for intermittent reinforcement. *Journal of the Experimental Analysis of Behavior, 21,* 463–473.

Kennedy, C. H., & Souza, G. (1995). Functional analysis and treatment of eye poking. *Journal of Applied Behavior Analysis, 28,* 27–37.

Kern, L., & Clemens, N. H. (2007). Antecedent strategies to promote appropriate classroom behavior. *Psychology in the Schools, 44,* 65–75.

Kern, L., Childs, K. E., Dunlap, G., Clarke, S., & Falk, G. D. (1994). Using assessment-based curricular intervention to improve the classroom behavior of a student with emotional and behavioral challenges. *Journal of Applied Behavior Analysis, 27,* 7–19.

Kodak, T., Northup, J., & Kelly, M. E. (2007). An evaluation of the types of attention that maintain problem behavior. *Journal of Applied Behavior Analysis, 40,* 167–171.

Kuhn, D. E., DeLeon, I. G., Fisher, W. W., & Wilke, A. E. (1999). Clarifying an ambiguous functional analysis with matched and mismatched extinction procedures. *Journal of Applied Behavior Analysis, 32,* 99–102.

Kurtz, P. F., Chin, M. D., Huete, J. M., Tarbox, R. S. F., O'Connor, J. T., Paclawsky, T. R., et al. (2003). Functional analysis and treatment of self-injurious behavior in young children: A summary of 30 cases. *Journal of Applied Behavior Analysis, 36*, 205–219.

Lerman, D. C., & Iwata, B. A. (1995). Prevalence of the extinction burst and its attenuation during treatment. *Journal of Applied Behavior Analysis, 28*, 93–94.

Lerman, D. C., Iwata, B. A., & Wallace, M. D. (1999). Side effects of extinction: Prevalence of bursting and aggression during the treatment of self-injurious behavior. *Journal of Applied Behavior Analysis, 32*, 1–8.

Lerman, D. C., & Vorndran, C. M. (2002). On the status of knowledge for using punishment: Implications for treating behavior disorders. *Journal of Applied Behavior Analysis, 35*, 431–464.

Lieving, G. A., Hagopian, L. P., Long, E. S., & O'Connor, J. (2004). Response-class hierarchies and resurgence of severe problem behavior. *The Psychological Record, 54*, 621–634.

Mace, F. C., & Belfiore, P. (1990). Behavioral momentum in the treatment of escape-motivated stereotypy. *Journal of Applied Behavior Analysis, 23*, 507–514.

Magee, S. K., & Ellis, J. (2000). Extinction effects during the assessment of multiple problem behaviors. *Journal of Applied Behavior Analysis, 33*, 313–316.

Matson, J. L., Mayville, S. B., & Laud, R. B. (2003). A system of assessment for adaptive behavior, social skills, behavioral function, medication side-effects, and psychiatric disorders. *Research in Developmental Disabilities, 24*, 75–81.

McCord, B. E., Thompson, R. J., & Iwata, B. A. (2001). Functional analysis and treatment of self-injury associated with transitions. *Journal of Applied Behavior Analysis, 34*, 195–210.

McLaren, E. M., & Nelson, C. M. (2009). Using functional behavior assessment to develop behavior interventions for students in Head Start. *Journal of Positive Behavior Interventions, 11*, 3–21.

Miltenberger, R. G. (2008). *Behavior modification: Principles and procedures* (4th ed.). Belmont: Thompson/Wadsworth.

Miltenberger, R. G., Flessner, C., Gatheridge, B. J., Satterlund, M., & Egemo, K. (2004). Evaluation of behavioral skills training to prevent gun play in children. *Journal of Applied Behavior Analysis, 37*, 513–516.

Moore, J. W., & Edwards, R. P. (2003). An analysis of aversive stimuli in classroom demand contexts. *Journal of Applied Behavior Analysis, 36*, 339–348.

Nahgahgwon, K. N., Umbreit, C., Liaupsin, C. J., & Turton, A. M. (2010). Function-based planning for young children at risk for emotional and behavioral disorders. *Education and Treatment of Children, 33*, 537–559.

Napolitano, D. A., Jack, S. L., Sheldon, J. B., Williams, D. C., McAdam, D. B., & Schroeder, S. R. (1999). Drug-behavior interactions in persons with mental retardation and developmental disabilities. *Mental Retardation and Developmental Disabilities Research and Reviews, 5*, 322–344.

Newcomer, L. L., & Lewis, T. J. (2004). Functional behavioral assessment: An investigation of assessment reliability and effectiveness of function-based interventions. *Journal of Emotional and Behavioral Disorders, 12*, 168–181.

Northup, J., Fussilier, I., Swanson, V., & Borrero, J. (1997). An evaluation of methylphenidate as a potential establishing operation for some common classroom reinforcers. *Journal of Applied Behavior Analysis, 30*, 615–625.

O'Neill, R. E., Horner, R. H., Albin, R. W., Sprague, J. R., Storey, K., & Newton, J. S. (1997). *Functional assessment and program development for problem behavior: A practical handbook* (2nd ed.). Pacific Grove: Brooks/Cole.

O'Reilly, M. F., Lacey, C., & Lancioni, G. E. (2000). Assessment of the influence of background noise on escape-maintained problem behavior and pain behavior in a child with Williams syndrome. *Journal of Applied Behavior Analysis, 33*, 511–514.

Patel, D. R., Pratt, H. D., & Patel, N. D. (2008). Team processes and team care for children with developmental disabilities. *Pediatric Clinics of North America, 55*, 1375–1390.

Pelios, L., Morren, J., Tesch, D., & Axelrod, S. (1999). The impact of functional analysis methodology on treatment choice for self-injurious and aggressive behavior. *Journal of Applied Behavior Analysis, 32*, 185–195.

Peterson, F. M., & Martens, B. K. (1995). A comparison of behavioral interventions reported in treatment studies and programs for adults with developmental disabilities. *Research in Developmental Disabilities, 16*, 27–41.

Piazza, C. C., Adelinis, J. D., Hanley, G. P., Goh, H., & Delia, M. D. (2000). An evaluation of the effects of matched stimuli on behaviors maintained by automatic reinforcement. *Journal of Applied Behavior Analysis, 33*, 13–27.

Piazza, C. C., Moes, D. R., & Fisher, W. W. (1996). Differential reinforcement of alternative behavior and demand fading in the treatment of escape-maintained destructive behavior. *Journal of Applied Behavior Analysis, 29*, 569–572.

Sarakoff, R. A., & Sturmey, P. (2004). The effects of behavioral skills training on staff implementation of discrete-trial teaching. *Journal of Applied Behavior Analysis, 37*, 535–538.

Scott, T. M., McIntyre, J., Liaupsin, C., Nelson, M., Conroy, M., & Payne, L. D. (2005). An examination of the relationship between functional behavior assessment and selected intervention. *Journal of Positive Behavior Interventions, 7*, 205–215.

Stenhoff, D. M., Davey, B. J., & Linugaris/Kraft, B. (2008). The effects of choice on assignment completion and percent correct by a high school student with a learning disability. *Education and treatment of Children, 31*, 203–211.

Sugai, G., Lewis-Palmer, T., & Hagan, S. (1998). Using functional assessments to develop behavior support plans. *Preventing School Failure, 43*, 6–13.

Thompson, R. H., & Iwata, B. A. (2007). A comparison of outcomes from descriptive and functional analysis of problem behavior. *Journal of Applied Behavior Analysis, 40*, 33–338.

Umbreit, J., Ferro, J., Liaupsin, C., & Lane, K. (2007). *Functional behavioral assessment and function-based intervention: An effective, practical approach.* Upper Saddle River: Prentice-Hall.

Underwood, M. A., Umbreit, J., & Liaupsin, C. (2009). Efficacy of a systematic process for designing function-based interventions for adults in a community setting. *Education and Training in Developmental Disabilities, 44*, 25–38.

Van Houten, R., Axelrod, S., Bailey, J. S., Favell, J. E., Foxx, R. N., Iwata, B. A., et al. (1988). The right to effective behavioral treatment. *The Behavior Analyst, 11*, 111–114.

Vollmer, T. R., Iwata, B. A., Zarcone, J. R., Smith, R. G., & Mazaleski, J. L. (1993). The role of attention in the treatment of attention-maintained self-injurious behavior: Noncontingent reinforcement and differential reinforcement of other behavior. *Journal of Applied Behavior Analysis, 26*, 9–21.

Wood, A. L., Luiselli, J. K., & Harchik, A. E. (2007). Training instructional skills with paraprofessional service providers at a community-based habilitation setting. *Behavior Modification, 31*, 847–855.

Wood, B. K., Ferro, J., Umbreit, J., & Liaupsin, C. J. (2011). Addressing the challenging behavior of young children through systematic function-based intervention. *Topics in Early Childhood Special Education, 30*, 221–232.

Worsdell, A. S., Iwata, B. A., Hanley, G. P., Thompson, R. H., & Kahng, S. W. (2000). Effects of continuous and intermittent reinforcement for problem behavior during functional communication training. *Journal of Applied Behavior Analysis, 33*, 167–179.

Ethical Issues and Considerations

13

Alan Poling, Jennifer L. Austin,
Stephanie M. Peterson, Amanda Mahoney,
and Marc Weeden

Functional behavioral assessment (FBA) refers to a range of methods designed to identify the environmental variables that control problematic behaviors. Methods for revealing these variables include indirect measures, such as interviews and questionnaires, or direct methods, such as narrative recording of the antecedents that precede responses of interest and the consequences that follow them. Many behavior analysts believe that the "gold standard" of FBA is experimental functional analysis (FA) (Iwata, Dorsey, Slifer, Bauman, & Richmond, 1982/1994), which systematically arranges consequences for problem behaviors to identify their functions, that is, the reinforcers that maintain those behaviors. FBA is one of several ways of collecting information about clients, and professional organizations such as the American Psychological Association (APA) and the Behavior Analyst Certification Board (BACB) have established general ethical guidelines regarding how assessments should be conducted and interpreted. For example, Standard 9 of the *Ethical Principles of Psychologists and Code of Conduct* promulgated by the APA (2010) is devoted entirely to assessment. The same is true of Standard 3.0 of the *Behavior Analyst Certification Board Guidelines for Responsible Conduct (BACB Guidelines, BACB, 2011).* That standard is presented in Table 13.1. Any practitioner who abides with the standards established there and elsewhere in the *Guidelines* is therefore behaving ethically, regardless of whether he or she is involved in functional assessment or another professional activity.

Because FBA can be an integral part of effective treatment, as other chapters in this book clearly illustrate, including it in treatment planning is ethical conduct. This perspective is evident in standard 3.02 of the current *BACB Guidelines* (BACB, 2011), which states: "The behavior analyst conducts a functional assessment, as defined below, to provide the necessary data to develop an effective behavior change program."

A. Poling (✉) • S.M. Peterson • A. Mahoney
Department of Psychology, Western Michigan University, Kalamazoo, MI 49008-5439, USA
e-mail: alan.poling@wmich.edu;
stephanie.peterson@wmich.edu;
mahoney.am@gmail.com

J.L. Austin
School of Psychology, University of Glamorgan, Pontypridd, CF37 1DL, UK
e-mail: jlaustin@glam.ac.uk

M. Weeden
Department of Psychology, Western Michigan University, Kalamazoo, MI 49008-5439, USA

Department of Special Education and Literacy Studies, Western Michigan University, Kalamazoo, MI 49008, USA
e-mail: marc.a.weeden@wmich.edu

J.L. Matson (ed.), *Functional Assessment for Challenging Behaviors,*
Autism and Child Psychopathology Series, DOI 10.1007/978-1-4614-3037-7_13,
© Springer Science+Business Media, LLC 2012

Table 13.1 Guidelines for responsible conduct with respect to assessing behavior[a]

3.0 Assessing behavior

Behavior analysts who use behavioral assessment techniques do so for purposes that are appropriate in light of research.

(a) Behavior analysts' assessments, recommendations, reports, and evaluative statements are based on information and techniques sufficient to provide appropriate substantiation for their findings.

(b) Behavior analysts refrain from misuse of assessment techniques, interventions, results, and interpretations and take reasonable steps to prevent others from misusing the information these techniques provide.

(c) Behavior analysts recognize limits to the certainty with which judgments or predictions can be made about individuals.

(d) Behavior analysts do not promote the use of behavioral assessment techniques by unqualified persons, i.e., those who are unsupervised by experienced professionals and have not demonstrated valid and reliable assessment skills.

3.01 Behavioral assessment approval

The behavior analyst must obtain the client's or client-surrogate's approval in writing of the behavior assessment procedures before implementing them. As used here, client-surrogate refers to someone legally empowered to make decisions for the person(s) whose behavior the program is intended to change; examples of client-surrogates include parents of minors, guardians, and legally designated representatives

3.02 Functional assessment

(a) The behavior analyst conducts a functional assessment, as defined below, to provide the necessary data to develop an effective behavior change program.

(b) Functional assessment includes a variety of systematic information-gathering activities regarding factors influencing the occurrence of a behavior (e.g., antecedents, consequences, setting events, or motivating operations) including interview, direct observation, and experimental analysis.

3.03 Explaining assessment results

Unless the nature of the relationship is clearly explained to the person being assessed in advance and precludes provision of an explanation of results (such as in some organizational consultation, some screenings, and forensic evaluations), behavior analysts ensure that an explanation of the results is provided using language that is reasonably understandable to the person assessed or to another legally authorized person on behalf of the client. Regardless of whether the interpretation is done by the behavior analyst, by assistants, or others, behavior analysts take reasonable steps to ensure that appropriate explanations of results are given.

[a]Published by the Behavior Analysis Certification Board (2011) in the *Behavior Analyst Certification Board Guidelines for Responsible Conduct* and reproduced by permission

It is, however, true that one can easily envision situations in which specific applications of FBA raise interesting ethical questions, as in the hypothetical case 3.02B presented by Bailey and Burch (2011) in a book devoted entirely to ethics for behavior analysts. In this case, the issue is whether an FA is necessary in situations where the person engages in self-injury, particularly when informal assessment methods have not led to an effective intervention. On the face of it, it appears that further discussion of the ethics of FBA, in general, and of FA, in particular, is merited. The purpose of this chapter is to initiate such discussion and to provide some general guidelines for ethical FBA. Our goal is not to dictate what is the right or wrong course in any one of the many decisions that must be made throughout the FBA process. Instead, we aim to identify applications of the analysis procedures that can give rise to important questions that behavior analysts should consider carefully. We begin our discussion with considerations regarding what might be considered "traditional" uses of FA; in other words, using FA to identify maintaining variables for self-injurious behavior (SIB) of individuals with developmental disabilities. We then discuss additional ethical considerations when expanding FBA to a broader range of populations and settings, using school-based FBA as an exemplar.

Special Considerations Regarding FA

Since the technique was first described by Iwata et al. (1982/1994), FA has been widely used to isolate controlling variables for self-injury and other challenging behaviors exhibited by people with intellectual and other developmental disabilities (e.g., Hanley, Iwata, McCord, 2003;; Hastings & Noone, 2005). Essentially, the procedure involves the systematic delivery of stimuli after the occurrence of problem behavior, whereby one of more of those stimuli is assumed to function as reinforcers. Decisions about functions of behavior are made by comparing rates of responding across different conditions. Those conditions that result in the highest rates of behavior are assumed to reveal the reinforcers for those behaviors. However, because it requires targeted behaviors to occur undercontrolled circumstances, FA in particular poses special ethical considerations.

FA and the Primum non Nocere Principle

The so-called Hippocratic injunction to first do no harm [in Latin, primum non nocere] has long been an axiom central to the education of medical and graduate students in the helping professions (Smith, 2005). Likewise, behavior analysts have a fundamental responsibility to not harm their clients or to allow harm to occur under their watch (Bailey & Burch, 2011). Iwata and his colleagues (1982/1994) were careful to uphold this principle in their seminal description of FA of SIB. In brief, Iwata et al. arranged five test conditions in an analogue setting to determine the conditions under which SIB regularly occurred, hence the variables that appeared to control such responding. They pointed out that the possibility of participants seriously injuring themselves during the assessment of controlling variables was a real concern. They were very careful to arrange protections to prevent this from occurring and they described those protections clearly and in detail. In fact, their article contains a section entitled "Human Subjects Protection" that comprises 56 lines. In it, Iwata and his colleagues indicated that procedures were approved by a human subjects committee (i.e., an Institutional Review Board, IRB), individuals who were at risk of severe physical harm were excluded from participation, and all potential participants received a complete medical exam, with neurological, audiological, and visual evaluations as appropriate "to assess current physical status and to rule out organic factors that might be associated with or exacerbated by self-injury" (p. 199). Criteria for terminating sessions were established through consultation with a physician. The physician or a nurse observed sessions intermittently to assess whether termination criteria needed to be adjusted. If termination criteria were met, participants were immediately removed from the therapy room and evaluated by a physician or nurse, who determined whether the sessions would continue. After every fourth session, each participant was examined by a nurse. Finally, each case was reviewed at least weekly both in departmental case conferences and in interdisciplinary rounds. Using safeguards such as those arranged by Iwata et al. and limiting the number and length of sessions to the minimum required to provide useful information minimizes harm to participants during FA.

Despite the possibility that harmful behavior will be temporarily reinforced (and thus increased) during FA sessions, it is important to point out that a properly conducted FA does not increase the risk of harm to participants relative to that they encounter in their everyday environment, a point made by Iwata et al. (1982/1994) in their seminal article. If it is ethically acceptable for a target behavior, such as SIB, to occur outside FA sessions, then the same should be true within such sessions, although safeguards to prevent serious harm might be required. Interestingly, published studies rarely mention such safeguards. Of 116 articles describing the FA of SIB recently reviewed by Weeden, Mahoney, and Poling (2010), 9 (7.7%) described session termination criteria and 23 (19.8%) described other procedural safeguards for reducing risk to participants. As Weeden et al. pointed out, it is possible, even probable, that appropriate safeguards to prevent harm to participants were in place in the other studies but were not described. Nevertheless, it is important for those implementing functional analysis procedures to consider the potential importance of having in place structured termination criteria and safeguards in place to protect individuals engaged in FAs.

Institutional Review Boards and Informed Consent

Having research approved by a Human Subjects Institutional Review Board is one way to ensure that procedures are ethically sound (Bailey & Burch, 2011), but only six of the articles (5%) reviewed by Weeden et al. (2010) indicated that such approval was obtained. Another safeguard is securing written informed consent. Section 3.01 in the *BACB Guidelines* (BACB, 2011) states that:

> The behavior analyst must obtain the client's or client-surrogate's approval in writing of the behavior assessment procedures before implementing them. As used here, client-surrogate refers to someone legally empowered to make decisions for the person(s) whose behavior the program is intended to change; examples of client-surrogates include parents of minors, guardians, and legally designated representatives

Although this datum was not reported by Weeden et al. (2010), only one of the 116 studies they evaluated (0.8%) specified that clients (or their surrogates) had provided written informed consent. Based on the information provided, one must presume that no harm was done in most of these studies. In fact, Weeden et al. assumed that protections generally were adequate and were careful not to accuse researchers of unethical conduct. They wrote:

> The present findings in no way suggest that FA procedures as arranged in studies of SIB are ethically or otherwise questionable. It is for that reason that we do not cite specific studies when making the case that high levels of SIB were sometimes present across many sessions with no safeguards reported. These findings do, however, clearly suggest that important information about safeguards arranged to protect participants is not included in many articles. If safeguards, such as criteria for terminating sessions and excluding participants, are in place—and we assume that

they are—describing them precisely and concisely would be easy. If safeguards are not in place, some explanation may be appropriate. We encourage authors of future articles to ensure, first and foremost, that the protections they arrange to prevent serious harm to participants are in fact adequate and to ensure as well that readers of those articles have sufficient information to evaluate and, if desired, to replicate those safeguards. We also encourage editors of relevant journals to require them to do so before their work is published. FA is an invaluable tool and these actions are suggested not to criticize what has been done in the past, but rather to improve that which is done in the future. (p. 302)

These recommendations appear prudent and we endorse them. From a methodological standpoint, however, it is important to note that the use of protective equipment could potentially alter the results of an FA. For example, Le and Smith (2002) found that FA of the SIB of three participants yielded different results when they did and did not wear protective equipment. When protective equipment was worn, very little SIB occurred and no clear functions were revealed. In the absence of protective equipment, however, SIB appeared to be maintained by negative reinforcement (escape from demands in one participant and escape from a wheel chair in a second participant) in two participants and by nonsocial (i.e., automatic) reinforcement in the third. Although other studies using FA have revealed clear functions in the presence of protective equipment (e.g., Iwata, Pace, Cowdery, & Miltenberger, 1994; Mace & Knight, 1986), the findings of Le and Smith call attention to the need to consider whether inconclusive FA results might be the result of protective equipment or other participant safeguards, such as very conservative session termination criteria that might prevent the collection of adequate data, and, if so, whether those safeguards could be safely and ethically withdrawn. Such decisions should be made by an informed team of individuals that includes a legal representative of, and an advocate for, the participant.

This example is an illustration of why there are not clear answers to questions as to the "right" and "wrong" course of action during an FA. While it may be considered "right" to include protective equipment in the analysis to protect the clients from harm during the analysis, if doing so calls into question the validity of the obtained results, then the inclusion of protective equipment may be less "right." The questions of if, when, and how protective equipment should be included in an FA is one the behavior analyst should be carefully consider before commencing an FA.

Brief FA and Harm Reduction

Because of the potential to strengthen harmful behavior temporarily during an FA, minimizing occurrences of the target behavior to the lowest number (and intensity) adequate to reveal controlling variables is an ethically sound goal. Brief FA (Northup et al., 1991) is one way to accomplish this goal. Brief FA is a modification to traditional FA procedures in which clients participate in fewer, truncated sessions and fewer types of sessions rather than the traditional five (alone, escape, control, tangible, and attention) described by Iwata et al. (1982/1994). Studies have shown that brief FAs are robust and can provide meaningful information about the variables that control target responses. For example, Kahng and Iwata (1999) compared data from 50 traditional FAs (35 with clear response patterns and 15 undifferentiated) with data from brief FAs constructed by isolating the first session of each condition from the rest of the complete analyses. They concluded that brief FA and within-session analysis (the examination of response rates within the isolated sessions to uncover within-session trends which may be obscured by overall session average) yielded results comparable to those of more lengthy evaluations in 66 and 68% of cases, respectively. Further analysis of the data revealed correspondence between brief and traditional methods in 27 of the 35 data sets (77%) where a function was clearly identified. However, it is important to note that when full FA outcomes were undifferentiated, correspondence for the within-session analysis was substantially higher (80% vs. 40%) than for the brief procedures.

More recently, another type of brief FA, termed *trial-based* FA, has gained considerable empirical support (e.g., Bloom, Iwata, Fritz, Roscoe, & Carreau, 2011; LaRue et al., 2010; Sigafoos & Saggers, 1995; Wallace & Knights, 2003; Wilder, Chen, Atwell, Pritchard, & Weinstein, 2006). Trial-based FAs involve comparing brief test conditions [motivational operation (MO) present] with control conditions (MO absent) of the same length. Trial-based FAs have the potential to yield the same results as extended FAs, thus reducing the time spent engaging in harmful behavior during the assessment. For example, Wallace and Knights (2003) compared the results of trial-based FA with extended FA and found that results were the same for two of the three participants. Further, they reported that the brief evaluations took an average of 36 min to complete, whereas the extended procedures took an average of 310 min (an 88.4% difference in session time). More recently, LaRue et al. (2010) found exact correspondence across trial-based and traditional FA models for the problem behaviors (e.g., aggression, self-injury, disruption, and inappropriate vocalization) of four of five participants, with partial correspondence obtained for the fifth participant. The authors also reported that traditional procedures took an average of 208 session minutes to complete, whereas the trial-based analysis took an average of only 31.6 (an 84.8% difference). Bloom et al. (2011) conducted their analyses in a more naturalistic classroom setting and found correspondence in six of the ten analyses they compared (with partial correspondence on a 7th case). However, their results revealed more modest savings in assessment time (271 min for traditional FA and 233 min for trial-based FA; a 14% difference).

Another potentially viable brief assessment technique involves measuring latency to the first response. In this arrangement, the participant is presented with conditions that resemble a typical FA, but the session ends following the first instance of problem behavior, and the latency to the problem behavior across conditions is measured. Call, Pabico, and Lomas (2009) compared results of a demand condition only latency FA and a standard FA with two participants who exhibited SIB and disruptive behavior. The latency FA yielded a hierarchy of demand aversiveness based on the latency to the first problem behavior. During subsequent functional analyses, the shorter latency demands produced more differentiated outcomes. Thomason-Sassi, Iwata, Neidert, and Roscoe (2011) conducted retrospective analyses of 38 FA data sets, in which data were graphed first as response rates (or, if appropriate, percentage of intervals) across sessions and secondly as latency to respond to the first target response within a session. Eighty six percent of the cases showed a high degree of correspondence between the two types of response measurement. Further, ten newly conducted FAs in which both traditional and latency analyses were performed showed correspondence in nine out of ten cases. These results suggest that latency may be a viable measure of responding in situations where repeated occurrences of behavior are dangerous or when response opportunities are limited. Despite these promising results, however, research on latency FA is currently somewhat limited. More research is needed to draw firm conclusions about the utility of this method.

Regardless of the particular method, brief, trial-based, and latency-to-first response functional analyses necessarily expose participants to fewer sessions or session types (e.g., Barretto, Wacker, Harding, Lee, & Berg, 2006; LaRue et al., 2010; Northup et al., 1991) and/or sessions of shorter duration (e.g., Barretto et al.; Kahng & Iwata, 1999; LaRue et al.; Northup et al.; Wallace & Iwata, 1999) than conventional FA. As a result, these forms of FA may limit opportunities to engage in harmful responses, reduce the likelihood that new topographies of harmful responses will occur, and make it unlikely that delivering putative reinforcers (e.g., attention and tangible items) will significantly strengthen target responses. Moreover, these forms of FA offer the possibility of quickly ascertaining the variables that control a targeted response and using this information to develop an effective intervention. All of these considerations are positive and a strong case can be made that from an ethical perspective these forms of FA are preferred to traditional functional assessment, whenever possible. It may be advisable to begin with more brief

forms of FA to identify behavioral function and to only proceed to the more traditional model when behavioral function cannot be identified by these methods (Vollmer, Marcus, Ringdahl, & Roane, 1995).

FA and Right to Effective Treatment

Behavior analysts strongly agree that their clients have a right to effective treatment (Van Houten et al., 1988). Inherent in this principle is the right to a treatment that is both appropriate and timely. A potential ethical issue with any form of FBA, but one especially likely to emerge when traditional FA is used, is that treatment is not designed and implemented until assessment is finished, which can require many hours or even days (Vollmer & Smith, 1996). Behavior analytic practitioners, as well as researchers, should consider whether time is better spent designing and evaluating an intervention based on other forms of FBA data (e.g., brief FA or descriptive analysis) or on collecting extensive FA data in the hope of eventually developing a superior intervention. In reality, it is likely that many practitioners do not have the time or resources needed to conduct an extensive experimental analysis of the variables that control a target behavior; they will of necessity prioritize assessing treatment effects, not accessing the functions of the target behavior. In our view, this strategy is defensible from both ethical and practical perspectives. In truth, behavior analysts use a relatively small number of behavior-change strategies and interventions formulated with and without FA data are often comparable (Schill, Kratochwill, & Elliott, 1998). FA, like FBA in general, is a useful tool but it can easily be overused. Moreover, FA that does not lead to an effective intervention does not benefit participants. More than a few published studies involving the FA of SIB do not even describe an intervention, but instead focus on delineating controlling variables per se. Such work is at best incomplete. In our view, the best (and most ethical) FA research delineates controlling variables, designs an intervention that takes those variables into account, and demonstrates that the intervention produces clinically significant changes in target behavior(s) in the participant's everyday environment, not just in short experimental sessions.

Issues in Expanding the Use of FBA Across Settings and Populations

FBA and Best Practice

Since its inception, FBA has been used to identify controlling variables for a range of problem behaviors in various populations and settings (Hanley et al., 2003). In 1991, a National Institutes of Health (NIH) consensus panel identified FA as a "best practice" for designing behavioral interventions for individuals with developmental disabilities. The value assigned to FBA in more recent years is evident in federal legislation dealing with the education of students with disabilities. When the Individuals with Disabilities Education Act (*IDEA*, P.L. 105–117) was reauthorized in 1997, FBA was specifically mandated for certain students. IDEA states:

> The [Individualized Education Program, IEP] team must address through a behavioral intervention plan any need for positive behavioral strategies and supports. In response to disciplinary actions by school personnel, the IEP team must within 10 days meet to develop a *functional behavioral assessment plan* [italics added] to collect information. This information should be used for developing or reviewing and revising an existing behavior intervention plan to address such behaviors. In addition, states are required to address the in-service needs of personnel (including professionals and paraprofessionals who provide special education, general education, related services, or early intervention services) as they relate to developing and implementing positive intervention strategies.

This mandate was retained in a second reauthorization, the Individuals with Disabilities Education Improvement Act of 2004 (P.L. 108–446), which states that whenever a child's educational placement is to be changed because of a violation of a code of student conduct, the IEP team must "conduct an FBA and develop a behavioral intervention plan for such child." Moreover, "a child with a disability who is removed from the child's current [educational] placement [because of a code violation] shall receive, as appropriate, a functional behavior assessment, behavioral intervention services, and modifications, that are designed to address the behavior so that it does not recur."

When FBA is applied in school settings, it is often applied across a wide range of problem behaviors and across a wide range of populations—reaching far beyond the population for which the methodology was originally pioneered (i.e., individuals with developmental disabilities in a highly controlled settings). The mandate set forth in IDEA required that FBAs be applied to a wide range of topographies of problem behavior other than self-injury, including aggression, noncompliance, off-task behavior, bullying, and bringing weapons to school, as these behaviors may all result in a placement change for an individual with disabilities.

Moreover, in addition to its being required by federal law in some instances, there is a growing consensus that FBA is in general "best practice" in developing behavioral interventions in school settings (e.g., Gresham, Watson, & Skinner, 2001; Steege & Watson, 2008), as well as a number of other settings, such as community mental health. For purposes of this discussion, we will focus on the application of FBA to school settings. One reason for the "best practice" view is that several authors have suggested conducting FBAs prior to selecting school-based intervention selection will produce better treatment outcomes than selecting interventions with no FBA data (e.g., Asmus, Vollmer, & Borrero, 2002; Crone & Horner, 2000; Vollmer & Northup, 1996). Given that "best" practices are (or should be) evidence-based, one would expect there are compelling data clearly showing that interventions based on FBAs are significantly superior to alternative interventions across a range of behaviors and educational settings. Reviewing the existing literature for school-based FBA, however, does not necessarily support such a simple and strong conclusion.

FBA in School Settings: Best Practice?

Despite the wealth of studies that employ FBA prior to designing treatments (for reviews, see Ervin et al., 2001; Hanley et al., 2003), few school-based studies *directly* compare function-based interventions to those selected without the benefit of FBA data. Several studies appear to support the use of FBA prior to intervention in school settings. However, some of the studies have produced conflicting results.

Much of the data confirming the effectiveness of function-based interventions have come from studies that evaluated the relative effectiveness of a given intervention when applied to behaviors maintained by different kinds of consequences (i.e., operant responses with different functions). For example, Taylor and Miller (1997) compared the effectiveness of time-out interventions with children whose problem behaviors were maintained by attention and with children whose problem behaviors were maintained by escape. Time-out generally was effective for attention-maintained behaviors but not for escape-maintained behaviors. In a similar but more complicated study, Meyer (1999) evaluated the effects of two interventions, one that allowed children to access assistance with tasks and a second that allowed children to access praise for working. Those children identified in an initial FA phase as exhibiting higher levels of problematic behavior in the presence of difficult tasks (regardless of the frequency of praise) responded more positively to the treatment that taught them how to recruit help appropriately. In contrast, those children whose behaviors were maintained by adult attention (regardless of task difficulty) exhibited fewer problem behaviors when taught to recruit praise. In a third study, Romaniuk et al. (2002) demonstrated that children whose behaviors were maintained by attention were less likely to benefit from choice-making interventions than those whose behaviors were maintained by escape. For the latter group of children, reductions in target behaviors were not observed until the implementation of differential reinforcement for on-task behavior. These studies and others (e.g., Carr & Durand, 1985) suggest that certain

interventions will be effective only if the target behaviors are maintained by specific kinds of reinforcers.

In the studies just described, the researchers implemented one or two general interventions across participants whose target behaviors were maintained by different kinds of events. Another strategy for illustrating the importance of FBA in developing effective interventions is to compare the effects of interventions based specifically on known functions with those of similar interventions without those specific components. This tack was taken by Ingram, Lewis-Palmer, and Sugai (2005) in a study in which relevant antecedents and consequences affecting the behavior of two boys in middle school initially were determined via informant and descriptive assessments. Following the FBA, two behavior intervention plans were designed for each child. One plan was designed to address specific variables identified in the FBA (e.g., task difficulty, escape from demands), whereas a second, similar plan omitted key elements related to function. Interventions were then rated by two experts not associated with the study for technical adequacy (i.e., level of research support for the intervention components) and match to hypothesis (i.e., how well the intervention addressed variables identified in the FBA). Technical adequacy was deemed to be high for both types of interventions. Match to hypothesis was rated higher for both function-based interventions as compared to their non-function-based counterparts. When the interventions were implemented, results clearly showed that problematic behaviors were less frequent under function-based interventions as compared to those that did not address relevant environmental events.

In a related study, Newcomer and Lewis (2004) compared the effects of function-based and non-function-based treatments on the behaviors of three elementary school students. Hypotheses about maintaining variables for the target behaviors were constructed using descriptive and experimental analyses. Following completion of the FBA, each child was exposed to a non-function-based intervention followed by a function-based intervention in a multiple baseline design. For all students, problematic behaviors were as high as or higher than baseline when non-function-based interventions were used. When the function-based treatment was introduced, problematic behaviors decreased immediately for two of the children and more gradually for the third. Ellingson, Miltenberger, Stricker, Galensky, and Garlinghouse (2000) also compared interventions based on hypothesized functions to those targeting a different function than that revealed by informant and descriptive assessments. For one of the three participants, results revealed that the function-based intervention was superior to the non-function-based alternative in reducing problematic behavior. Results were less compelling for the remaining participants, but suggested that the function-based interventions were more effective.

Although these direct comparison studies appear to suggest that function-based interventions produce more favorable outcomes that non-function-based treatments in school settings, a few methodological cautions are warranted. In each of the three studies just described (Ellingson et al., 2000; Ingram et al., 2005; Newcomer & Lewis, 2004), the non-function-based treatments for some of the participants included components that were contraindicated by the FBAs. Specifically, baseline and nonfunctional treatment conditions in Ellingson et al.'s study reinforced problem behavior using stimuli that the FBA suggested maintained those behaviors (i.e., teacher attention). Likewise, one of the children in Newcomer and Lewis's study engaged in behaviors that appeared to be maintained by escape from peer interactions. During the non-function-based treatment, the child was exposed to a dependent group contingency that effectively put him in closer contact with his peers. It is, therefore, not surprising that his behavior worsened during the implementation of the intervention, as it occasioned more opportunities for escape. Similarly, Ingram and her colleagues used teacher ignoring as part of the non-function-based treatment package for a behavior maintained by escape from demands.

As suggested by Iwata et al. (1994), extinction interventions based on form instead of function can potentially make problems worse. If the strategies compared to FBA-informed treatments reinforce responses targeted for reduction or increase their probabilities in other ways, it is not surprising that function-based strategies would prove more effective. Granted, it is possible that these authors intentionally used interventions contraindicated by the FBAs in an attempt to approximate the relatively common error among school personnel of using interventions that are based on form, not function (Vollmer & Northup, 1996). It is unclear, however, whether the outcomes would have been the same if the comparison interventions had not reinforced problem behavior.

Most investigations within this limited literature suggest that function-based interventions produce better treatment outcomes, but the findings are not universally positive. For instance, Schill et al. (1998) compared treatments based on FBAs to standard treatment packages (i.e., those developed without a preceding assessment of relevant antecedents and consequences of behavior). Nineteen children in Head Start who displayed persistent problem behaviors were randomly assigned to one of two groups. Teachers of children in Group 1 met with trained consultants to functionally assess problem behaviors and develop interventions based on hypothesized functions (functional approach). Teachers of children in Group 2 met with trained consultants to describe the topography of problem behaviors (technological approach). Behaviors were classified as externalizing (e.g., aggression, noncompliance) or internalizing (e.g., social withdrawal), and then Group 2 teachers were given a self-help manual that described strategies for intervening with both categories of behaviors. Analysis of effect sizes between groups revealed no significant differences between function- and non-function-based treatments; both types of interventions were equally effective. It is important to note, however, that one potential reason there were no significant differences between treatments is that the interventions used in the two conditions were often identical. For example, differential reinforcement, goal-setting, and praise featured prominently as intervention components in both the functional and techno-logical approaches. Failure to observe significant differences in treatment outcomes potentially could be accounted for by the inadvertent use of function-based treatments in the technological condition. Because function was not assessed for the children in the technological group, it is impossible to discern whether the treatments selected for those children did or did not address functions of behaviors.

Given the extant literature, drawing strong conclusions regarding the utility of conducting FBAs prior to designing school-based interventions for problem behavior is somewhat difficult. One reason for this difficulty is that the database is relatively sparse and based primarily on small n research designs. This is not to suggest that single-case designs cannot reveal phenomena that hold widely, but only to emphasize that to do so requires sufficient replications of their results. As of yet, the data are simply too limited to draw firm conclusions. Further, and importantly, Gresham et al.'s (2004) review of 150 school-based intervention studies published in the *Journal of Applied Behavior Analysis* over a 9-year period (1991–1999) revealed that treat-ments preceded by FBAs were no more effective than those in which FBAs were absent (or at least not reported). Blakeslee, Sugai, and Gruba (1994) found a similar pattern across intervention stud-ies reported over a wider range of settings in journals considered to be primarily or exclusively behavior analytic in nature.

Limitations within the existing literature lead to the conclusion that a good deal more research is needed to provide a firm empirical base for the use of FBAs prior to school-based treatment planning. This is not to suggest that FBAs should not be used in school settings. It is, however, a call to researchers to conduct additional studies in the utility of school-based FBA to broaden our literature base and the evidence upon which best practices can be made. Specifically, investiga-tions that directly compare interventions indi-cated, contraindicated, and unrelated to behavioral function should be conducted to assess the relative effectiveness and efficiency of different intervention approaches. Comparisons of function-based interventions to alternative interventions commonly used in school settings and favored by teachers (e.g., token economies) and often imple-mented without the benefit of a FBA would be of particular practical value. In all comparisons, it is essential that a legitimate attempt is made to develop maximally effective interventions and to ensure that those interventions are implemented with sufficient integrity. Until further research is conducted, in our view there are not sufficient data to conclude with confidence that interven-tions tied to FBA are always, or even typically, more effective than alternative interventions for reducing undesired target behaviors in school settings.

To say this is not to disparage FBA or to deny its usefulness, but it is to suggest that if taken lit-erally to imply that behavior analysts working in school settings must *always* conduct FBA before developing an intervention, then Standard 3.02 of the current *BACB Guidelines* (BACB, 2011) is inconsistent with Standard 1.01, which reads: "Behavior analysts rely on scientifically and pro-fessionally derived knowledge when making scientific or professional judgments in human service provision, or when engaging in scholarly or professional endeavors." In fact, there may be several instances where an FBA is simply not warranted for effective intervention, and in these cases, ethical conduct might involve behavioral interventions that are *not* preceded by an FBA.

Effective Intervention in the Absence of FBA

Research data and our professional experience certainly indicate that FBA can play an invalu-able role in developing effective treatments for reducing undesired behavior in school settings. But they also indicate that FBA is not always needed. Consider, for example, a situation in which a behavior analyst is called in to help a special education teacher develop an interven-tion that the teacher can use to reduce the disrup-tive behavior of students to acceptable levels. The consultant's first visit to the classroom reveals that the teacher lacks basic behavior management skills. Clear rules for appropriate student conduct are lacking as are meaningful consequences for inappropriate or appropriate behavior. Activities are poorly organized and the overall impression is one of chaos. In such a situation, FBA is not a pressing priority. Regardless of the variables that control the undesired behaviors of the students, establishing effective strategies for general classroom management is the obvious first step and a prerequisite to reducing disruptive behavior.

The same can occur when consulting with individuals with developmental disabilities. For example, consider another example we recently experienced. One of the authors was asked to provide an FA for a 26-year-old young man who was reported to engage in elopement from his home and aggression toward his mother. Upon the behavior analyst's first visit to the home, the behavior analyst learned that the young man was only allowed out of his house for therapy 6 h per week. During these times, he displayed appropriate behavior in the community and never eloped. The rest of the week he was required to stay in his house, because no services were available, and his mother did not feel she could handle him in the community. She also did not allow him in the yard, because he often eloped from the yard. Observations within the home revealed a rather sterile environment, For example, all of the cupboards were locked to keep him from getting into them. Rather than conducting an FA, the behavior analyst focused on identifying ways to increase the client's access to community activities, as it was hypothesized that this would decrease the motivation for elopement and addressed an underlying problem of limited services that resulted in the client's restricted access to functional activities. In addition, the behavioral intervention focused on teaching him skills he could use to be even more successful in the community.

Good interventions are those which produce desired and lasting effects, and ethical professional conduct comprises actions that lead to such interventions, regardless of how the interventions are selected or their modality (Poling, 1994; Poling, Ehrhardt, Wood, & Bowerman, 2010). In our view, in interpreting standard 3.02 of the

current *BACB Guidelines,* "the behavior analyst conducts a functional assessment … to provide the necessary data to develop an effective behavior change program," it is important to acknowledge that "the necessary data" sometimes means limited if any FBA data. FBA is a useful tool, not a panacea, for improving the behavior of school children. The same is true with respect to other populations, where studies similar to those conducted in schools suggest that treatments tied to FBA data generally are more successful than alternative treatments (Carr et al., 1999; 2009; Kurtz et al., 2003), although it is beyond our purpose to review the relevant data. Given the extant literature, in our opinion the widespread use of FBA is easily justified on both ethical and practical grounds, but it is inappropriate to elevate its use to an ethical imperative.

The Competent Use of FBA

Although FBA is not always required to develop an effective behavior-change intervention, it is often of real and significant value. For that value to be realized, however, FBA data must be collected and interpreted appropriately and interventions skillfully crafted in view of those data. Standard 1.02 (a) of the *BACB Guidelines* (BACB, 2011) dictates that, "behavior analysts provide services, teach, and conduct research only within the boundaries of their competence, based on their education, training, supervised experience, or appropriate professional experience," and this convention obviously applies to the use of FBA. It is essential than any behavior analyst who uses FBA ensures that he or she is competent with respect to FBA in general and with respect to the specific information-gather strategies that she or he uses. Given the recognized importance of FBA in behavior analysis, graduate training programs in the area typically provide appropriate instruction and useful information about the topic can be obtained at workshops, such as those held at the Association for Behavior Analysis International conference, and in written works such as this book. Given these considerations, it appears that most legitimate applied behavior analysts currently possess, or could easily acquire, expertise in FBA.

The same is not true, however, for school personnel. Although the majority of educators are not trained in behavior analysis, legislative mandates may require that they conduct FBAs, despite their reservations regarding skills for doing so. Pindiprolu, Peterson, and Bergloff (2007) surveyed special education teachers, administrators, support staff, and general educators and found that the vast majority of them reported that developing interventions for problem behavior and conducting FBAs were among the areas in which they most desired professional development. In addition, when specifically asked about their skill level in conducting FBAs, special education teachers stated they felt especially weak in (1) testing hypotheses regarding the purpose of problem behaviors, (2) interviewing caregivers regarding problem behaviors, (3) devising procedures for measuring problem behaviors, and (4) developing intervention plans to decrease problem behaviors or increase desired behaviors.

If schools are to use FBAs effectively to inform treatment selection, then ensuring these assessments are done with integrity is a critical issue. Further, if school personnel are to conduct FBAs, then it may be up to behavior analysts to train them how to assess and analyze behavioral functions appropriately. It is incumbent upon these behavior analysts not only to *teach* school personnel to use best practices in FBA and intervention selection, but also to *use* best practices in the training procedures used to teach these skills.

Ethics and FBA Training

Given the relative scarcity of behavior analysts in schools, teaching others to conduct FBAs is often necessary to attenuate resource deficits. Therefore, several researchers have endeavored to develop effective training strategies for school personnel and to evaluate the effects of those procedures. In an early study, Sasso et al. (1992) showed that with minimal training two special education teachers could be taught to conduct descriptive assessments and classroom-based FAs, as well as simultaneously collect data on behavior. Training consisted of providing a written description of the FBA procedures combined with approximately 2 h of instruction and practice for each procedure. Data from teacher-conducted assessments and analyses were compared to data yielded by a "conventional" FA conducted by Sasso. Results revealed a high degree of similarity in teacher- and experimenter-collected data, suggesting teachers could accurately identify controlling variables and descriptive assessments produced the same results as FAs. One potential limitation of this investigation was that the procedures for training teachers were not described in sufficient detail to allow for replication. Fortunately, later investigations have supplied more clearly specified protocols for teaching FA and other FBA skills to people with limited or no training in behavior analysis.

The most notable among these is Iwata et al. (2000), who provided a detailed account of procedures used to train undergraduate students to conduct attention, demand, and play conditions of an FA (Iwata et al., 1982/1994) using a combination of written instructions, video modeling, and feedback. Consistent with the results of Sasso et al. (1992), Iwata et al. noted that training procedures could be completed in about 2 h (assuming that the written materials had been read prior to the start of face-to-face training). Interestingly, Iwata et al. (2000) observed that their participants were fairly accurate in implementing conditions after simply reading the written descriptions and instructions. Although these results could imply that learning to conduct an FA is a relatively simple process, several factors caution against this conclusion. First, the participants in the study were upper-level undergraduate psychology majors who had completed a course in behavior analysis. The ease of training observed by Iwata et al. probably was at least partially the result of participants' prior knowledge of behavior analytic principles, which seemingly exceeded the knowledge teachers would have garnered from their training programs. Remarkably, many teachers fail to receive even the most basic information on managing problematic behaviors, much less on identifying how classroom variables affect student responding (Latham, 2002). Second, data on accuracy of performance were collected during role play situations with a graduate student assuming the role of a student/client. Accurate implementation in more naturalistic settings might have proved more challenging, and thus might have required additional training.

In an attempt to extend the findings of Iwata et al. (2000), Moore et al. (2002) showed that similar procedures could be used to train three general education teachers to implement attention and demand FA conditions. Consistent with the procedures of Iwata et al., the initial phase of the study required teachers to read materials pertaining to FA and answer questions with the researchers. Unlike Iwata and colleagues' participants, however, teachers' accuracy during this phase was relatively low (thereby supporting the hypothesis that prior exposure to behavior analysis might bolster the effectiveness of written training materials). With the addition of individualized feedback, however, performance of all three participants increased substantially and maintained during classroom probes.

Other studies also have shown that teachers could be quickly trained to conduct FA sessions. For example, Wallace, Doney, Mintz-Resudek, and Tarbox (2004) demonstrated that teachers could accurately arrange conditions after a 3-h workshop that included opportunities to role play each condition and receive feedback on performance. Similarly, Moore and Fisher (2007) showed that staff at a center for treatment of severe behavior disorders could be trained to conduct attention, demand, and play conditions via written materials, lecture, and video modeling. Although exact times spent in training were not reported, Moore and Fisher speculated that successful staff training could potentially be accomplished with video models in as little as 15 min, assuming the videos showed sufficient exemplars.

Although these studies have demonstrated effective strategies for training people who are not behavior analysts to conduct the experimental conditions of an FA, they have not addressed many of the other skills that are required for carrying out school-based FBAs. The FBA process requires a much broader repertoire, including selecting the appropriate assessment/analysis strategies to match available resources and competence, correctly carrying out selected strategies, appropriately scoring and graphing data, accurately analyzing data, and effectively using data to inform intervention selection. Therefore, additional research has been undertaken to address some of these issues.

One example is Pindiprolu, Peterson, Rule, and Lignugaris/Kraft (2003), who provided web-based, experiential cases as a training tool for preservice special education teachers, and then used pre- and posttests to evaluate the effects of the case study instruction on students' knowledge and application of FBAs. Participants were taught to conduct FBA interviews, and design FAs based on their interviews. Different methods of teaching were used: reading materials only that summarized client information, reading the results of an FBA interview, and being able to conduct their own interview. Students in all three groups improved significantly from pre- to posttest, but no differences in effectiveness of the different teaching tactics among groups were observed. Further, differences in pre- and post scores for all groups revealed that mean scores for groups did not exceed 67% for declarative knowledge or 59% for application of skills. Therefore, although the improvements were statistically significant, the scores suggest that the students still failed to master much of the basic information pertaining to FBAs and the skills required to conduct them. This study suggests that teaching the *analytic* skills involved in *designing* effective FBAs (as opposed to conducting experimental session) may be more challenging than initially meets the eye.

Unlike Pindiprolu et al. (2003), who focused on teaching the assessment portion of FBA, Scott et al. (2005) examined the effects of FBA training on school staff's abilities to identify effective interventions for problem behavior. The researchers provided FBA training to five staff members from four elementary schools. Training lasted 6 h, and included descriptions of procedures for both conducting FBAs and developing function-based interventions. Participants also practiced skills using three video case studies, both with the trainer and in small groups, and were provided feedback on their performance. Each participant subsequently was assigned the role of facilitator in their school's intervention team, ensuring that at least one member of each team had been trained in conducting FBAs and linking interventions to FBA outcomes. The authors then reviewed the teams' behavior plans for 31 students and compared the suggested strategies with those of experts who were asked to develop interventions based on each student's case and the teams' FBAs.

Both experts and teams selected a range of intervention strategies from a district-generated list (e.g., antecedent manipulation, instructional techniques, consequences for positive behavior and misbehavior), but that teams were much more likely than experts to select punitive and exclusionary intervention components, regardless of the identified function. Although intervention plans prior to FBA training were not evaluated, these results suggest that FBA training did not necessarily produce a bias toward reinforcement-based interventions. Scott et al. (2005) did not assess whether the hypotheses generated by the teams were reasonable given the data or whether the strategies selected matched the hypothesized functions of the behaviors, it is impossible to assess the effectiveness of their training strategy in teaching these two very important skills.

Dukes, Rosenberg, and Brady (2007) also evaluated the effects of FBA training on special educators' knowledge of behavioral function and subsequent intervention selection. Teachers were trained over 3 full days, with the second and third training days separated by 6 weeks. Teachers, trained in groups of 45–100, were exposed verbal instruction, a written manual, case studies, and role plays. Training was specifically designed to teach teachers to identify functions of behaviors and then link functions to intervention selections. Several weeks after the completion of training, participants were given an assessment comprising five scenarios. Participants were asked to identify the likely function of the behaviors described in each scenario from a list of functions, and then to

provide a description of interventions strategies that would likely result in "effective (i.e., rapid and semi-permanent) control of [the student's] problem behavior" (p. 167) in an open-ended question format. In addition, the assessment required participants to answer five multiple choice questions about FBA strategies and purposes. Identical assessments also were sent to teachers who had not completed the training.

Although trained participants answered more questions about function correctly, they were no more likely than untrained participants to suggest interventions that matched behavioral function. It is interesting that this study employed a longer period of training than other studies (i.e., three 7-h days of training), yet participants still did not achieve one of the primary goals of the in-service. Although it is difficult to discern what might have accounted for these negative results (e.g., quality of training, treatment integrity, effects of 6 week delay), they nonetheless raise concerns about the outcomes produced by the training strategies commonly employed by behavioral researchers and practitioners alike.

In addition to the often discouraging results of studies aimed at training broad FBA skill repertoires, another important issue concerns measurement of learning outcomes. Specifically, it is unclear whether identifying functions from written scenarios and designing corresponding interventions is analogous to engaging in these behaviors in more authentic contexts. Van Acker, Boreson, Gable, and Potterton (2005) presented a compelling and disconcerting portrait of FBAs and behavior intervention plans (BIPs) in Wisconsin schools, finding that 70% of the FBAs/BIPs failed to identify or define the target behavior, 25% failed to identify a function for the behavior, and 46% proposed the use of aversive strategies as the sole means of changing behavior. Further, the results showed that school personnel with substantial training in the FBA process were no more likely to define target behaviors clearly or to design interventions to modify the physical or social context than those with no training. These findings clearly show the potential for disconnect between training and practice. On a more positive note, the authors found that FBA/BIP teams with at least one trained member were more likely to verify the hypothesized function through some sort of testing, to incorporate behavioral function into the design of the behavior intervention plan, to use reinforcement based strategies, and to plan for treatment monitoring. These latter findings bode well for the potential to train school personnel to identify functions and develop corresponding interventions, but there is still much left to do if we are to effectively and consistently train sufficient repertoires of FBA and intervention skills across a broad population of learners.

As noted, the results of some studies might suggest that teaching others, including teachers, to conduct FBAs is a relatively easy endeavor that takes minimal time and resources (e.g., Iwata et al., 2000; Moore et al., 2002; Moore & Fisher, 2007; Wallace et al., 2004). Perhaps this finding explains the propensity of some behavior analysts to agree to teach functional assessment and analysis to school personnel during relatively short in-services or workshops. Before making such agreements, they should recognize that these studies were designed to assess training methods for a very limited scope of FBA skills (i.e., arranging FA sessions), not for establishing broad FBA competencies. Clearly, training this relatively limited skill set does not address the skills required to collect and interpret FBA data.

Moreover, outside the realm of research, FA (and in particular, analogue analyses) are not likely to be recommended as viable FBA strategies in schools (Bambara & Kern, 2005; Chandler & Dahlquist, 2010). It is much more likely that FBAs will be conducted via informant and descriptive assessments (Van Acker et al., 2005), and much less is known about how to teach school personnel to collect these types of data in a valid and reliable manner (see Neef & Peterson, 2007) than is known about teaching FA. Although some researchers have attempted to provide evaluations of a broader scope of training (e.g., Dukes et al., 2007; Pindiprolu et al., 2003; Sasso et al., 1992; Scott et al., 2005), their contributions have produced mixed results that make it impossible to establish clear training guidelines. Current gaps in the existing literature also make it difficult

to know whether a complex range of skills can be effectively taught and maintained, and if so, how much and what type of training is required to do so.

Given the relative paucity of information regarding the strategies needed to teach the full complement of FBA skills puts practitioners in somewhat of an ethical conundrum: Schools want effective training in FBA and intervention design, but our own literature makes it difficult to know exactly how meet these needs. Further, we want our science and technology to be accessible to others, but we want procedures to be implemented with integrity by those who are fully competent. Standard 3.0(d) of the *BACB Guidelines for Responsible Conduct* (BACB, 2011) states that "(b)ehavior analysts do not promote the use of behavioral assessment techniques by unqualified persons, i.e., those who are unsupervised by experienced professionals and have not demonstrated valid and reliable assessment skills." Behavior analysts who provide training in FBA for teachers or other care providers should recognize that their efforts will not necessarily provide trainees with adequate, including valid and reliable, assessment skills. Even though a conservative interpretation of standard 3.0(d) might provide a basis for doing so, in our view it is pointless and inappropriate to accuse behavior analysts who provide such training of unethical conduct. However, it is appropriate to call attention to the need to develop and use empirically-validated training procedures that maximize the likelihood that trainees acquire the repertoire of complex and inter-related skills needed to use FBA successfully.

Potentially Effective Models for Collaboration to Increase FBA Competence

Given the current status of our training literature, practitioners should perhaps focus on training school personnel (or any other relevant stakeholders) to be good collaborators in the FBA process, as opposed to attempting to train a very complex skill repertoire with little evidence about which training methods are most effective. Peck Peterson, Derby, Berg, and Horner (2002) suggested a collaborative model for conducting home-based FBAs with family members who may have little background in behavior analysis. This model involves family members and behavior analysts assuming different roles during each stage of the functional behavior assessment process (i.e., problem identification and hypothesis development, hypothesis testing, design of intervention, evaluation and adjustment, and efficiency redesign).

The overall role of the behavior analyst in this process is to "improve the technology, expand the science, and make more effective the design of environments that reduce problem behavior and increase prosocial behavior" (Peck Peterson et al., 2002, p. 19). Complementing the behavior analyst's role is that of the family, which provides "the context for the most efficient FA and ongoing intervention" (Peck Peterson et al., p. 19). Perhaps this model could be adapted to describe the appropriate roles of school personnel and behavior analysts in conducting functional behavior assessments in school settings. This adapted model is outlined in Table 13.1 and may provide the cooperative, on-site training model preferred by school personnel (Pindiprolu et al., 2007), as well as the collaboration between school districts, state departments of education, and institutes of higher education recommended by Shellady and Stichter (1999). Table 13.2 also provides information about collaboration between school personnel and behavior analysts for functional analyses and behavioral interventions.

The preceding discussion has focused on the use of FBA in school settings, but similar considerations apply in all circumstances where people are trained to use FBA and put that knowledge to use in an attempt to improve behavior. "Benefitting others" is one of the core ethical principles that guide the practice of psychology (Koocher & Keith-Spiegel, 1998) and of applied behavior analysis (Bailey & Burch, 2011). For example, Standard 2.0 of the *BACB Guidelines* (BACB, 2011) reads: "The behavior analyst has a responsibility to operate in the best interest of clients." "Pursuit of excellence" is another core ethical principle (Bailey & Burch, 2011). Our discussion

of FBA in school settings is intended to illustrate that there is substantial room for improvement with respect to how FBA is used in school settings and to offer strategies for increasing the likelihood that FBA eventually will be used to the maximum benefit of teachers and students, thereby approaching the excellence that all concerned individuals value.

Concluding Comments

"Doing FBA" is not ethical conduct. "Doing FBA" in a manner that produces maximum benefit and minimal harm for the people whose behaviors are of concern is ethical conduct and should be the goal of behavior analysts. It is, for example, not enough for members of an IEP team to conduct a poor FBA and design a weak intervention for a student with a developmental disability who is facing disciplinary action, although doing so might meet the requirements of IDEA. In a 1994 discussion of the ethics of using psychotropic drugs to manage behavior in people with developmental disabilities, Poling wrote:

> It is critical that decisions concerning [medication] use are individualized and data-based to the fullest extent possible. Because we can never know a priori how a given person will respond to medication, we must always determine what the medication is intended to do and whether this goal is accomplished. Moreover, we must take care to ensure that observed benefits are evaluated relative to real and possible costs to the patient, and that all decisions are made in her or his best interests. If this is done, treatment is rational and ethical as well. (p. 171)

To capture the essence of the ethical use of FBA, "FBA-based intervention" can simply be substituted for "medication" in the foregoing passage.

No reasonable person argues that it is fundamentally wrong, hence unethical, for applied behavior analysts or others in the helping professions to try to determine why their clients emit inappropriate behaviors or fail to emit appropriate behaviors, and then use this knowledge to help the clients. From a conceptual perspective FBA is perfectly acceptable as a general approach for designing behavior-change interventions and from an empirical perspective it is a general

Table 13.2 Collaboration between school personnel and behavior analysts for functional analyses and behavioral interventions (adapted from Peck Peterson et al., 2002)

Stage of functional behavior assessment	Role of school personnel	Role of behavior analyst
Problem identification and hypothesis development (interviews and naturalistic observations)	1. Broadly define the problem and the goals for intervention 2. Describe antecedents and consequences associated with problem behavior	1. Guide organization of information 2. Clarify patterns 3. Determine what conditions will be used in experimental manipulations
Hypothesis testing (experimental manipulations)	1. Implement experimental conditions with guidance 2. Take data; perhaps check interobserver agreement	1. Coach personnel as they conduct experimental conditions 2. Assist personnel in determining what stimuli will be used in experimental conditions 3. Check fidelity of implementation; perhaps conduct interobserver agreement 4. Assist personnel in interpreting results of experimental manipulations
Design of intervention	1. Identify intervention methods that fit within classroom routines and/or modify classroom routines so intervention is a good fit 2. Identify external supports needed (if any)	1. Identify intervention methods that are consistent with best practice and research in behavior analysis 2. Predict expected patterns and rates of behavior change
Evaluation and adjustment	1. Collect data on problem and/or replacement behaviors 2. Identify aspects of the intervention that are problematic for implementation and participate in intervention redesign (if necessary)	1. Assist in designing practical data collection procedures 2. Provide checks to ensure data are being collected 3. Assist personnel in interpreting results of intervention implementation 4. Monitor intervention fidelity and provide feedback to school personnel on fidelity 5. Ensure that intervention redesign (if necessary) is consistent with best practice and research in behavior analysis
Maintenance and generalization	1. Implement prompt fading and reinforcement schedule thinning procedures 2. Continue collecting data on problem and/or replacement behaviors 3. Identify stimuli (i.e., settings, people, materials, cues) for which generalization programming is necessary 4. Identify maintenance and generalization problems and participate in intervention redesign (if necessary)	1. Assist school personnel with recommendations for prompt fading and reinforcement schedule thinning 2. Continue monitoring intervention fidelity and providing feedback to school personnel on fidelity as intervention changes over time 3. Continue providing checks to ensure data are being collected 4. Assist personnel in interpreting results of intervention implementation

approach of demonstrated value. As we point out, however, successful interventions can be designed in the absence of FBA data and collecting such data does not ensure that a treatment will be effective. Moreover, support for the contention that interventions based on FBA are generally more effective than alternative interventions is less than overwhelming and further research is certainly needed. At present, there is

no compelling conceptual or empirical basis for claiming that ethical or effective behavior analysis *always* begins with FA or another form of FBA. To date, FBA has been used primarily in the context of developing interventions to decelerate inappropriate behaviors in people with developmental disabilities. FBA has rarely been used to delineate the variables responsible for the non-occurrence of desired responses or to ascertain why low-rate, high-intensity behaviors occur (Irwin et al., 2001). Moreover, the utility of FBA for understanding rule-governed behavior is unclear (Irwin et al., 2001). None of these considerations should be taken as criticisms of FBA, but they should serve as cautions against overenthusiastic and naïve endorsements. As Irwin, Ehrhardt, and Poling (2001) pointed out, "The logic and methods of functional assessment are evident in Skinner's writings, and many early researchers and practitioners influenced by his ideas employed functional assessment [although it was not labeled as such] in designing interventions in school and other settings" (p. 173). Contemporary behavior analysts—including us—continue to use FBA to the great benefit of those they serve.

Certain applications of FBA, however, notably those involving FA of seriously harmful responses, raise interesting ethical issues and we attempted to illustrate some of these issues. Although some general guidelines were suggested, it is important to recognize that ethical treatment of clients is inevitably individualized treatment. As Johnston and Sherman (1993) emphasize in a discussion of the Least Restrictive Alternative (LRA) principle, a cornerstone for protecting people with disabilities, "to be an effective constitutional safeguard, the LRA must be a subjective and dynamic principle tailored to individual needs (Parry, 1985). Likewise, in determining the needs of [people with developmental disabilities], treatment decisions cannot be made in isolation from the individual's personal preferences, values, and circumstances" (p. 112). This statement holds true regardless of whether FBA is or is not being consider as part of or is being used in the treatment.

In closing, we should acknowledge that framing a discussion in terms of ethical issues may render emotion-laden what would otherwise be innocuous points. It is, for example, one thing to say that it is better practice to arrange a few short FA sessions than to arrange many long ones, quite another to claim that a person who does the latter is unethical. We have attempted to avoid making ethical judgments and apologize in advance if our suggestions strike a reader as accusatory. Our hope was not to cause offense, but to call attention to the kinds of variables that behavior analysts and laypeople consider in determining whether or not a professional's actions relevant to FBA are or are not "ethical." As behavior analysts, we see this as a matter of stimulus control, not morality. In other words, there often may not be a "right" or "wrong" thing to do at certain points in time. Rather, specific stimulus conditions (e.g., type of curriculum being used with an individual, other behavioral supports and rules in place, type and severity of problem behavior displayed) frequently interact to create a variety of interesting dilemmas for the behavior analyst. The behavior analyst must constantly evaluate these stimulus conditions in order to determine the best course of action for completing an FBA in order to make decisions that comply with both the letter and spirit of the ethical codes of conduct guiding our field.

References

American Psychological Association. (2010). *Ethical principles of psychologists and code of conduct: 2010 Amendments*. Washington, DC: Author.

Asmus, J. M., Vollmer, T. R., & Borrero, J. C. (2002). Functional behavioral assessment: A school based model. *Education and Treatment of Children, 25*, 67–90.

Bailey, J. S., & Burch, M. R. (2011). *Ethics for behavior analysts* (2nd ed.). Mahway: Lawrence Erlbaum.

Bambara, L. M., & Kern, L. (2005). *Individualized supports for students with problem behaviors: Designing positive behavior plans*. New York: Guilford.

Barretto, A., Wacker, D. P., Harding, J., Lee, J., & Berg, W. K. (2006). Using telemedicine to conduct behavioral assessments. *Journal of Applied Behavior Analysis, 39*, 333–340.

Behavior Analysis Certification Board. (2011). *Guidelines for responsible conduct for behavior analysts*. Retrieved from http://www.bacb.com/index.php?page=57.

Blakeslee, T., Sugai, G., & Gruba, J. (1994). A review of functional assessment use in data-based intervention studies. *Journal of Behavioral Education, 4*, 397–413.

Bloom, S. E., Iwata, B. A., Fritz, J. N., Roscoe, E. M., & Carreau, A. B. (2011). Classroom application of a trial-based functional analysis. *Journal of Applied Behavior Analysis, 44*, 19–31.

Call, N. A., Pabico, R. S., & Lomas, J. E. (2009). Use of latency to problem behavior to evaluate demands for inclusion in functional analyses. *Journal of Applied Behavior Analysis, 42,* 723–728.

Carr, E. G., & Durand, V. M. (1985). Reducing behavior problems through functional communication training. *Journal of Applied Behavior Analysis, 18,* 111–126.

Carr, E. G., Horner, R. H., Turnbill, A. P., Marquis, J. G., McLaughlin, D. D., McAtee, M. L., et al. (1999). *Positive behavior support for people with developmental disabilities: A research synthesis.* Washington, DC: American Association for Mental Retardation.

Carr, J. E., Severtson, J. M., & Lepper, T. L. (2009). Noncontingent reinforcement is an empirically supported treatment for problem behavior exhibited by individuals with developmental disabilities. *Research in Developmental Disabilities, 30,* 44–57.

Chandler, L. K., & Dahlquist, C. M. (2010). *Functional assessment: Strategies to prevent and remediate challenging behavior in school settings* (3rd ed.). Columbus: Prentice Hall.

Crone, D. A., & Horner, R. H. (2000). Contextual, conceptual, and empirical foundations of functional behavioral assessment in schools. *Exceptionality, 8,* 161–172.

Individuals with Disabilities Education Improvement Act, 20 U.S.C. § 1400 (2004).

Dukes, C., Rosenberg, H., & Brady, M. (2007). Effects of training in functional behavior assessment. *International Journal of Special Education, 22,* 163–173.

Ellingson, S. A., Miltenberger, R. G., Stricker, J., Galensky, T. L., & Garlinghouse, M. (2000). Functional assessment and intervention for challenging behaviors in the classroom by general classroom teachers. *Journal of Positive Behavior Interventions, 2,* 85–97.

Ervin, R. A., Radford, P. M., Bertsch, K., Piper, A. L., Ehrhardt, K. E., & Poling, A. (2001). A descriptive analysis and critique of the empirical literature on school-based functional assessment. *School Psychology Review, 30,* 193–210.

Gresham, F. M., McIntyre, L. L., Olson-Tinker, H., Dolstra, L., McLaughlin, V., & Van, M. (2004). Relevance of functional behavioral assessment research for school-based interventions and positive behavioral support. *Research in Developmental Disabilities, 25,* 19–37.

Gresham, F., Watson, T. S., & Skinner, C. H. (2001). Functional behavioral assessment: Principles, procedures, and future directions. *School Psychology Review, 30,* 156–172.

Hanley, G. P., Iwata, B. A., & McCord, B. E. (2003). Functional analysis of problem behavior: A review. *Journal of Applied Behavior Analysis, 36,* 147–185.

Hastings, R. P., & Noone, S. J. (2005). SIB and FA: Ethics and evidence. *Education and Training in Developmental Disabilities, 40,* 335–342.

Individuals with Disabilities Education Act Amendments of 1997, 20 U.S.C. (1997)

Ingram, K., Lewis-Palmer, T., & Sugai, G. (2005). Function-based intervention planning: Comparing the effectiveness of FBA function-based and non-function-based intervention plans. *Journal of Positive Behavior Interventions, 7,* 224–236.

Irwin, R. A., Ehrhardt, K. E., & Poling, A. (2001). Functional assessment: Old wine in new bottles. *School Psychology Review, 30,* 173–179.

Irwin, R. A., Radford, P. M., Bertsch, K., Piper, A. L., Ehrhardt, K. E., & Poling, A. (2001). A descriptive analysis and critique of the empirical literature on school-based functional assessment. *School Psychology Review, 30,* 193–210.

Iwata, B. A., Dorsey, M. F., Slifer, K. J., Bauman, K. E., & Richman, G. S. (1982/1994). Toward a functional analysis of self-injury. *Journal of Applied Behavior Analysis, 27,* 197–209. Reprinted from *Analysis and Intervention in Developmental Disabilities, 2,* 3–20 (1982).

Iwata, B. A., Pace, G. M., Cowdery, G. E., & Miltenberger, R. G. (1994). What makes extinction work: An analysis of procedural form and function. *Journal of Applied Behavior Analysis, 27,* 131–144.

Iwata, B. A., Wallace, M. D., Kahng, S. W., Lindberg, J. S., Roscoe, E. M., Conners, J., et al. (2000). Skill acquisition in the implementation of functional analysis methodology. *Journal of Applied Behavior Analysis, 33,* 181–194.

Johnston, J. M., & Sherman, R. A. (1993). Applying the least restrictive alternative principle to treatment decisions: A legal and behavioral analysis. *The Behavior Analyst, 16,* 103–115.

Kahng, S., & Iwata, B. A. (1999). Correspondence between outcomes of a brief and extended FA. *Journal of Applied Behavior Analysis, 32,* 149–160.

Koocher, G. P., & Keith-Spiegel, P. (1998). *Ethics in psychology: Professional standards and cases.* New York: Oxford University Press.

Kurtz, P. F., Chin, M. D., Huete, J. M., Tarbox, R. S. F., O'Connor, J. T., Paclawskyj, T. R., et al. (2003). Functional analysis and treatment of self-injurious behavior in young children a summary of 30 cases. *Journal of Applied Behavior Analysis, 36,* 205–219.

LaRue, R. H., Lenard, K., Weiss, M. J., Bamond, M., Palmieri, M., & Kelley, M. E. (2010). Comparison of traditional and trial-based methodologies for conducting functional analyses. *Research in Developmental Disabilities, 31,* 480–487.

Latham, G. I. (2002). *Behind the schoolhouse door: Managing chaos with science, skills, and strategies.* North Logan: P & T Ink.

Le, D. D., & Smith, R. G. (2002). FA of self-injury with and without protective equipment. *Journal of Developmental and Physical Disabilities, 14,* 277–290.

Mace, F. C., & Knight, D. (1986). FA and treatment of severe pica. *Journal of Applied Behavior Analysis, 19,* 411–416.

Meyer, K. A. (1999). Functional analysis and treatment of problem behavior exhibited by school children. *Journal of Applied Behavior Analysis, 32,* 229–232.

Moore, J. W., Edwards, R. P., Sterling-Turner, H. E., Riley, J., Dubard, M., & McGeorge, A. (2002). Teacher acquisition of functional analysis methodology. *Journal of Applied Behavior Analysis, 35,* 72–77.

Moore, J. W., & Fisher, W. W. (2007). The effects of videotape modeling on staff acquisition of functional analysis methodology. *Journal of Applied Behavior Analysis, 40*, 197–202.

National Institutes of Health. (1991). *Treatment of destructive behaviors in persons with developmental disabilities*. Washington, DC: U. S. Department of Health and Human Services.

Neef, N. A., & Peterson, S. M. (2007). Functional behavior assessment. In J. O. Cooper, T. E. Heron, & W. Heward (Eds.), *Applied behavior analysis* (pp. 500–524). Columbus: Merrill-Prentice Hall.

Newcomer, L. L., & Lewis, T. J. (2004). Functional behavioral assessment: An investigation of assessment reliability and effectiveness of function-based interventions. *Journal of Emotional and Behavioral Disorders, 12*, 168–181.

Northup, J., Wacker, D., Sasso, G., Steege, M., Cigrand, K., Cook, J., et al. (1991). A brief FA of aggression and alternative behavior in an outclinic setting. *Journal of Applied Behavior Analysis, 24*, 509–522.

Parry, L. (1985). Least restrictive alternative: An overview of the concept. *Mental and Physical Disabilities Law Reporter, 9*, 963–972.

Peck Peterson, S. M., Derby, K. M., Berg, W. K., & Horner, R. H. (2002). Collaboration with families in the functional behavior assessment and intervention for severe behavior problems. *Education and Treatment of Children, 25*, 5–25.

Pindiprolu, S. S., Peterson, S. M., & Bergloff, H. (2007). School personnel's professional development needs and skill level with functional behavior assessments in ten midwestern states in the United States: Analysis and issues. *Journal of the International Association of Special Education, 8*, 31–42.

Pindiprolu, S. S., Peterson, S. M. P., Rule, S., & Lignugaris/Kraft, B. (2003). Using web-mediated experiential case-based instruction to teach functional behavioral assessment skills. *Teacher Education and Special Education, 26*, 1–16.

Poling, A. (1994). Pharmacological treatment of behavioral problems in people with mental retardation: Some ethical considerations. In L. J. Hayes, G. J. Hayes, S. C. Moore, & P. M. Ghezzi (Eds.), *Ethical issues in developmental disabilities* (pp. 149–177). Reno: Context.

Poling, A., Ehrhardt, K., Wood, A., & Bowerman, R. (2010). Psychopharmacology and behavior analysis in autism treatment. In J. A. Matson & E. A. Mayville (Eds.), *Behavioral foundations of effective autism treatment*. New York: Sloan.

Romaniuk, C., Miltenberger, R., Conyers, C., Jenner, N., Jurgens, M., & Ringenberg, C. (2002). The influence of activity choice on problem behaviors maintained by escape versus attention. *Journal of Applied Behavior Analysis, 35*, 349–362.

Sasso, G. M., Reimers, T. M., Cooper, L. J., Wacker, D., Berg, W., Steege, M., et al. (1992). Use of descriptive and experimental analyses to identify the functional

properties of aberrant behavior in school settings. *Journal of Applied Behavior Analysis, 25*, 809–821.

Schill, M. T., Kratochwill, T. R., & Elliott, S. N. (1998). Functional assessment in behavioral consultation: A treatment utility study. *School Psychology Quarterly, 13*, 116–140.

Scott, T. M., McIntyre, J., Liaupsin, C., Nelson, C. M., Conroy, M., & Payne, L. D. (2005). An examination of the relation between functional behavior assessment and selected intervention strategies with school-based teams. *Journal of Positive Behavior Interventions, 7*, 205–215.

Shellady, S., & Stichter, J. P. (1999). Training preservice and inservice educators to conduct functional assessments: Initial issues and implications. *Preventing School Failure, 43*, 154–159.

Sigafoos, J., & Saggers, E. (1995). A discrete-trial approach to the functional analysis of aggressive behaviour in two boys with autism. *Australia & New Zealand Journal of Developmental Disabilities, 20*, 287–297.

Smith, C. M. (2005). Origin and uses of *primum non nocere*—above all, do no harm! *The Journal of Clinical Pharmacology, 45*, 371–377.

Steege, M. W., & Watson, T. S. (2008). Best practices in functional behavioral assessment. In A. Thomas & J. Grimes (Eds.), *Best practices in school psychology V* (pp. 347–248). Washington, DC: National Association of School Psychologists.

Taylor, J., & Miller, M. (1997). When timeout works some of the time: The importance of treatment integrity and functional assessment. *School Psychology Quarterly, 12*, 4–22.

Thomason-Sassi, J. L., Iwata, B. A., Neidert, P. L., & Roscoe, E. M. (2011). Latency as an index of response strength during functional analysis of problem behavior. *Journal of Applied Behavior Analysis, 44*, 51–67.

Van Acker, R., Boreson, L., Gable, R. A., & Potterton, T. (2005). Are we on the right course? Lessons learned about current FBA/BIP practices in schools. *Journal of Behavioral Education, 14*, 35–56.

Van Houten, R., Axelrod, S., Bailey, J. S., Foxx, R. M., Iwata, B. A., & Lovaas, O. I. (1988). The right to effective behavioral treatment. *Journal of Applied Behavior Analysis, 28*, 381–384.

Vollmer, T. R., Marcus, B. A., Ringdahl, J. E., & Roane, H. S. (1995). Progressing from brief assessments to extended experimental analyses in the evaluation of aberrant behavior. *Journal of Applied Behavior Analysis, 28*, 561–576.

Vollmer, T. R., & Northup, J. (1996). Some implications of functional analysis for school psychology. *School Psychology Quarterly, 11*, 76–92.

Vollmer, T. R., & Smith, R. G. (1996). Some current themes in functional analysis research. *Research in Developmental Disabilities, 17*, 229–249.

Wallace, M. D., Doney, J. K., Mintz-Resudek, C. M., & Tarbox, R. S. F. (2004). Training educators to implement functional analyses. *Journal of Applied Behavior Analysis, 37,* 89–92.

Wallace, M. D., & Iwata, B. A. (1999). Effects of session duration on functional analysis outcomes. *Journal of Applied Behavior Analysis, 32,* 175–183.

Wallace, M. D., & Knights, D. J. (2003). An evaluation of a brief functional analysis format within a vocational setting. *Journal of Applied Behavior Analysis, 36,* 125–128.

Weeden, M., Mahoney, A., & Poling, A. (2010). SIB and FA: Where are the descriptions of participant protections? *Research in Developmental Disabilities, 31,* 299–303.

Wilder, D. A., Chen, L., Atwell, J., Pritchard, J., & Weinstein, P. (2006). Brief functional analysis and treatment of tantrums associated with transitions in preschool children. *Journal of Applied Behavior Analysis, 39,* 103–107.

About the Editor

Johnny L. Matson is Professor and Distinguished Research Master, and Director of Clinical Training in the Department of Psychology at Louisiana State University in Baton Rouge, LA. Prior to his 25-year tenure at LSU, Dr. Matson was a professor of Psychiatry at the University of Pittsburgh School of Medicine. He is the author of over 600 publications including 34 books and is editor-in-chief of two journals, *Research in Developmental Disorders* and *Research in Autism Spectrum Disorders.*

J.L. Matson (ed.), *Functional Assessment for Challenging Behaviors,*
Autism and Child Psychopathology Series, DOI 10.1007/978-1-4614-3037-7,
© Springer Science+Business Media, LLC 2012

Index

A
ABA. *See* Applied behavior analysis (ABA)
A–B–C data. *See* Antecedent–behavior–consequence
    (A–B–C) data
Adaptive skills, 93
Aggression
    adverse consequences, 36
    definition, 33
    forms and classification, 33–34
    populations and problems, 73–74
    prevalence, 34–35
    risk factors, 35–36
Alone condition, 128
American Psychological Association (APA), 213
Antecedent–behavior–consequence (A–B–C) data
    analysis, 101
    charts, 160–161
    contingency event recording, 109–111
    description, 65
    recording form, 101
Antecedent intervention, 201–202
APA. *See* American Psychological Association (APA)
Applied behavior analysis (ABA)
    after 1982, 13
    behavior observation, 91–92
    birth of, 6–7
    challenging behaviors
        automatic reinforcement, 10–11
        function of, 7–8
        negative reinforcement, 9–10
        positive reinforcement, 8–9
    ecological validity, 20–21
    expansion across behaviors
        access to stereotypy, 17
        across settings, 15–16
        control, 17
        low-rate behaviors, 15
        multiple topographies, 14–15
        precursor behaviors, 15
        tangible function, 16–17
    expansion across populations, 14
    experimental designs, 18
    experimentation with humans, 5–6
    functional analysis
        antecedent-only, 19
        data interpretation, 19
        duration, 18–19
        training, 19–20
    historical roots, 4–5
    idiosyncratic variables, 17–18
    nonexperimental methods, 20
Attention alone/in combination behaviors
    for bizarre speech, 51
    inappropriate sexual behavior, 50
    intellectual disability, 51–52
    Prader–Willi syndrome, 52
    task analysis, 50–51
Attention condition, 127
Autism spectrum disorders (ASD), 25–26.
        See also Challenging behavior
Automatic reinforcement
    ABA, challenging behaviors, 10–11
    challenging behaviors
        auditory masking, 58
        with autism patient, 58–59
        dangerous behavior, 57
        intervention program, 56–57
        oral stimulation, 59
        positive effects, 57
        sensory extinction, 57
    description, 187
    differential reinforcement, 189–190
    extinction, 187–188
    response-independent delivery of alternate
        sources, 188–189

B
BACB Guidelines. *See* Behavior Analyst Certification
        Board Guidelines for Responsible Conduct
        (BACB Guidelines)
Behavioral skills training, 207–208